Contents

Contributors   *xi*
Preface   *xv*

Part I: Foundations for Practice

Chapter 1   An Overview of Complementary/Alternative   3
             Therapies
             Mariah Snyder and Ruth Lindquist

Chapter 2   Cultural Diversity and Complementary Therapies   15
             Kathleen Niska and Mariah Snyder

Chapter 3   Self as Healer   25
             Barbara Leonard and Sue Towey

Chapter 4   Presence   35
             Mariah Snyder

Chapter 5   Therapeutic Listening   45
             *Shigeaki Watanuki, Mary Fran Tracy, and
             Ruth Lindquist*

Part II: Mind–Body Therapies

Chapter 6   Imagery   59
             Janice Post-White and Maura Fitzgerald

Chapter 7   Music Intervention   79
             Linda Chlan

Chapter 8   Humor   93
Kevin Smith

Chapter 9   Yoga   107
Miriam E. Cameron

Chapter 10   Biofeedback   117
Marion Good

Chapter 11   Meditation   129
Mary Jo Kreitzer

Chapter 12   Prayer   143
Mariah Snyder

Chapter 13   Storytelling   153
Roxanne Struthers

Chapter 14   Journaling   165
Mariah Snyder

Chapter 15   Animal-Assisted Therapy   175
Jennifer Jorgenson

Part III: Energy and Biofield Therapies

Chapter 16   Magnet Therapy   191
Corjena K. Cheung

Chapter 17   Healing Touch   203
Alexa W. Umbreit

Chapter 18   Therapeutic Touch   225
Janet F. Quinn

Chapter 19   Reiki   243
Debbie Ringdahl and Linda L. Halcón

Chapter 20   Acupressure   255
Pamela Weiss

Chapter 21   Reflexology   271
Thora Jenny Gunnarsdottir

Complementary/ Alternative Therapies in Nursing

5th Edition

Mariah Snyder
PhD, RN, FAAN

Ruth Lindquist
PhD, RN, FAAN, APRN, BC

Editors

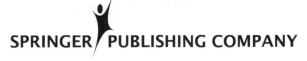

SPRINGER PUBLISHING COMPANY

New York

Springer Publishing Company, Inc.
11 West 42nd Street
New York, NY 10036

Acquisitions Editors: Sally J. Barhydt and Ruth Chasek
Production Editor: Sara Yoo
Cover design by Joanne Honigman
Typeset by International Graphic Services, Newtown, PA

07 08 09 10 / 5 4 3 2

Library of Congress Cataloging-in-Publication Data

Complementary/alternative therapies in nursing / editors, Mariah Snyder, Ruth Lindquist.—5th ed.
    p. ; cm.
  Includes bibliographical references and index.
  ISBN 0-8261-1447-4
  1. Holistic nursing.   2. Nurse and patient.   3. Alternative medicine.
  [DNLM: 1. Complementary Therapies—nursing.   2. Holistic Nursing.
WY 86.5 C737 2006]
I. Snyder, Mariah.   II. Lindquist, Ruth.
RT41.I53 2006
610.73—dc22   2005027206

Printed in the United States of America by Bang Printing.

To our late parents

Agnes and Peter Snyder
Elsie and Warren Dennis

Part IV: Manipulative and Body-Based Therapies

Chapter 22   Massage   285
              Mariah Snyder

Chapter 23   Exercise   295
              Diane Treat-Jacobson, Daniel L. Mark, and
              Ulf Bronäs

Chapter 24   Tai Chi   313
              Kuei-Min Chen

Chapter 25   Muscle Relaxation Techniques   323
              Mariah Snyder, Elizabeth Pestka, and
              Catherine Bly

Part V: Biologically Based Therapies

Chapter 26   Aromatherapy   335
              Linda L. Halcón and Jane Buckle

Chapter 27   Herbal Medicines   351
              Gregory A. Plotnikoff with Yun Lu

Chapter 28   Functional Foods and Nutraceuticals   367
              Bridget Doyle and Melissa Frisvold

Part VI: Perspectives on Future Research and Practice

Chapter 29   Perspectives on Future Research and Practice   383
              Ruth Lindquist and Mariah Snyder

Index   *395*

Contributors

Catherine Bly, BSN, RN
Neuroscience Care Coordinator
Lutheran Hospital
LaCrosse, WI

Ulf Bronäs, MS, ATC-R
Doctoral Student
Department of Kinesiology
University of Minnesota
Minneapolis, MN

Jane Buckle, PhD, RN
Director, R.J. Buckle Associates,
  LLC
and Complementary and
  Alternative Medicine Research
  Fellow
Center for Clinical Epidemiology
  and Biostatistics (CCEB)
School of Medicine
University of Pennsylvania
Philadelphia, PA

Miriam E. Cameron, PhD, MNS,
  MA, RN
Faculty
Center for Spirituality and Healing
University of Minnesota
Minneapolis, MN

Kuei-Min Chen, PhD, RN
Associate Professor
Fooyin University
Kaoshiung, Taiwan

Corjena K. Cheung, PhD, RN
Assistant Professor
Department of Nursing
College of St. Catherine
St. Paul, MN

Linda Chlan, PhD, RN
Associate Professor
School of Nursing, Center for
  Spirituality and Healing
University of Minnesota
Minneapolis, MN

Bridget Doyle, PhD, MPH, RD,
  LD
Retired
Minneapolis, Minnesota

Maura Fitzgerald, MS, RN, MA,
  CNS
Clinical Nurse Specialist
Children's Hospital and Clinics of
  Minnesota
Integrative Medicine Project
St. Paul, MN

Melissa Frisvold, MS, RN, CNM
Doctoral Student
University of Minnesota
Minneapolis, MN

Marion Good, PhD, RN, FAAN
Professor
Frances Payne Bolton School of
    Nursing
Case Western Reserve University
Cleveland, OH

Thora Jenny Gunnarsdottir, PhD
    Candidate, MS, RN
School of Nursing
University of Minnesota
Minneapolis, MN

Linda L. Halcón, PhD, MPH, RN
Associate Professor
School of Nursing
University of Minnesota
Minneapolis, MN

Jennifer Jorgenson, BSN, RN
Doctoral Student
University of North Carolina at
    Chapel Hill
Chapel Hill, NC

Mary Jo Kreitzer, PhD, RN
Director, Center for Spirituality
    and Healing,
Associate Professor, School of
    Nursing
University of Minnesota
Minneapolis, MN

Barbara Leonard, PhD, RN, FAAN
Professor
Director, Children with Special
    Health Care Needs
School of Nursing
University of Minnesota
Minneapolis, MN

Yun Lu, Pharm D, MS, BCPS,
    R.Ph
Clinical Specialist, Cardiology
Hennepin County Medical Center
Minneapolis, MN

Daniel L. Mark, MD, ABMS
Medical Orthopedics
St. Mary's/Duluth Clinic Health
    System
Duluth, MN

Kathleen Niska, PhD, RN
Associate Professor
Department of Nursing
College of St. Scholastica
Duluth, MN

Elizabeth Pestka, MS, APRN, RN
Nursing Education Specialist
Coordinator of Department of
    Nursing Orientation
Genomics Liaison for Department
    of Nursing
Mayo Clinic
Rochester, MN

Gregory A. Plotnikoff, MD
Associate Professor
University of Minnesota
Minneapolis, MN

Janice Post-White, PhD, RN,
    FAAN
Associate Professor
Academic Health Center for
    Spirituality and Healing
University of Minnesota
Minneapolis, MN

Janet F. Quinn, PhD, RN, FAAN
Haelen Works
Boulder, CO

Debbie Ringdahl, MS, CNM, RN
Teaching Specialist
School of Nursing
University of Minnesota
Minneapolis, MN

Kevin Smith, MSN, RN, CNP
Senior Teaching Specialist
School of Nursing
University of Minnesota
Minneapolis, MN

Roxanne Struthers, PhD, RN
(Deceased)
Assistant Professor
School of Nursing
University of Minnesota
Minneapolis, MN

Sue Towey, MS, RN, CNS, LP
Private Practice, Integrative Health
  Consultants
Faculty, Center for Spirituality and
  Healing
University of Minnesota
Minneapolis, MN

**Mary Fran Tracy, PhD, RN,
  FAAN, CCRN**
Critical Care Clinical Nurse
  Specialist
University of Minnesota Hospital
Minneapolis, MN

Diane Treat-Jacobson, PhD, RN
Assistant Professor
School of Nursing
University of Minnesota
Minneapolis, MN

**Alexa W. Umbreit, MS, RNC,
  CHTP**
Patient Learning Center
University of Minnesota Medical
  Center—Fairview
Minneapolis, MN

Shigeaki Watanuki, PhD
Associate Professor
Aino University
Osaka, Japan

**Pamela Weiss, PhD, MPH, RN,
  Dip.Ac., L.Ac**
Associate Professor
Department of Nursing
Augsburg College
Minneapolis, MN

Preface

Fifth edition! Saying this phrase is both daunting and exciting. Daunting in identifying new information and approaches that can be included to make *Complementary/Alternative Therapies in Nursing* appealing and helpful to nursing students and practitioners. Exciting, in that like Beethoven's Fifth Symphony, the appeal of independent nursing interventions and complementary therapies to nursing and health care has not only persisted over time but has continued to grow. The holistic and caring aspects of these therapies have been and continue to be valued both by nurses and those to whom care is provided whether this is in the United States or in countries around the world. Roles of nursing continue to evolve, but within all of these varied roles and places in which nurses practice, concern for the comfort and healing of patients remains foremost in their minds.

Complementary therapies assume a key role in the promotion of healing, comfort, and care. More than 1,800 complementary/alternative therapies and systems of care have been identified. Many of these therapies have been used by nurses for centuries, and an increasing number that have been a part of systems of care across the world are receiving attention in the United States. The increasing mobility of society, whether through immigration, travel, or attendance at international conferences, requires that nurses be knowledgeable about ancient therapies used by many persons around the world. Attention to health care practices of other cultures is given throughout this book. Although nurses may not necessarily administer these therapies, knowledge is required so that respect for the practices of others can be shown and use of these therapies can be reflected in the total plan of care.

The previous editions of this book have focused largely on the use of complementary/alternative therapies with adults. Studies have shown that these therapies are also being used by children and adolescents.

Therefore, material that addresses the use of these therapies with children and adolescents is included in many chapters.

When the first edition of *Independent Nursing Interventions* was published (the book's original title), computers were just coming into vogue and the Internet was an idea that had not yet evolved. As noted throughout the book, content is now being retrieved from web sites, and so we include web sites for obtaining the most recent information about specific therapies. Caution is needed in using web sites as many do not receive the scrutiny for scientific accuracy and safety that is given to journal publications.

As has been the tradition in this book, the scientific basis for use of therapies is provided. In the practice realm, evidence-based practice is being emphasized. Various groups, including the National Academy of Science, have proposed goals to achieve in relation to research on complementary therapies. In addition to continuing to include research studies related to the therapy covered in each chapter, a chapter dedicated solely to research has been added. Developing a research base for complementary therapies is a goal in which nurses can be integrally involved.

As in previous editions, some therapies have been deleted and others added. Our goal has been to include those therapies that nurses frequently use. To assist readers in accessing information about each therapy, a similar format exists across all chapters. A description of the therapy, the scientific basis for use of the therapy to the extent that it exists, the inclusion of one or two techniques that can be used to implement the therapy, conditions and patient populations in which the therapy has been used, and suggestions for research are found in each chapter. Precautions to be aware of when using a therapy are noted in the intervention section. Renewed attention is required as a commonly held fallacy is that all complementary therapies are benign.

As the consumer demand for and use of complementary therapies continue to increase, it is critical that nurses have knowledge about complementary therapies so that they can include selected ones in their practice, provide patients with information about therapies, be informed about research and practice guidelines related to complementary therapies, alert patients to possible contraindications with traditional medicines, and incorporate some of these therapies into their own self-care. Nurses can also direct consumers to reliable sources for obtaining additional information.

We wish to thank the many students across the years who, through the interest they have shown in complementary therapies, have prompted us to continue our quest to obtain new information about complementary therapies that can be used by nurses. We wish to thank our colleagues at the University of Minnesota School of Nursing and the Center for Spirituality and Healing for their continued support and for helping to develop the knowledge base for complementary therapies and educate students about these therapies.

Mariah Snyder PhD, RN, FAAN
Ruth Lindquist PhD, RN, FAAN, APRN, BC

PART I

Foundations
for Practice

Complementary/alternative therapies (often referenced as complementary/alternative medicine) encompass more than 1,800 therapies and systems of care (Kreitzer & Jensen, 2000). Nurses have used a number of these therapies for centuries in providing care to patients in diverse settings. However, there are many therapies that are less familiar to nurses as these are a part of health care systems other than the Western biomedical model. It is important for nurses to be aware of the broad spectrum of therapies as they provide care to persons from many cultures. Chapter 2 introduces nurses to health care practices in several cultures that use some non-biomedical therapies.

Part I provides an overview of complementary therapies including two in particular, presence and active listening, that are part of the underlying philosophy of complementary therapies. Although it is important for nurses to be competent in a specific therapy before administering it to a patient, it is equally important that they incorporate the philosophy into their practice. The caring, holistic philosophy of nursing is also the philosophy underlying many complementary therapies.

Modeling the holistic, caring philosophy to patients and coworkers is important to the success of complementary therapies. Chapter 3 provides nurses with strategies they can use to "take care of self," incorporating self-care practices in their lives to renew their energy and to be more present to patients and colleagues. Readers can explore the therapies described in subsequent chapters and select those that they can use in their personal lives as well as in caring for patients.

Presence and therapeutic listening are an integral part of the underlying, holistic, caring philosophy of complementary therapies. The content in the chapters on therapies may not specifically refer to presence and listening, but these are integrated into the administration of all complementary therapies.

REFERENCE

Kreitzer, M. J., & Jensen, D. (2000). Healing practices: Trends, challenges, and opportunities for nurses in acute and critical care. *AACN Clinical Issues, 11*, 7–16.

CHAPTER 1

An Overview of Complementary/ Alternative Therapies

Mariah Snyder and Ruth Lindquist

Complementary/alternative therapies have become an important part of health care in the United States and other countries. Although we will use the term *complementary therapies* primarily in this book, numerous other designations have been used for therapies that have not been a part of the traditional Western medicine system of care. The term *complementary* is preferred by some as it conveys the idea that a therapy is used as an adjunct to Western therapies whereas *alternative* indicates a therapy that is used in place of a Western medicine approach. Both terms are used by the National Center for Complementary and Alternative Medicine (NCCAM) of the National Institutes of Health. More recently the term *integrative medicine* indicates that the care provided blends Western medicine, complementary therapies, and therapies from other systems of health care. NCCAM notes that complementary therapies used in integrative medicine must have "some high-quality scientific evidence of safety and effectiveness" (National Center for Complementary and Alternative Medicine, 2004).

DEFINITION AND CLASSIFICATION

Much debate has occurred over defining complementary therapies. Nursing and other health professions frequently call the area *complementary therapies* whereas NCCAM refers to them as *complementary medicine*. The broad scope of these therapies and the many health professionals and therapists who are involved in delivering them create challenges for finding a definition that captures the scope of this field.

The definition for complementary/alternative therapies put forth by NCCAM is: "Complementary and alternative medicine is a group of diverse medical and health care systems, practices, and products that are not presently considered to be part of conventional medicine" (NCCAM, 2004).

Conventional refers to Western biomedicine. In an earlier NCCAM definition (Panel, 1997), it was noted that complementary medicine included a broad domain of healing practices that were not part of the dominant health system in a society or culture. Thus, Western medicine would be the complementary system of care in a non-Western country.

The ambiguity within the definition of complementary therapies poses challenges when comparing findings from the various surveys that have been conducted on their use. Some surveys have included multiple therapies and others have limited their number. For example, when the NCCAM/National Center for Health Statistics removed the category of prayer, the percent of persons using complementary therapies fell from 62% to 36%. Many studies have focused on persons who speak English, thus excluding recent immigrants who are believed to use many therapies from their native cultures.

According to Kreitzer and Jensen (2000), more than 1,800 therapies have been identified as complementary. NCCAM has classified these multiple therapies and systems of care into five categories, which are shown in Table 1.1. Some of these have been highly publicized and are widely used whereas others are not familiar to anyone who has traditionally used Western medicine. Table 1.1 includes a number of therapies that have been a part of nursing for many years.

USE OF COMPLEMENTARY THERAPIES

Interest in and use of complementary/alternative therapies has increased exponentially during the past quarter century. Numerous surveys have attempted to determine the percent of use in the United States and other countries (Barnes, Powell-Griner, McFann, & Nahin, 2004; Eisenberg et

TABLE 1.1 NCCAM Classification for Complementary Therapies and Examples of Therapies

Alternative Systems of Care

Systems of health care that have been developed separate from the Western biomedical approach to care

Examples: Traditional Chinese Medicine, Ayurvedic, Native American medicine, curanderismo, homeopathy, naturopathy

Mind–Body Therapies

Interventions that employ a variety of techniques to facilitate the mind's capacity to impact physical symptoms and body functions

Examples: imagery, meditation, yoga, music therapy, prayer, journaling, biofeedback, humor, tai chi, art therapy

Biologically Based Therapies

Natural and biologically based practices and products

Examples: plant-derived preparations (herbs), special diets such as the Pritikin and the Ornish, orthomolecular medicine (nutritional and food supplements), other products such as cartilage

Manipulative and Body-Based Systems

Therapies that are based on manipulation and movement of the body

Examples: chiropractic medicine, the many types of massage, body work such as Rolfing, light and color therapies, hydrotherapy

Energy Therapies

Therapies that focus on energy emanating from within the body (biofields) or energy coming from external sources

Examples: healing touch, therapeutic touch, Reiki, external Qi Gong, magnets

---

al., 1998; O'Brien, 2004; Rhee, Barg, & Hershey, 2004; Rosen, Azzam, Levi, Braun, & Krivoy, 2003). The percent of persons using complementary therapies varied from 21% (Rosen et al.) to 85.4% (Rhee et al.). NCCAM and the National Center for Health Statistics reported that 62% of American adults used some type of complementary therapy (NCCAM, 2004). A survey by Eisenberg and colleagues (1998) found that the percent of Americans using complementary therapies increased from 31% in 1991 to 42% in 1997.

The use of complementary therapies is not limited to adults. Bruener, Barry, and Kemper (1998) found that 70% of a sample of homeless teens reported using them. The percent of children and adolescents using

complementary therapies was lower in a study by Yussman, Ryan, Auinger, and Weitzman (2004), with only 2% using these therapies. However, the study asked about visits to complementary therapists as
contrasted with overall use of therapies.

Some researchers have attempted to identify the characteristics of
persons who use complementary therapies. Rosen and colleagues (2003)
found that more females used these therapies than did males. Also, a
higher percent of users had academic degrees, as contrasted with a non-
user group. These findings were further validated in the national survey
conducted by the NCCAM and the National Center for Health Statistics
(2004). Struthers and Nichols (2004) reviewed studies on the use of
complementary therapies in racial and ethnic minority populations; in
seven studies, persons in minority groups did not use more complementary
therapies than did persons in other groups.

Currently, third-party payers, such as insurance companies, pay for
a limited number of complementary therapies. Those most frequently
covered are chiropractic, acupuncture, and biofeedback. In most instances, physician referral is required for reimbursement. Some states,
such as Washington, require the inclusion of complementary therapists
in private, commercial insurance products (Lafferty et al., 2004). According to NCCAM (2004), Americans spent between $36 and $47 billion
on complementary therapies in 1997 with $12 to $20 billion paid directly
by the consumer. People must feel that complementary therapies produce
positive results if they continue to pay for these therapies when insurance
companies or HMOs do not pay for them.

What has prompted this rapidly growing interest in complementary
therapies? First, the holistic philosophy underlying complementary therapies differs significantly from the dualistic or Cartesian philosophy that
for several centuries has permeated Western medicine. In Cartesian philosophy, the mind and body are viewed as separate and non-interacting
entities. In complementary therapies the total person is considered: physically, emotionally, mentally, and spiritually. The goal is to create harmony
or balance within the person. An individual seeks care from complementary therapists or facilities because he/she wants to be treated as a whole
person and not as a heart attack or a fractured hip. Another reason is
that people want to be involved in decision making; they want to be
empowered. In a study by Mitzdorf and colleagues (1999), 64% of patients stated that they were given minimal time to discuss their health
concerns with their physicians, and 42% noted that they were not afforded
time to ask questions. The increasing pressure of cost containment in
health care has reduced the amount of time physicians and nurses spend
with their patients. Physicians, nurses, and others provide assistance to

persons to attain health, but true healing can only come from within the patient. A third reason cited for seeking care from complementary therapists relates to quality of life. Patients have reported they do not want the treatment for a health problem to be worse than the health problem itself. The focus of Western medicine has been on curing problems whereas the philosophy underlying complementary therapies is on harmony within the person and promotion of health. Mitzdorf and colleagues found that 82% of patients reported the side effects of medications as a reason for using complementary therapies.

The personal qualities of the complementary therapist (whether a nurse, physician, or other health care professional) are key in the healing process. Caring, which has received considerable attention in nursing across the years, is a vital component in the administration of complementary therapies. Two therapies that will be covered in subsequent chapters—presence and active listening—illustrate this caring. Remen (2000), a physician who is involved in cancer care, stated:

> I know that if I listen attentively to (sic) someone, to their essential self, their soul, as it were, I often find that at the deepest, most unconscious level, they can sense the direction of their own healing and wholeness. If I can remain open to that, without expectations of what the (sic) someone is supposed to do, how they are supposed to change in order to be better, or even what their wholeness looks like, what can happen is magical. By that I mean that it has a certain coherency or integrity about it, far beyond any way of fixing their situation or easing their pain that I can devise on my own. [p. 90]

The heightened interest in complementary therapies prompted the National Institutes of Health (NIH) to establish the Office of Alternative Medicine in 1992, which was elevated to the National Center for Complementary/Alternative Medicine (NCCAM) in 1998. What was significant in establishing this NIH office was that consumers, rather than health professionals, lobbied for it. The purposes of the NCCAM are:

1. to facilitate the evaluation of therapies,
2. to investigate and evaluate the efficacy of therapies,
3. to serve as an information clearinghouse on complementary therapies, and
4. to support research training.

NCCAM has funded studies for individual researchers and for centers that explore the efficacy of a number of specific complementary therapies, such as acupuncture and Saint John's wort. Other centers explore the use of complementary therapies in the treatment of specific conditions such as addictive disorders, arthritis, cardiovascular disease, and neurological disorders.

IMPLICATIONS FOR NURSING

Complementary therapies (although this term was not originally used) and their basic philosophies have been a part of nursing since its beginnings. In *Notes on Nursing* (1859/1936) Florence Nightingale stressed the importance of creating an environment in which healing could occur and the importance of therapies such as music in the healing process.

Although it is indeed gratifying to see medicine and other professions recognizing the importance of listening and presence in the healing process, nursing needs to assert the fact that many of these therapies have been taught in nursing programs and have been practiced by nurses for centuries. Therapies such as meditation, imagery, support groups, music therapy, humor, journaling, reminiscence, caring-based approaches, massage, touch, healing touch, active listening, and presence have been practiced by nurses throughout time.

Complementary therapies are receiving increasing attention within nursing. Journals such as the *Journal of Holistic Nursing* and *Complementary Therapies in Nursing & Midwifery* are devoted almost exclusively to complementary therapies and their use. Many journals have devoted entire issues to exploring them.

Because of their increasing use by patients to whom they provide care, and because patients expect health professionals to possess knowledge about complementary therapies, it is critical that nurses have this knowledge in order to

1. provide guidance in obtaining health histories and assessing patients,
2. answer basic questions about the use of complementary therapies and refer patients to reliable sources of information,
3. refer patients to competent therapists, and
4. administer a selected number of complementary therapies.

Information about the use of complementary therapies must be a routine part of a complete health history. Many patients may not volunteer information about using complementary therapies unless they are specifically asked; others may be reluctant to share this information unless the practitioner displays an acceptance of their use. Although information about all complementary therapies is needed, it is especially critical to obtain information about use of herbal preparations. Interactions between certain prescriptive drugs and herbal preparations may pose a threat to health unless complete information is obtained.

The vast number of complementary therapies makes it impossible for nurses to be knowledgeable about all of them, but knowledge about the more common ones will assist nurses in answering basic questions. Many organizations, professional associations, individuals, and groups have excellent web sites that provide information about specific therapies. Caution is needed, however, in accepting information from any web site. Walji and colleagues (2004) found that 25% of the web sites on St. John's wort contained information that could be harmful if a person acted upon it. One of the functions of NCCAM is to provide consumer information. Web sites for specific therapies are identified in chapters in this book.

Referring patients to competent therapists or helping patients to identify competent therapists is another role for nurses, and this is not an easy task. Because many complementary therapists are not members of a health profession, licensure and regulation often do not apply to them, and regulation varies greatly from state to state. In 2000 the Minnesota legislature passed a bill placing unlicensed complementary and alternative therapies under the auspices of the Department of Health (Alternative Health Care Bill, H. F. 3839). Notably, this bill contains a patient bill of rights. If clients have concerns, they can make them known to the commissioner for complementary and alternative therapies. This law is a beginning in the protection of clients.

The area of practice and nurses' own preferences will assist in determining those therapies in which they wish to become proficient. As with any treatment or procedure, the nurse must have competence in administering the therapy before using it in practice. This may require education beyond that received in basic or advanced education programs. An increasing number of nurses are being certified to administer specific therapies such as healing touch and aromatherapy. Certification shows patients and colleagues that the nurse has the knowledge and expertise necessary to administer the therapy competently.

Education

Inclusion of complementary therapies into nursing curricula at all levels is needed if nurses are to be expected to incorporate these therapies into their practices. Halcón, Chlan, Kreitzer, and Leonard (2003) reported that 95% of faculty and students in one school believed that complementary

therapies should be incorporated into patient care. In a survey of baccalaureate nursing programs in the United States, Richardson (2003) found
that 77% included content and/or experiential learning in the teaching
of these therapies. This figure is very encouraging and reflects the fact
that nurse educators have made efforts to prepare students for contemporary practice.

Little discussion has taken place about which therapies should be
taught in basic nursing programs and which should be included in master's
curricula. The therapies taught vary across schools of nursing. Therapies
such as music intervention, imagery, massage, prayer, aromatherapy, and
healing touch could be logically included in baccalaureate curricula, as
research exists to support their use in practice. Conveying these therapies
within an evidenced-based approach will help students grasp their legiti-
macy. In addition to content on specific therapies, information about
their underlying philosophy is also needed.

Attention to content on complementary therapies in graduate education is also required. Programs preparing advanced nurse practitioners
need to ensure that graduates are asking patients about their use of these
therapies. Based on the faculty expertise, programs may include courses
on selected therapies such as healing touch or aromatherapy that will
prepare the graduate to take the certification examination for that therapy. Research courses could focus on helping students examine studies
that have been conducted on a specific therapy to evaluate the evidence
that exists for its use in practice settings.

Continuing education offerings are needed to help practicing nurses
gain basic information about complementary therapies and to update
their knowledge and expertise about specific therapies. Some therapies,
such as aromatherapy, have self-study modules available. The University
of Minnesota Center for Spirituality and Healing has a number of online
courses available (www.csh.umn.edu). Other institutions that offer online
courses on complementary therapies can be accessed at http://
www.nursece.com.

Practice Settings

On an individual basis and in facilities, nurses are incorporating complementary therapies into their practice. Some facilities have developed practice guidelines for the use of specific therapies. In some instances this
may mean that only nurses who are certified or who have had additional
preparation can administer the therapy. It is critical not only that guidelines for specific therapies be addressed, but also that the philosophy
underlying complementary therapies, holism, and caring be emphasized.
Adding therapies without their underlying philosophy may result in
nurses' viewing complementary therapies as just another task to complete.

Patient demand for complementary therapies has resulted in more and more hospitals and clinics integrating them into the care provided. Some facilities, such as the Woodwinds Health Campus in Woodbury, Minnesota, are based on a holistic philosophy of care with complementary therapies part of the warp and woof of the facility. The Institute for Health and Healing at Abbott Northwestern Hospital in Minneapolis offers a number of therapies to patients including massage, reflexology, guided imagery, relaxation techniques, acupuncture, nutrition consultations, healing touch, Reiki, reconnective healing, QiGong, and therapeutic touch. Clients, of course, receive information about the cost of each therapy.

Some concerns have been voiced about nurses implementing complementary therapies as part of their practice. Sparber (2001) found that 47% of boards of nursing had statements about nurses' use of these therapies but 40% had not formally addressed the topic. Seven states (13%) were exploring it. An individual nurse's knowledge about and competence in implementing a specific therapy are key to the administration of a therapy in practice.

The New York State Nurses Association (2003) has developed a position statement on the inclusion of complementary therapies in the practice of nursing. This statement includes a number of recommendations regarding nurses' use of complementary therapies. These include:

- have the appropriate education, experience, and supervision to be competent;

- discuss options with the patient;

- become familiar with state practice acts, particularly as they relate to acupuncture and massage;

- incorporate the American Holistic Nurses Association Standards of Practice and the American Nurses Association's Code of Ethics in one's practice;

- participate in research about the effectiveness of specific therapies;

- advocate for the inclusion of complementary therapies in care settings and for coverage by third-party payers.

Research

As emphasis on evidence-based practice grows, concerns about the lack of studies to support the use of complementary therapies are being voiced.

Although the body of knowledge on some complementary therapies is increasing, few have been studied extensively using the gold standard of Western medicine, the double-blind clinical trial. However, research has been conducted outside the United States. For example, scientists in Germany have conducted many studies on herbs. Anecdotal evidence and case studies provide support for their efficacy. But there is a need for significantly more research on these therapies.

Over the years, nurses have conducted their own research on a number of the complementary therapies, as can be noted in the references provided for the therapies in this book. Experience with the administration of complementary therapies places nurses in a prime position for assuming leadership roles on interdisciplinary teams that are investigating them. Numerous challenges exist in conducting research on many complementary therapies because current designs and measurement techniques may not be appropriate for therapies whose philosophical basis differs from the traditional Western therapies for which these methods were developed. Chapter 29 will address this issue further.

REFERENCES

Alternative Health Care Bill. H. F. 3839. Minnesota State Legislature. (2000).

Barnes, P. M., Powell-Griner, E., McFann, K., & Nahin, R. L. (2004, May 27). Complementary and alternative medicine use among adults: United States, 2002. *Advance Data, 343*, 1–19.

Bruener, C., Barry, P., & Kemper, K. (1998). Alternative medicine use by homeless youth. *Archives of Pediatric and Adolescent Medicine, 152*, 1071–1075.

Eisenberg, D. M., Davis, R. B., Ettner, S. L., Appel, S., Wilkey, S., Van Rommapy, M., et al. (1998). Trends in alternative medicine use in the United States, 1990–1997. *Journal of the American Medical Association, 280*, 1569–1575.

Halcón, L. L., Chlan, L. L., Kreitzer, M. J., & Leonard, B. J. (2003). Complementary therapies and healing practices: Faculty/student beliefs and attitudes and the implications for nursing education. *Journal of Professional Nursing, 19*, 387–397.

Kreitzer, M. J., & Jensen, D. (2000). Healing practices: Trends, challenges, and opportunities for nurses in acute and critical care. *AACN Clinical Issues, 11*, 7–16.

Lafferty, W. E., Bellas, A., Corage Baden, A., Tyree, P. T., Standish, L. J., & Patterson, R. (2004). The use of complementary and alternative medical providers by insured cancer patients in Washington state. *Cancer, 100*, 1522–1530.

Mitzdorf, U., Beck, K., Horton-Hausknecht, J., Weidenhammer, W., Kindermann, A., Takaxc, M., et al. (1999). Why do patients seek treatment in hospitals of complementary medicine? *Journal of Alternative and Complementary Medicine, 5*, 463–473.

National Center for Complementary and Alternative Medicine. (2004). What is complementary and alternative medicine (CAM)? Retrieved December 1, 2004, from http://nccam.nih.gov/health/whatiscam

New York State Nurses Association. (2003). Complementary therapies in the practice of nursing. Retrieved December 8, 2004, from http://www.nysna.org/programs/practce/positions/position14.htm

Nightingale, F. (1859/1936/1992). *Notes on nursing.* Philadelphia: Lippincott.

O'Brien, K. (2004). Complementary and alternative medicine: The move into mainstream health. *Clinical & Experimental Optometry, 87,* 110–120.

Panel on Definition and Description, CAM Research Methodology Conference. (1997). Defining and describing complementary and alternative medicine. *Alternative Therapies in Health and Medicine, 3*(2), 49–57.

Remen, R. N. (2000). *My grandfather's blessings.* New York: Riverhead Books.

Rhee, S. M., Barg, V. K., & Hershey, C. O. (2004). Use of complementary and alternative medicines by ambulatory patients. *Archives of Internal Medicine, 164,* 1004–1009.

Richardson, S. F. (2003). Complementary health and healing in nursing education. *Journal of Holistic Nursing, 21,* 20–35.

Rosen, I., Azzam, A. S., Levi, T., Braun, E., & Krivoy, N. (2003). Patient approach and experience regarding complementary medicine: Survey among hospitalized patients in a university hospital. *Pharmacoepidemiology & Drug Safety, 12,* 679–685.

Sparber, A. (2001). State boards of nursing and scope of practice of registered nurses performing complementary therapies. *Online Journal of Issues in Nursing, 6*(2). Retrieved January 28, 2002, from http://www.nursingworld.org/ojin/topic15/tpc15_6.htm

Struthers, R., & Nichols, L. A. (2004). Utilization of complementary and alternative medicine among racial and ethnic minority populations: Implications for reducing health care disparities. *Annual Review of Nursing Research, 2,* 285–313.

Walji, M., Sagaram, S., Sagaram, D., Meric-Gernstam, F., Johnson, C., Mirza, N. Q., et al. (2004, June 29). Efficacy of quality criteria to identify potentially harmful information: A cross-sectional survey of complementary and alternative medicine web sites. *Journal of Medical Internet Research, 6,* e21.

Yussman, S. M., Ryan, S. A., Auinger, P., & Weitzman, M. (2004). Visits to complementary and alternative medicine providers by children and adolescents in the United States. *Ambulatory Pediatric, 4,* 429–435.

CHAPTER 2

Cultural Diversity and Complementary Therapies

Kathleen Niska and Mariah Snyder

Culture refers to the shared way of life of a group of people. Medical anthropologists McElroy and Townsend (2004) specified, "the culture of a group is an information system transmitted from one generation to another through nongenetic mechanisms" (p. 110). The use of symbols, categories, rules, rituals, and other learned behaviors enhances the adaptation of the group, enabling its members to survive within their ecological setting. While people transform their healing systems in the process of adapting, they also maintain fidelity to long-standing traditions (Rogoff, 2003). Traditional healing systems that have persisted over thousands of years and are still alive today are Traditional Chinese Medicine (TCM), Tibetan medicine, Ayurvedic medicine, Samoan medicine, and native medicine of the aboriginal peoples of Australia and the Americas (Selin, 2003). Although differences among these systems exist, a common theme is that health is based on harmony within the person and between the person and the universe. This chapter examines the contribution of these ancient healing systems to the current medical pluralism within American health care that is evident in the coexistence of biomedicine and complementary/alternative therapies. Knowledge about these systems will help nurses be aware of the many healing practices patients may be using. Table 2.1 presents therapies found in the healing systems discussed.

TRADITIONAL CHINESE MEDICINE (TCM)

For more than 4,000 years, TCM has consisted of two cosmological principles (yin and yang); five elements (wood, fire, earth, metal, and air); theories about energy channels, viscera, and pathogenesis; and principles of treatment. Yan and Jingfeng (2003) explained: "The underlying basis of TCM is that all of creation is born from the interdependence of two opposite principles, yin and yang. These two opposites are in constant motion, creating a fluctuating balance in the healthy body. Disease results when either yin or yang is in a state of prolonged excess or deficiency" (p. 56). Qi is the pervasive energy of the universe produced when polar opposites are harmonized within the body (Cohen, 1997).

TCM focuses on prevention of diseases as well as prevention of new complications or the worsening of existing diseases. Diet therapy aims to balance the polar opposites of yin/yang, hot/cold, and deficiency/excess. Acupuncture restores harmony by relieving pain, anxiety, and nausea. Herbal medicines are complex blends of plant, animal, and mineral substances.

Young (2001) emphasized: "A healthy individual lives in harmony with the universe and seasons of nature with a balanced diet, calm mind, and energetic body" (p. 100). A healthy person attends to responsibilities

TABLE 2.1 Complementary/Alternative Therapies Rooted in Ancient Healing Systems

Traditional Chinese Medicine	Tibetan Medicine	Ayurvedic Medicine	Samoan Medicine	Native Medicine of the Americas
Acupuncture	Acupuncture	Aromatherapy	Herbal medicine	Drum circle
Diet therapy	Diet therapy	Diet therapy	Massage	Herbal medicine
Herbal medicine	Herbal medicine	Herbal medicine	Prayer	Massage
Massage	Hot/cold compresses	Massage		Prayer
Qi Gong	Massage	Meditation		Singing
Tai Chi	Meditation	Spiritual advice		Storytelling
Visualization	Yoga	Yoga		Sweat lodge purification
				Talking circle

of his or her intergenerational family (Tung, 2000), meditates daily (Chen, 2001), and exercises doing Qi Gong to maintain an energetic body (Cohen, 1997). Qi Gong is disciplined daily exercise consisting of graceful movements, meditative breathing, and focused concentration. The search for longevity is a respected endeavor within TCM.

TRADITIONAL TIBETAN MEDICINE

Buddhism was introduced to Tibet in the seventh century CE. The first formal Tibetan medical texts, *Four Medical Tantras,* emerged in the twelfth century CE. In 1696, Tibetans created their first medical college. Medical education of seven years combined memorization of medical texts with practical patient care. In 1959, Tibet was invaded by Communist China, causing many Tibetans to flee to northern India for refuge. The fourteenth Dalai Lama set up a new medical school in northern India.

Steiner (2003) elucidated the spiritual core of Tibetan medicine stating, "Through the discipline of mindfulness, generosity, and compassion, suffering can be transformed. Thus, healing is synonymous with complete awakening or enlightenment" (p. 103). Cameron (2001) stressed, "Tibetan Buddhism encourages intensive spiritual practice to produce a calm mind, good heart, and enlightenment in one lifetime" (p. 45).

Integral to this spiritual core, the strong and healthy person has a balance of three humors (wind, bile, and phlegm) whereas the person suffering from disease and mental illness has lost the balance of these humors (Young, 2001), which are made up of the five elements of the cosmos: earth, water, fire, air, and space. Diseases are categorized by the type of humoral imbalance. Tibetan physicians use questioning, observation, palpation, pulse taking, and urinalysis to diagnose disease (Loizzo & Blackhall, 1998). Treatments focus on using diet modification, prayer, herbal medicines, massage, and moxibustion (burning the herbs gerbera, nutmeg, and ginger in the dried moxa herb). Tibetan herbal pills may contain 3 to 150 herbs per formula.

Self-care is based on modifying one's diet, improving one's virtue, and seeking natural beauty by looking at beautiful scenery, smelling pleasant odors, and listening to pleasing sounds. Meditation promotes relaxation and inner peace. Yoga offers mental calm arising from disciplined breathing, meditation, and coordinated exercise.

AYURVEDIC MEDICINE

In Ayurveda, health-seeking endeavors were a religious obligation (Desai, 2000). The healthy body was seen as a microcosm of the universe composed of primordial elements of earth, water, fire, air, and ether, which combined to form three humors, or doshas. The relative balance of the three doshas (pitta, vata, and kapha) regulated physiological processes of the body. If the equilibrium of the body were to be upset, disease resulted. Ayurvedic physicians observed the tongue, eyes, skin, tone of voice, pulse, and general appearance, and evaluated urine and feces (Young, 2001). The physician might recommend dietary treatment to restore the equilibrium of the body through rebalancing the doshas. Using food as medicine, warming foods (sour, salty, and pungent) would be digested easily and cooling foods (sweet, bitter, and astringent) would be digested slowly. Ayurvedic massage used essential oils according to the state of balance of the doshas. For example, almond oil was used when vata predominated, sandalwood when pitta regulated, and sesame oil when kapha dominated the physiological processes. Herbal medicines came in the form of pills, powders, pastes, teas, and medicated oils.

Introducing the Ayurvedic tradition to Western people, Chopra (1990) explained a fundamental approach to wellness: "The guiding principle of Ayurveda is that the mind exerts the deepest influence on the body and freedom from sickness depends upon contacting our own awareness, bringing it into balance, and then extending that balance to the body" (p. 6). Meditation was a way of finding calm awareness as part of a daily routine (Chopra, 1991). Yoga practice blended meditation, chanting, and postures of the body, giving the practitioner relaxation, flexibility, and strength. Spiritual advice as an avenue to wellness called for lifestyle improvements, fasts, purification, ritual prayers, and pilgrimages. Cultivating good habits extended to living in harmony with the seasons, and eating and exercising according to the seasons to ensure health.

SAMOAN MEDICINE

Ancient Samoans taught that all humans were descendants of gods, known as atua and aitu. Illnesses were the result of the gods' anger at the lack of respect shown by individuals and families (Macpherson & Macpherson, 2003). Traditional Samoan medicine consisted of prayers, incantations, herbal medicine, massage using scented oils, and simple surgery.

Samoans distinguished new illnesses brought to them by contact with European explorers and merchants who introduced influenza, measles, mumps, whooping cough, and syphilis. Botanical fieldworkers found 336 plants in Samoa in 1868, even though the Samoans were using only nine at the time. With education, Samoans learned how to use many more native plants for medicinal purposes (Macpherson & Macpherson, 2003). When Margaret Mead (1928) lived among the Samoans she noted, "There is no specialization among women, except in medicine and midwifery, both the prerogatives of very old women who teach their arts to their middle-aged daughters and nieces. The only other vocation is that of the wife of an official orator, and no girl will prepare herself for this one type of marriage which demands special knowledge, for she has no guarantee that she will marry a man of this class" (p. 25). Folk remedies employed by women were herbal medicines and massage. With contact with Western visitors, a hybrid healing system emerged. Samoan healers continued to diagnose and treat intrinsically Samoan illnesses that had their root cause in social or spiritual imbalance related to pre-Christian gods (Ishida, Toomata-Mayer, & Mayer, 1996). Samoan healers diagnosed and treated illnesses caused by trauma, effects of the ecosystem, and germs, using Western diagnostic categories and biomedicine for treatment.

NATIVE TRADITIONS OF THE AMERICAS

To present a broad view of North American native healing, Mehl-Madrona (2003) observed, "Traditional Native American cultures perceive health as a state of balance of spirit, mind, and body; illness is the result of disharmony or imbalance. Illness requires treatment at many levels, including personal, family, community, and spiritual. Traditional medicine has included herbalists, shamans, purification ceremonies, healing rituals, emotional therapies, manipulative medicine, teas, herbs, and special foods" (p. 211). To present a broad view of Mesoamerican and South American healing, Mendoza (2003) stated, "Mexica Aztec, Inca or Quechua, Aymara or Kalawaya, and other American Indian doctors and physicians were required to balance herbal and surgical treatments with interpretive models of causation ranging from the supernatural and magical to the natural and physical" (p. 234). Botanists have documented the native use of more than 1,500 species of medicinal plants, among which the Indians especially valued coca, mescaline, curare, quinine, belladonna, and dopamine (Stark, 1981).

In North America, the land has been a source of healing. The first step for an Indian doctor was to learn to walk in balance with the Earth Mother, and then to seek the power that came from the Great Spirit (Steiger, 1984). Indian doctors organized the power to heal through songs, stories, and ritual acts (McMaster & Trafzer, 2004). Lame Deer and

Erdoes (1992) described the typical medicine man among the Lakota as knowing the right songs to go with every medicine he used in every ceremony he performed. Ritual acts among the First Nations of Canada were the talking circle, the drum circle, smudging, and the sweat lodge ceremony (Hunter, Logan, Barton, & Goulet, 2004). Massage was a healing procedure among the Cherokees and Pawnees (Vogel, 1970). The Cree healing ceremony had five parts: ritual to purify and open the door to the spiritual world, petition of the patient and the healer, treatment with herbal medicine and a sweat lodge ceremony, education of the patient, and closure of the ceremony, emphasizing that the Great Spirit would continue the healing already underway (Morse, Young, & Swartz, 1991). Among the Ojibway, Johnston (1976) noted, "Initially, healers were herbalists. . . . Eventually herbalists became medicine men; and the medicine men became philosophers concerned not only with preserving life and mitigating pain, but also with offering guidance and principles for living the good life whose end was to secure general well being" (p. 71). Peacock and Wisuri (2002) affirmed, "Medicine people sometimes still come all the way from Canada to visit Ojibwe communities. They travel throughout Ojibwe country via an informal network of traditional people, who let each other know when the medicine person will be in town. . . . They are among the most highly respected members of our communities because they are the purveyors and keepers of ancient sacred knowledge" (p. 102).

In the context of Mesoamerica, Lipp (2001) clarified, "In Mesoamerican traditional medicine, illnesses are signs of natural disequilibrium or disorder, and therapeutic treatment is fundamentally concerned with restoring harmonious relations between internal body processes and the physical, social, and cosmological order" (p. 109). When a family member became ill, household remedies consisted of medicinal plants, fright-illness rituals, massage, and sweat baths. If no relief resulted, the shaman joined the family and relatives for a curing ceremony of prayer, sacrificial offerings, ritual meals, and a pilgrimage to local shrines. Divine intervention was the rule that pervaded all facets of life. Health, recovery from illness, and effective use of medicine depended upon divine assistance for healing (Viesca, 2003). In colonial Mexico, the Moorish influence in Spanish medicine blended into indigenous healing practices, creating a strong herbal base, an emphasis on balance between light/dark and hot/cold, and Christian belief that healing came from the power of God through prayer and ritual (Torres, 1983, 1984). In the mid-twentieth century, good health in the Mexican American family was associated with the ability to work (Baca, 1969), whereas illness was associated with sadness, because illness prevented members from working in ways that sustained the family (Ulibarri, 1978). Samora (1978) identified a conceptualization of health in which being healthy was attributed to the beneficence of God. Hayes-Bautista (1998) noted that for Latinos the strong emotions of fright, shame, sorrow, rejection, and disillusionment were perceived to be triggers for illness. Compassionate listening conveyed respect, and problem solving was facilitated by the use of analogies, wisdom sayings, and stories.

IMPLICATIONS FOR NURSES AND THE HEALTH CARE TEAM

Numerous complementary/alternative therapies have originated within ancient healing systems of other cultures. Entire systems of health care have survived for thousands of years among neighboring cultures around the globe, whose immigrants have come to live in the United States and have shared healing traditions with health care workers in this country. Through clinical and scholarly work, nurses have learned to extend nursing care in culturally competent ways, have been alert to investigate the scientific foundation for the therapeutic success of specific complementary/alternative therapies belonging to these ancient healing traditions, and have formed collegial bonds with practitioners of diverse ways of healing.

Although they may not be familiar with the minute details, it is helpful for nurses to understand the worldview of these ancient healing traditions that have survived to the present day. Only then can nurses ask patients and family members about specific needs and preferences that are a natural part of their healing tradition.

REFERENCES

Baca, J. (1969). Some health beliefs of the Spanish speaking. *American Journal of Nursing, 69,* 2172–2176.

Cameron, M. (2001). *Karma & happiness.* Minneapolis, MN: Fairview.

Chen, Y. (2001). Chinese values, health and nursing. *Journal of Advanced Nursing, 36,* 270–273.

Chopra, D. (1990). *Perfect health.* New York: Harmony Books.

Chopra, D. (1991). *Unconditional life: Mastering the forces that shape personal reality.* New York: Bantam.

Cohen, K. (1997). *The way of Qigong: The art and science of Chinese energy healing.* New York: Ballantine.

Desai, P. (2000). Medical ethics in India. In R. Veatch (Ed.), *Cross-cultural perspectives in medical ethics* (pp. 240–258). Boston: Jones and Bartlett.

Hayes-Bautista, D., & Chiprut, R. (1998). *Healing Latinas: Reslidad y fantasia.* Los Angeles: Cedars-Sinai Health System.

Hunter, L., Logan, J., Barton, S., & Goulet, J. (2004). Linking aboriginal healing traditions to holistic nursing practice. *Journal of Holistic Nursing, 22,* 267–285.

Ishida, D., Toomata-Mayer, T., & Mayer, J. (1996). Samoans. In J. Lipson, S. Dibble, & P. Minarik (Eds.), *Culture & nursing care* (pp. 250–263). San Francisco: UCSF Nursing Press.

Johnston, B. (1976). *Ojibway heritage.* Lincoln: University of Nebraska Press.

Lame Deer, A., & Erdoes, R. (1992). *Gift of power: The life and teaching of a Lakota medicine man.* Santa Fe, NM: Bear.

Lipp, F. (2001). Southern Mexican and Guatamalan shamans. In B. Huber & A. Sandstrom (Eds.), *Mesoamerican healers* (pp. 95–116). Austin: University of Texas Press.

Loizzo, J., & Blackhall, L. (1998). Traditional alternatives as complementary sciences: The case of Indo-Tibetan medicine. *The Journal of Alternative and Complementary Medicine, 4,* 311–319.

Macpherson, C., & Macpherson, L. (2003). When healing cultures collide: A case from the Pacific. In H. Selin (Ed.), *Medicine across cultures* (pp. 191–207). Boston: Kluwer Academic Publishers.

McElroy, A., & Townsend, P. (2004). *Medical anthropology in ecological perspective.* Boulder, CO: Westview.

McMaster, G., & Trafzer, C. (Eds.). (2004). *Native universe: Voices of Indian America.* Washington, DC: The Smithsonian Institution.

Mead, M. (1928). *Coming of age in Samoa.* New York: HarperCollins, 2001.

Mehl-Madrona, L. (2003). Native American medicine: Herbal pharmacology, therapies, and eldercare. In H. Selin (Ed.), *Medicine across cultures* (pp. 209–224). Boston: Kluwer Academic Publishers.

Mendoza, R. (2003). Lords of the medicine bag: Medical science and traditional practice in ancient Peru and South America. In H. Selin (Ed.), *Medicine across cultures* (pp. 225–257). Boston: Kluwer Academic Publishers.

Morse, J., Young, D., & Swartz, L. (1991). Cree Indian healing practices and western health care: A comparative analysis. *Social Science & Medicine, 32,* 1361–1366.

Peacock, T., & Wisuri, M. (2002). *Ojibwe waasa inaabidaa—We look in all directions.* Afton, MN: Afton Historical Society Press.

Rogoff, B. (2003). *The cultural nature of human development.* New York: Oxford University Press.

Samora, J. (1978). Conceptions of health and disease among Spanish-Americans. In R. Martinez (Ed.), *Hispanic culture and health care* (pp. 65–74). St. Louis, MO: Mosby.

Selin, H. (Ed.). (2003). *Medicine across cultures.* Boston: Kluwer Academic Publishers.

Stark, R. (1981). *Guide to Indian herbs.* Blaine, WA: Hancock House.

Steiger, B. (1984). *Indian medicine power.* Gloucester, MA: Para.

Steiner, P. (2003). Cultural perspectives on traditional Tibetan medicine. In H. Selin (Ed.), *Medicine across cultures* (pp. 85–113). Boston: Kluwer Academic Publishers.

Torres, E. (1983). *Green medicine*. Kingsville, TX: Nieves.

Torres, E. (1984). *The folkhealer: The Mexican-American tradition of curanderismo*. Kingsville, TX: Nieves.

Tung, M. (2000). *Chinese Americans and their immigrant parents*. New York: Haworth Clinical Practice Press.

Ulibarri, H. (1978). Social and attitudinal characteristics of Spanish-speaking migrant and ex-migrant workers in the Southwest. In N. Wagner & M. Haug (Eds.), *Chicanos: Social and psychological perspectives* (pp. 164–170). St. Louis, MO: Mosby.

Viesca, C. (2003). Medicine in ancient Mesoamerica. In H. Selin (Ed.), *Medicine across cultures* (pp. 259–283). Boston: Kluwer Academic Publishers.

Vogel, V. (1970). *American Indian medicine*. Norman: University of Oklahoma Press.

Yan, Z., & Jingfeng, C. (2003). Medicine in ancient China. In H. Selin (Ed.), *Medicine across cultures* (pp. 49–73). New York: Springer.

Young, J. (2001). *The healing path*. London: Thorsons.

CHAPTER 3

Self as Healer

Barbara Leonard and Sue Towey

For nursing students and practitioners of complementary and alternative therapies, the process of developing an authentic self is as integral to practice as learning the technical skills for administering these therapies. An individual's explorations into self-knowledge, self-awareness, consciousness, and spiritual development are an ongoing dialogue between the inner and outer parts of one's being. A nurse must balance being in the moment and fully present with a patient while also taking the self-healing journey. Living an undivided life facilitates the journey toward wholeness (Palmer, 2004). Kabat-Zinn (2005) describes healing as a process of recognizing our wholeness "even when we are terrified or broken apart in life" (p. 336). Nurses integrating complementary therapies into their practice need to embark on the path of personal inner and outer development as part of their professional journey. The student and the practitioner must be aware that they need to care for the self.

Self-awareness and self-care are an integral part of reflective holistic nursing practice. In its Code of Ethics, the American Holistic Nurses Association states that "the nurse has a responsibility to model healthy behaviors. Holistic nurses strive to achieve harmony in their own lives and assist others striving to do the same" (American Holistic Nurses Association, 1992, p. 275). Janet Quinn (as cited in Horrigan, 1996) notes that each nurse needs to do his or her own work in order to become a healing energy for patients. They need to become whole persons and live authentic lives. The physical, emotional, and spiritual health of practitioners is experienced in their relationship with patients. Commitment to the use of self as an instrument of healing and understanding is the focus of this chapter.

A metaphor from the reductionistic biomedical health care system helps to understand issues associated with self as healer. Just as surgical instruments are washed and sterilized before being used for another procedure, professionals who are instruments of healing must identify therapies that will ensure the cleansing of self so as to provide a personal energy field and space that facilitate healing for self and patients.

In the literature on energy-healing therapies, Brennan (1987) describes the human energy field as the "manifestation of universal energy that is intimately involved with human life" (p. 41). Energetic healing is a term for healing that occurs at the electromagnetic level of a person (Slater, 1995). How do we care for ourselves as "instruments of healing" in our work with patients? Barbara Dossey, a leader in holistic nursing, stated that self-care includes activities that promote an awareness of self that facilitates being an instrument of healing (Horrigan, 1999).

SELF-CARE

Becoming a healer is a very individual process, one that grows from the inside (Brennan, 1987). Each person is unique and must assess his or her individual strengths and talents in order to move toward wholeness. There are many ways to create a plan for self-care and intentional personal healing. Therapies that will help a person to increase self-knowledge, become more aware of transpersonal experiences, and accept the paradoxical mysteries in life need to be explored.

Several concepts and techniques that are widely accepted as important in self-care are:

- a balanced diet appropriate to current health needs,

- exercise appropriate to the individual,

- adequate sleep and rest,

- social support systems,

- stress management skills,

- meditation and prayer, and

- an active sense of humor (Towey, 1995, p. 11).

Many of the therapies included in this book may be used singly or in combination to heal the self (Gunnarsdottir & Peden-McAlpine, 2004). Santorelli (2000) suggested use of mindfulness meditation, a mind–body intervention, to heal the self. Nature is another therapy frequently used in self-healing (Gunnarsdottir & Peden-McAlpine). Spending time outdoors is innately renewing, restorative, and healing. According to Lewis (1996), "as we garden, tramp through field or forest, we may come to an unexpected door that opens inward to self" (p. xix). Two other interventions that can be used in the healing of self, spiritual direction and dreams, will be discussed later.

TRANSFORMATIONAL JOURNEY

Healing is a key element of the transformational journey. Keegan (1994) defines healing as the integration of the totality of humankind in body, mind, and spirit. The healer is one who is capable of producing and catalyzing integration within self and patients. Keegan further notes that "the spiritual journey involves the process an individual undergoes in the search of the meaning and purpose of life" (p. 4).

Becoming a Healer

The initiation of a healer in ancient cultures was a rigorous process that included a personal journey of inner development and transformation. For centuries, cultures have treated inner transformation as a necessary and desired component of life. The universal aspects of shamanism work with the inner aspects of healing through the use of altered states of consciousness (Grof & Grof, 1990). Like the Greek mythological figure Chiron, shamans, as wounded healers, have the gift for healing others while remaining unable to heal themselves. A nurse's transformational healing journey is a living out of both the woundedness of Chiron and current knowledge about one's ability and need to connect with the inner healer (Santorelli, 2000).

Barriers, Stressors, and Needs

As the 21st century begins, the rapid transformation of our health care systems and health profession education has placed great demands on the time, energy, spirit, and health of professionals and students. Nurses and other health care employees are often caught in the crossfire of mergers, downsizing, redesign, and other changes that create uncertainty and anxiety in the work environment (Disch & Towey, 1998). The current national nursing shortage is making work environments more stressful, and professionals must rapidly acquire new information in order to accomplish their work. Limits of time and economic resources in health care create many challenges to health professionals and require new approaches in educating students.

Viewing time as the enemy creates stress that is not conducive to a healing environment in the workplace (Lofy, 2000). Bailey (1999) identifies the loss of quality relationships among workers as an unhealthy factor in many workplaces. However, healing requires interactions with others. Quiet times are also necessary so that a person is able to listen to the voice of inner wisdom. Silence may help reduce stress (Rubin, 2000), and yet silent reflection is difficult to attain without intentionally setting aside time for quiet. Uncertainty is another stressor in current health care settings. Finding ways to maintain hope and to develop resiliency are needed in the face of uncertainty (Towey, 1995).

The Dalai Lama (1999) described the ethics he regarded as necessary in the 21st century. In addition to restraint, virtue, and compassion, he identified a need for discerning the truth in the unseen world; this requires a healthy level of spiritual development, discipline, and practice.

SPIRITUAL DIRECTION

Spiritual direction is a time-honored tradition of accompanying other persons as they seek to grow in their relationship with God or a Higher Being. It is journeying with the person as they become more aware of their relationship with God or Higher Being. Spiritual direction is not psychotherapy or counseling, but rather focuses on the spiritual aspect of a person's life. Spiritual directors are professionals who have completed specialized education in the field. As with counseling and other professions, the director maintains professional boundaries when interacting with the directee. Persons may seek spiritual direction during time of spiritual distress or on an ongoing basis.

Some form of spiritual direction is found in many of the major religions of the world. Among traditional Native Americans a medicine person will guide a vision quest and interpret the dreams and visions of the seeker. A Zen master gives spiritual guidance to a seeker in the Buddhist tradition. In Christianity, spiritual direction has existed since the 4th century CE. Until recently spiritual direction was exclusive to those in religious life; laypersons rarely sought direction (Moon, 2002).

Today it is found in many Protestant denominations as well as in the Roman Catholic Church. Benner (2002) states that although large sectors within Christianity have never heard of spiritual direction until recently, seminaries and colleges of many denominations are now busy refashioning departments of Christian education into programs of spiritual formation. Clergy and laity alike are seeking opportunities to learn about spiritual direction.

The modern spiritual director has received education in the art and practice of spiritual direction and adheres to professional ethics such as those specified by Spiritual Directors International. This organization is a global organization of persons from many faiths who share a common concern and passion for the practice of spiritual direction. Opportunities are available for sharing of resources and ideas online (http://www.sdi world.org). The profession strongly recommends that directors receive their own ongoing direction and supervision. A person seeking direction should inquire about a director's educational preparation, supervision, and practice. A spiritual director, with permission of the directee, may collaborate with other professional persons working with a directee. When a directee is in crisis, working with both a counselor and a director may be very beneficial; for others it may be best to work with a counselor first and then with a director.

Nurses would seek spiritual direction to reflect on how God or the sacred is present in their lived experience as a nurse and a person. The focus of spiritual direction is on the inward movement of the spirit in the nurse's life. A nurse may seek direction during life transitions or crises or during ordinary times to gain a deeper relationship with God or the sacred. All of life's experiences can be brought to direction but always at the discretion of the person seeking it (Birmingham & Connolly, 1994). In the course of receiving direction, some of the circumstances of one's life may appear unchanged, but the inner transformation will be evident in professional work, personal relationships, and even in one's environment. Problems may resolve as a side benefit of direction. A nurse, for example, working with a group of women in transition from prison to society, said of herself, "I no longer say prayers; I am prayer." She went on to describe how she had become less judgmental and more accepting, patient, peaceful, relaxed, and joyful. The work was still the same, the women's problems as serious, but she is different and as a result she has become much more present to the women she works with.

Spiritual direction is especially useful to nurses whose working lives are spent in high-stress health care environments dealing with ultimate human questions on a regular basis. Spiritual direction is about reflection on one's life in all of its complexity. At the heart of direction is one's unique relationship with God or a Higher Being. Direction can help nurses become more sensitive to God's presence in their work and God's desire to "partner" with them. Developing an awareness of this partnership with God provides a serenity that can prevent emotional and spiritual burnout so that relationships with patients, families, and colleagues are healthy and healing.

Spiritual direction typically occurs monthly or more frequently if the individual desires it. Spiritual directors may meet with individuals over several years or months, depending upon the circumstances of the directee. Group spiritual direction is also available. The director and directee assess their work together periodically. For access to a spiritual director, individuals can contact their religious denomination or Spiritual Directors International. Directors are usually willing to see people from any religious tradition.

DREAMS

The ancients asserted the relationship of health and dreams. Greek temples served as places to receive a dream. The given dream would reveal the nature of a person's illness or need, enabling the physician to prescribe appropriate treatment. In the West, until the 5th century, dreams were respected by all religions as revealing the divine. Subsequently, Christians were admonished to ignore dreams because their religious leaders considered them linked to the occult. This thinking prevailed until the 20th century but changed with the discovery of a mistranslation 15 centuries earlier of Scripture from the Greek to the Latin. Fortunately, dreams are once again recognized for their importance to human health (Kelsey, 1974). Jungian psychology has contributed greatly to the restoration of dreams as part of health and healing.

Dreams serve many functions for the psyche in healing and maintenance of health. They give emotional compensation, reveal truths about life situations that the ego resists, provide warnings, and uncommonly provide what Jung called archetypal understanding (Kelsey, 1974). An archetype is a term used to denote an idea or image that is part of the collective unconscious of persons across time. An example of emotional healing occurred through a dream a woman had following her husband's death. She was in deep grief until her husband appeared to her in a dream, reassuring her that he was happy and wanted her to be as well. She was freed to move on with her life. After the recent tsunami disaster, a young physician had a dream in which an androgynous figure used hand signals to broadcast God's unconditional love to those who had died.

Experts claim that few dreams are prophetic. Nightmares occur when an issue needs to be brought into the person's consciousness. Dreams are specific to the individual and correct interpretations may be difficult. Friends, spiritual directors, or therapists may be helpful as the person tries to understand his or her dreams. For example, a dreamer with a new diagnosis of cancer saw herself riding a bicycle, hitting a bump in the road, falling off the bicycle, and then dusting herself off and riding on happily. Her trusted friend helped her see the relationship between the bump in the road and her cancer. The dream gave her hope that she would be able to continue her journey and that her cancer was not the end.

All human beings and animals dream, but unless dreams are recorded, they are not remembered. A time-tested way to remember dreams is to jot them down even in the middle of the night (a pad and pencil at bedside aids this process). When one awakens, the dream fades quickly and is not easily recalled unless it recurs. It is important to rewrite the dream in as much detail as possible without interpreting it. Then one notes the words, the feeling state, and the sequence of events in the dream. Once the dream is recorded without editing, interpretation can begin. Words may be looked up in the dictionary, and the dream can be meditated upon for further understanding. Dreams often have many levels of interpretation. If one keeps a journal and reviews it from time to time, the meaning of particular dreams may become clear as the person's life experience is seen in retrospect. For example, a woman dreamed about marine life displays in an aquarium. The next day, she made an unplanned visit to an aquarium and recognized the marine displays from her dream even though she had never seen them either live or in pictures before the dream. The journal serves as a record and years later, new awareness of meaning may occur to the individual.

Dreams are gifts that help us find direction and resolve emotional and other life issues. They teach us about our lives and ourselves. Dreams do not lie. They are presented in images tailored exclusively for us. Recording one's dreams honors the gift that they are.

FUTURE RESEARCH

Research in the following areas will contribute to knowledge about self-care and the nurse as healer:

1. qualitative studies on the transformational journeys of healers,
2. studies about the effects of the energy field of the healer on patients and colleagues, and
3. a survey of healers to identify the therapies they use in self-care.

REFERENCES

American Holistic Nurses Association. (1992, September). Code of ethics for holistic nurses. *Journal of Holistic Nursing, 10,* 275–276.

Bailey, J. (1999). *The speed trap: How to avoid the frenzy of the fast lane.* San Francisco: HarperCollins.

Benner, D. G. (2002). Nurturing spiritual growth. *Journal of Religion and Theology, 30,* 355–361.

Birmingham, M., & Connolly, W. J. (1994). *Witnessing to the fire: Spiritual direction and the development of directors: One center's experience.* Kansas City, MO: Sheed & Ward.

Brennan, B. (1987). *Hands of light: A guide to healing through the human energy field.* New York: Bantam.

Dalai Lama. (1999). *Ethics for the new millennium.* New York: Riverhead.

Disch, J., & Towey, S. (1998). Unit III case study: The healthy work environment as core to an organization's success. In D. Mason & J. Leavitt (Eds.), *Policy and politics in nursing and health care* (pp. 332–346). Philadelphia: Saunders.

Grof, S., & Grof, C. (1990). *The stormy search for the self.* New York: Tarcher-Putnam.

Gunnarsdottir, T., & Peden-McAlpine, C. (2004). The experience of using a combination of complementary therapies: A journey of balance through self-healing. *Journal of Holistic Nursing, 222,* 116–132.

Horrigan, B. (1996). Interview: Janet Quinn, RN, PhD: Therapeutic touch and a healing way. *Alternative Therapies in Health and Medicine, 2*(4), 68–75.

Horrigan, B. (1999). Interview: Barbara Dossey, RN, MS, on holistic nursing, Florence Nightingale, and the healing rituals. *Alternative Therapies in Health and Medicine, 5*(1), 79–86.

Kabat-Zinn, J. (2005). *Coming to our senses: Healing ourselves and the world through mindfulness.* New York: Hyperion.

Keegan, L. (1994). *The nurse as healer.* Albany, NY: Delmar.

Kelsey, M. T. (1974). *God, dreams & revelation: A Christian interpretation of dreams.* Minneapolis, MN: Augsburg.

Lewis, C. (1996). *Green nature/human nature: The meaning of plants in our lives.* Urbana & Chicago: University of Illinois Press.

Lofy, M. (2000). *A matter of time: Power, control, and meaning in people's everyday experience of time.* Unpublished doctoral dissertation, The Fielding Institute: Santa Barbara, CA.

Moon, G. W. (2002). Spiritual direction: Meaning, purpose, and implications for mental health professionals. *Journal of Religion and Theology, 30,* 264–275.

Moon, G. W., & Benner, D. G. (2004). *Spiritual direction and the care of souls: A guide to Christian approaches and practices.* Downers Grove, IL: InterVarsity Press.

Palmer, P. (2004). *A hidden wholeness: The journey toward an undivided life.* San Francisco: Jossey-Bass.

Rubin, A. (2000). *The power of silence: Using technology to create free structure in organizations.* Unpublished master's thesis, The Fielding Institute: Santa Barbara, CA.

Santorelli, S. (2000). *Heal thyself: Lessons on mindfulness in medicine.* New York: Bell Tower.

Slater, V. (1995). Toward an understanding of energetic healing: Part I: Energetic structures. *Journal of Holistic Nursing, 13,* 209–224.

Towey, S. (1995). Personal and professional skills for living with uncertainty. *Creative Nursing, 1*(1), 9–11.

CHAPTER 4

Presence

Mariah Snyder

Presence is an intervention that is integral to the administration of all complementary therapies, though it can be used independently of other therapies. It is closely related to the therapy of active listening, and the two share many characteristics. Although presence has been recognized for centuries within nursing, research on the subject has been initiated only recently. This research has largely been conducted in conjunction with the concept of caring.

DEFINITION

Two of the pioneers in this field, Paterson and Zderad (1976), described presence as the process of being available with the whole of oneself and open to the experience of another through a reciprocal interpersonal encounter. Gardner (1992) expanded on this definition by adding specifics related to physical and psychological presence. She defined presence as "the physical being there and the psychological being with a patient for the purpose of meeting the patient's health care needs" (p. 191). According to Liehr (1989), the nurse needs to genuinely engage with the patient for true presence to occur. From the perspective of patients, presence requires an emotional, subjective interaction with nurses in which the nurses convey genuine concern for patients, not just as patients but as human beings (Paulson, 2004).

Benner (1984) chose the verb *presencing* to denote the existential practice of being with a patient. *Presencing* is one of the eight competencies Benner identified as constituting the helping role of the nurse. This view of presence in nursing is supported by Parse (1992), who characterized presence as "the primary mode of nursing practice" (p. 40).

Presence is reciprocal. The interaction must be meaningful to both the patient and the nurse. According to Pettigrew (1990), nurses must be involved in the interaction, and the interaction must be deemed meaningful by the patient for presence to produce positive patient outcomes. This transactional characteristic of presence was emphasized by McKivergin and Day (1998): In presence, the nurse is available to the patient with the wholeness of his or her unique individual being. Presence can be characterized as a process that consists of an exchange in which meaningful awareness on the part of the nurse helps to bring integration and balance to the life of the patient (Snyder, Brandt, & Tseng, 2000).

Two classifications of presence have been developed (McKivergin & Daubenmire, 1994; Osterman & Schwartz-Barcott, 1996). The continuum in both classifications extends from merely being physically present with the patient to being available with the wholeness of self. Table 4.1 describes the categories of presence and provides an example of each type of presence. It is only the transcendent (Osterman & Schwartz-Barcott) or therapeutic presence (McKivergin & Daubenmire) that constitutes the complementary therapy designated as presence.

The universality of presence and caring has been documented (Endo, 1998; Jonsdottir, Litchfield, & Pharris, 2004). Presence transcends cultures. Even if the nurse and patient are unable to communicate verbally, the patient perceives the presence of a caring nurse. Paulson (2004) noted that nurses need to focus on positive concern for their patients and not on their personality, race, or socioeconomic status.

SCIENTIFIC BASIS

Paterson and Zderad (1976) recognized presence as an integral component of their theory of humanistic nursing. Presence implies an openness, a receptivity, a readiness, or an availability on the part of the nurse. Many nursing situations require close proximity to another person, but that in itself does not constitute presence. In order to experience the lived dialogue of nursing, the nurse responds with an openness to a "person-with-needs" and with an "availability-in-a-helping way" (Paterson & Zderad). Reciprocity often emerges through the dialogue.

TABLE 4.1 Examples of Use of the Various Types of Presence

Types of Presence	Example
Presence/partial presence (Osterman & Schwartz-Barcott, 1996); physical presence (McKivergin & Daubenmire, 1994)	Routine tasks such as taking vital signs and administering medications; nurse enters a patient's room to check the blood pressure, doing so deftly but failing to notice the tears slipping from the patient's eyes; nurse is absorbed in own thoughts.
Full presence (Osterman & Schwartz-Barcott, 1996); psychological presence (McKivergin & Daubenmire, 1994)	Nurse enters a patient's room to check the ventilator. The nurse greets the patient by name and uses personalized ways of interacting with the patient. The nurse is attentive to nonverbal responses of the patient and will occasionally touch the patient. Needs are assessed and a plan of care is developed in conjunction with the patient.
Transcendent presence (Osterman & Schwartz-Barcott, 1996); therapeutic presence (McKivergin & Daubenmire, 1994)	The nurse uses centering before entering the patient's room. The nurse greets the patient by name while simultaneously holding the patient's hand or arm. The nurse uses all of her personal resources of body, mind, emotions, and spirit in being present and available to the patient. The nurse is attentive to responses of the patient and directs attention to specific concerns. All of these can be done while simultaneously regulating the IV or doing other care activities.

Note: From "Use of Presence in the Critical Care Unit," by M. Snyder, C. Brandt, and Y. Tseng, 2000, *AACN Clinical Issues: Advanced Practice in Acute and Critical Care*, 11(1), pp. 27–33. Copyright 2000 by Lippincott. Reprinted with permission.

Presence is closely aligned with caring. It involves the nurse as "co-participant" in the caring process (Watson, 1985). Caring requires the nurse to be keenly attentive to the needs of the patient, the meaning the patient attaches to the illness or problem, and how the patient wishes to proceed. According to Watson, "a truly caring nurse/artist is able to destroy in the consciousness of the recipient the separation between him- or herself and the nurse" (p. 68). The use of presence helps lead the patient to healing, discovery, and finding meaning.

The body of knowledge documenting patients' perceptions of the value of presence is evolving. Much of the research on presence is found within studies on caring. Nurse researchers have sought to elicit patients' views of the caring behaviors of nurses. In a study of hospitalized patients and their nurses, presence was validated as a caring behavior in a study by Hegedus (1999). In a study by Nelms (1996), nurses revealed that presence was the essence of nursing.

Similar findings have been reported in other studies. In a qualitative study by Riemen (1986) of patients' perceptions of nurses' behaviors, noncaring actions included having minimal contact with the patient and being physically present but emotionally distant. Availability, kindness, and consideration were desired characteristics identified by patients in a study by Cronin and Harrison (1988). Engaging in a reciprocal process with the nurse was one of the caring behaviors identified by patients who had been discharged from a critical care unit (Burfitt, Greiner, Miers, Kinney, & Branyon, 1993).

Studies on the expert practice of critical-care nurses have demonstrated the importance of presence. Minick (1995) found that connectedness with the patient was important not only as a caring behavior but also because it assisted the nurse in the early identification of postoperative problems. Therapeutic presence may help nurses to be more attentive and to detect subtle changes that may not be evident in its absence. Nurses who lacked this connectedness were perceived by their patients as detached. Hanneman (1996) explored the effects of expert nurses on care outcomes and found that these nurses displayed two characteristics: presence with and focused assessment of a patient's situation. Wilkin and Slevin (2004) further validated the fact that the importance of the critical-care nurse being present to the patient was as essential a part of nursing care as were the skills needed to reach unresponsive and intubated patients.

Mohnkern (1992) asked 15 nurses to identify the antecedents, defining attributes, and consequences of presence. Antecedents included a patient who trusts the nurse and has a need to have her or his life processes facilitated, and a nurse who possesses a sense of mission, has an altruistic desire to help the patient, and is willing and strong enough to be open to the experience of the patient. Attributes of presence were physical closeness between the nurse and the patient, a metaphysical connection between the nurse and patient in which energy is exchanged, and the nurse's use of a range of skills to facilitate the patient's experience. Perspectives of patients were not reported.

The importance of presence in care has been recognized for centuries. Documentation of why it plays a role in health outcomes is slowly evolving.

INTERVENTION

The description of presence related by Mitch Albom (1997) in *Tuesdays with Morrie* succinctly captures its essential elements. Albom is reporting how Morrie, a man with advanced amyotrophic lateral sclerosis, viewed presence:

> I believe in being fully present. That means you should be with the person you're with. When I'm talking with you now, Mitch, I try to keep focused only on what is going on between us. I am not thinking about something we said last week. I am not thinking about what's coming up this Friday. I am not thinking about doing another Koppel show, or about medications I'm taking. I am talking to you, I am thinking about you. [pp. 135–136]

Centering

Presence entails conscious attention to the upcoming interaction with the patient. The nurse must be available with the whole of self and be open to the personal and care needs of the patient. This process is called centering, a meditative state. The nurse takes a short time, sometimes only 10 or 20 seconds, to eliminate distractions, so that the focus can be on the patient. Some people find that taking a deep breath and closing the eyes helps in freeing them of distractions and becoming centered. This may be done outside the room or setting in which the encounter will occur. Centering may also be as simple as the nurse's pausing before contact with the patient and repeating the patient's name to help focus attention on that person.

Technique

Table 4.2 lists the key components of presence and the skills necessary for practicing it. Sensitivity to the other requires the nurse to be an

TABLE 4.2   Presence: Key Components and Necessary Skills

Key Components	Necessary Skills
Whole person to whole person interaction	Centering
Intersubjectivity	Sensitivity and openness
Direction of self toward other	Communication and active listening
Attentiveness	
Accountability	

Note: From "Use of Presence in the Critical Care Unit," by M. Snyder, C. Brandt, and Y. Tseng, 2000, *AACN Clinical Issues: Advanced Practice in Acute and Critical Care*, 11(1), pp. 27–33. Copyright 2000 by Lippincott. Reprinted with permission.

excellent listener and observer. (Active listening is addressed in chapter 5.) Good observation skills assist nurses in identifying nuances in expression and communication that may reveal the real concerns of the patient. Presence often means periods of silence in which subtle interchanges occur. Continuing attentiveness on the part of the nurse is a critical aspect of this therapy. Both the nurse and the client experience a sense of union or joining for a moment in time.

Little is known about the length of a therapy session or when therapeutic presence should be used. Often the nurse identifies it intuitively: "It just seems like this patient truly needs me now." Because of the intense nature of the interaction, the length of time the nurse is present to the patient may seem greater even though only a minute or two may have passed. Although presence is often used in conjunction with another therapy or treatment, identifying when a patient needs someone to just be present for a few minutes may be the most effective therapy.

Measurement of Effectiveness

Measuring outcomes of presence interventions will involve both the patient and the nurse because of their reciprocal interaction. Comments from the patient about feeling cared for, being able to express concerns, and feeling understood are some outcome measures that can be used. The consequences of presence identified by Mohnkern (1992) included improved psychosocial, spiritual, and emotional functioning; improved physical functioning or a peaceful death; and an appreciation of more interaction with the nurse. According to Mohnkern, one consequence noted by nurses was an affirmation of their role as nurses. Because of the intangibles that often occur with the use of presence, finding words or indices to measure presence may be challenging.

Precautions

The major precaution in the use of presence is to take one's cue from the patient and not force an encounter. A true presence encounter considers the wants and needs of the patient and is not for the nurse's primary benefit. If the nurse is "available with the whole of oneself and open to the experience" of the client, as the definition states, the nurse will act in accordance with the wishes and needs of the patient.

One negative consequence of presence identified by Mohnkern was nurses reporting that colleagues were critical about the time they spent with patients and families. Certainly this should not be a deterrent to the use of presence, but rather a concern that should be discussed and resolved by nursing staff.

USES

Presence can be used in any nursing situation. Persons struggling with a new diagnosis, an exacerbation of a condition, or a loss are especially in need of moments of presence. Moch (1995) included presence as part of a psychosocial intervention for women diagnosed with breast cancer and found the intervention to be helpful to these women. Presence is of particular value with hospice patients (Zerwekh, 1995).

Presence is also needed with patients in critical-care settings (Wilkin & Slevin, 2004) and emergency departments (Wiman & Wikblad, 2004). Patients and their families often feel lost in high-tech critical-care settings. The use of presence helps prevent critical-care nurses from being viewed by their patients as emotionally distant and focusing only on the machines and technology (Marsden, 1990). Research suggests that incorporating the therapy of presence in critical-care settings can reduce anxiety for patients and their families (Mohnkern, 1992).

FUTURE RESEARCH

Nurses chart assessments made and treatments administered, but rarely do they document the use of presence and the outcomes of this therapy. Despite the challenges in identifying and documenting outcomes of presence, current interest in complementary therapies provides an opportunity for nurses to validate the positive outcomes from the use of presence. Areas in which research are needed include the following:

1. Although every patient could benefit from presence, large caseloads often place restrictions on nurses' time. What are assessments that would alert nurses to patients who most need the therapy of presence?

2. What are strategies that can be used to teach nursing students and other health professionals how to implement presence?

3. With the advent of telemedicine, how can presence be introduced into these contacts with patients? Is physical presence essential or is presence a non-local phenomenon like prayer?

REFERENCES

Albom, M. (1997). *Tuesdays with Morrie*. New York: Doubleday.

Benner, P. (1984). *From novice to expert: Excellence and power in clinical nursing practice*. Menlo Park, CA: Addison-Wesley.

Burfitt, S. N., Greiner, D. S., Miers, L. J., Kinney, M. R., & Branyon, M. E. (1993). Professional nurse caring as perceived by critically ill patients: A phenomenologic study. *American Journal of Critical Care, 2,* 489–499.

Cronin, S. N., & Harrison, B. (1988). Importance of nurse caring behaviors as perceived by patients after myocardial infarction. *Heart and Lung, 17,* 374–380.

Endo, E. (1998). Pattern recognition as a nursing intervention with Japanese women with ovarian cancer. *Advances in Nursing Science, 20*(4), 49–51.

Gardner, D. L. (1992). Presence. In G. M. Bulechek & J. C. McCloskey (Eds.), *Nursing interventions: Essential nursing treatments* (2nd ed., pp. 191–200). Philadelphia: Saunders.

Hanneman, S. K. (1996). Advancing nursing practice with a unit-based clinical expert. *Image: Journal of Nursing Scholarship, 28,* 331–337.

Hegedus, K. S. (1999). Providers' and consumers' perspective of nurses' caring behaviors. *Journal of Advanced Nursing, 30,* 1090–1096.

Jonsdottir, H., Litchfield, M., & Pharris, M. D. (2004). The relational core of nursing practice in partnership. *Journal of Advanced Nursing, 47,* 241–248.

Liehr, P. R. (1989). The core of true presence: A loving center. *Nursing Science Quarterly, 2*(1), 7–8.

Marsden, C. (1990). Ethical issues in critical care. *Heart and Lung, 19,* 540–541.

McKivergin, M., & Daubenmire, J. (1994). The essence of therapeutic presence. *Journal of Holistic Nursing, 12*(1), 65–81.

McKivergin, M., & Day, A. (1998). Presence: Creating order out of chaos. *Seminars in Perioperative Nursing, 7,* 96–100.

Minick, P. (1995). The power of human caring: Early recognition of patient problems. *Scholarly Inquiry for Nursing Practice: An International Journal, 9,* 303–317.

Moch, S. D. (1995). *Breast cancer: Twenty women's stories*. New York: National League for Nursing Press.

Mohnkern, S. M. (1992). *Presence in nursing, its antecedents, defining attributes, and consequences*. Doctoral dissertation, University of Texas, Austin.

Nelms, T. P. (1996). Living a caring presence in nursing: A Heideggerian hermeneutical analysis. *Journal of Advanced Nursing, 24,* 368–374.

Osterman, P., & Schwartz-Barcott, D. (1996). Presence: Four ways of being there. *Nursing Forum, 31,* 23–30.

Parse, R. R. (1992). Human becoming: Parse's theory of nursing. *Nursing Science Quarterly, 5,* 35–42.

Paterson, J. G., & Zderad, L. T. (1976). *Humanistic nursing*. New York: Wiley.

Paulson, D. S. (2004). Taking care of patients and caring for patients are not the same. *AORN Online, 79,* 359–360, 362, 365–366.

Pettigrew, J. (1990). Intensive nursing care: The ministry of presence. *Critical Care Nursing Clinics of North America, 2,* 503–508.

Riemen, D. J. (1986). Noncaring and caring in the clinical setting: Patients' descriptions. *Topics in Clinical Nursing, 8,* 30–36.

Snyder, M., Brandt, C. L., & Tseng, Y. (2000). Use of presence in the critical care unit. *AACN Clinical Issues, 11,* 27–33.

Watson, J. (1985). *Nursing human science and human care: A theory of nursing.* Norwalk, CT: Appleton-Century-Crofts.

Wilkin, K., & Slevin, E. (2004). The meaning of caring to nurses: An investigation into the nature of caring work in an intensive care unit. *Journal of Clinical Nursing, 13,* 50–59.

Wiman, E., & Wikblad, K. (2004). Caring and uncaring encounters in nursing in an emergency department. *Journal of Clinical Nursing, 13,* 422–429.

Zerwekh, J. V. (1995). A family caregiving model for hospice nursing. *Hospice Journal, 10,* 27–44.

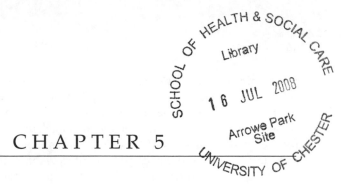

CHAPTER 5

Therapeutic Listening

Shigeaki Watanuki, Mary Fran Tracy, and Ruth Lindquist

> The most basic of all human needs is the need to understand and be understood. The best way to understand people is to listen to them.
>
> —Ralph Nichols

Listening is an active and dynamic process of interaction with a client requiring intentional effort to attend to a client's verbal and nonverbal cues. Listening is an integral part of nurse–client relationships. In fact, it is one of the most effective therapeutic techniques available to nurses (Sundeen, Stuart, Rankin, & Cohen, 1998). The theoretical underpinnings of listening can be traced back to counseling psychology and psychotherapy. Rogers (1957) used counseling and listening to foster independence and promote growth and development and stressed that empathy, warmth, and genuineness with clients were necessary and sufficient for therapeutic changes to occur. Listening has been identified as a significant component of therapeutic communication with patients and therefore fundamental to a therapeutic relationship between nurse and patient (Foy & Timmins, 2004).

DEFINITION

A variety of modifiers are used with the word *listening*, including active, therapeutic, empathic, and holistic. The choice of modifier seems to depend more on an author's paradigm than on differences in the descriptions of listening (Fredriksson, 1999). Unless active listening was explicitly used by researchers in the articles reviewed, the term *therapeutic listening* is used in this chapter to focus on the formal, deliberate actions of listening for therapeutic purposes (Lekander, Lehmann, & Lindquist, 1993). Therapeutic listening is defined as "an interpersonal confirmation process involving all the senses in which the therapist attends with empathy to the client's verbal and nonverbal messages to facilitate the understanding, synthesis, and interpretation of the client's situation" (Kemper, 1992, p. 22).

SCIENTIFIC BASIS

Therapeutic listening is a topic of interest and concern to a variety of disciplines. There are studies or clinical trials of therapeutic listening or communication in the literature; however, anecdotal reports and editorial articles (descriptive or reflective) comprise the main body of nursing literature (Fredriksson, 1999). A number of studies provide a scientific basis of intervention effects in relation to process (e.g., behavioral changes of providers that foster communication) and outcomes (e.g., client satisfaction, improved clinical indicators).

A systematic literature review of 20 intervention studies that aimed at improving patient–doctor communication revealed the effectiveness of interventions that typically increased patient participation and clarification (Harrington, Noble, & Newman, 2004). Although few improvements in patient satisfaction were found, significant improvements in perceptions of control over health, preferences for an active role in health care, adherence to recommendations, and clinical outcomes were achieved. Likewise, preferable client outcomes were found in several studies in nursing. A survey of 195 parents of hospitalized pediatric patients showed that health care provider use of immediacy and perceived listening were positively associated with satisfaction with care and communication (Wanzer, Booth-Butterfield, & Gruber, 2004). Clients of a community mental health center who perceived that the practitioner used skills of empathy, listening, openness, and genuineness were very satisfied with the care received (Sheppard, 1993). In another study, client distress was inversely associated with nurse-expressed and client-perceived empathy (Olson & Hanchett, 1997).

Studies evaluating training of health care providers in therapeutic communication skills have shown varying results. Training of nurses was effective in improving their therapeutic communication skills. Twenty-six registered nurse graduates attended a 6-hour communication skills training module. An analysis of the attendees' audiotaped responses to clinical vignettes revealed that active-listening scores increased significantly, whereas attempts to suppress or discount clients' feelings decreased significantly when compared to pretraining scores (Olson & Iwasiw, 1987). Conversely, the level of patient satisfaction did not significantly improve after a system-wide training program for physicians to improve their communication styles with patients although the physicians' self-assessed scores of confidence and communication style improved significantly (Brown, Boles, Mullooly, & Levinson, 1999). Such inconclusive results are likely attributed to the complexities of disentangling relationships among training interventions, empathic interpersonal and therapeutic listening skills, and client outcomes.

The helping styles of psychotherapists, crisis intervenors, and untrained individuals were compared with those of nursing school seniors who were completing a course in interpersonal relationships. The students were similar to trained psychotherapists in their use of empathic listening, as evidenced by statements reflecting affect and content (Ryden, McCarthy, Lewis, & Sherman, 1991). An irony, however, is that primary nurses with more years of education or professional experience were rated by the clients as less empathic, perceptive, or effective as listeners than nurses with fewer years of education or professional experience (Reid-Ponte, 1992). Such results may reflect the realities of busy clinical settings or the fact that experienced nurses may rely more on their intuitive sense rather than therapeutically listening to clients in order to elicit their feelings and needs.

Biophysiological instruments can be useful in capturing the process changes of clients and nurses. Electroencephalography (EEG) changes were observed during client-centered interviews conducted by a nurse trained with Rogers' psychotherapy techniques (Minamisawa & Mitoh, 1997). An increased frequency of nurses' alpha wave activity (implying a relaxed state) was observed when they perceived that they established empathic rapport and active presence with their clients. Clients' EEG patterns also showed occasional increased frequency of alpha wave activity at about the same time as those of the nurse interviewers.

Qualitative methodologies provide rich understanding of the nature of therapeutic listening and explore the meaning and experience of being listened to in the context of real-world settings. Self-expression opportunities that enable clients to be listened to and understood can promote their self-discovery, meaning reconstruction, and healing (Myers, 2000; Sandelowski, 1994).

Sources of contradictory or inconclusive findings of studies on therapeutic listening may include lack of a clear theoretical framework, limitations in design and measurement sensitivity, and deficiencies of sample size (Kruijver, Kerkstra, Francke, Bensing, & van de Wiel, 2000). Further systematic studies are needed to enhance knowledge as to evidence of intervention effectiveness, especially the link between client characteristics and type of interventions.

INTERVENTION

Therapeutic listening enables clients to better understand their feelings and to experience being understood by another caring person. Effective engagement in therapeutic listening requires nurses to be aware of verbal and nonverbal communication that conveys explicit and implicit messages. When expressed words contradict nonverbal messages, communicators rely more often on nonverbal cues; facial expression, tone of voice, and silence are as important as words in determining the meaning of a message (Kacperek, 1997). Nonverbal communication is inextricably linked to verbal communication and can change, emphasize, or distract from the words that are spoken (Bush, 2001).

Guidelines

Listening is an active process, incorporating explicit behaviors as well as attention to choice of words, quality of voice (pitch, timing, and volume), and full engagement in the process (Burnard, 1997). Therapeutic listening requires the receiver to tune in to the client and to use all the senses in analyzing, inferring, and evaluating both the stated and the underlying meaning of the client's message. Therapeutic listening requires concentration and an ability to differentiate between what is actually being said and what one wants or expects to hear. Listeners are cautioned to avoid making assumptions that might lead them to hear what they think the client ought to say (Schlesinger, 1994). It may be difficult to listen accurately and interpret messages they find difficult to relate to or to listen to information they may not want to hear, therefore making therapeutic listening both a cognitive and an emotional process (Arnold & Underman Boggs, 1999). When one is not fully engaged, it can be easy to become distracted or to start formulating a response rather than to stay focused on the message. Three components have been identified by De Vito (1995) as being key to listening:

1. rephrasing the patient's words and thoughts to ensure clarity and accuracy,

2. conveying an understanding of the speaker's perceptions, and

3. asking questions and prompting in order to clarify.

These and other techniques are presented in Table 5.1 for this type of intervention.

Therapeutic listening with pediatric patients can be even more complex as it frequently becomes triangular among the nurse, child, and caregiver (Whaley & Wong, 1996). This may take particular skill on the part of the nurse as she attends to both the spoken and nonverbal messages and the reactions of two persons simultaneously. In addition, the nurse

TABLE 5.1 Therapeutic Listening Techniques

Active Presence: Active presence involves focus on the clients to interpret the messages they are trying to convey, recognition of themes, and hearing what is left unsaid.

Accepting Attitude: An accepting attitude will allow clients to feel comfortable expressing themselves. This can be demonstrated by short affirmative responses or gestures.

Clarifying Statements: Clarifying statements and summarizing can help the listener verify message interpretation and create clarity. Encourage specificity rather than vague statements to facilitate communication. Rephrasing and reflection can assist the client in self-understanding.

Use of Silence: Use of silence can encourage the client to talk, facilitate the nurse's focus on listening rather than the formulation of responses, and reduce the use of leading questions.

Tone: Tone of voice can express more than the actual words through empathy, judgment, or acceptance. Match the intensity of the tone appropriately to the message received to avoid minimizing or overemphasizing.

Nonverbal Behaviors: Clients relaying sensitive information may be very aware of the listener's body language and the listener will be viewed as either accepting of the message or closed to it, judgmental, and/or uninterested. Eye contact is essential to convey true interest. Maintaining a conversational distance and judicious use of touch may increase the client's comfort. Cultural and social awareness are important to avoid undesired touch.

Environment: Distractions should be eliminated to encourage the therapeutic interchange. Therapeutic listening may require careful planning to provide time for undivided attention or may occur spontaneously. Some clients may feel comfortable having family present whereas others may feel inhibited when others are present.

must be sensitive to the clarification of information and cues in front of either the child or the caregiver, depending on the child's age.

Adolescents may especially appreciate talking with an adult outside their family (Whaley & Wong, 1996). They may, however, respond quickly and abruptly to any perceived indications of judgment, indifference, or disrespect on the part of the listener. It is especially important with adolescents to be fully attentive, allow for complete expression of thoughts, and avoid statements or facial expressions that imply disapproval or can be misinterpreted.

Because therapeutic listening involves both cognitive and emotional processes, it is important that nurses recognize the role of emotional intelligence in their therapeutic interactions. Emotional intelligence is defined as an ability to recognize emotions in self and others and to understand and utilize these emotions in thinking processes and interactions with others (Vitello-Cicciu, 2002). Nursing requires a significant amount of emotional labor, resulting in expectations of caring, understanding, and empathy from patients and families. Strategies such as reflection, empathizing, and skilled therapeutic listening can promote a healing environment (Molter, 2003).

Recently, a new type of listening intervention has been described and tested; this intervention is referred to as *change-oriented reflective listening* (Rollnick et al., 2002). The technique has been piloted on general practitioners to motivate them to intervene with opiate users and as part of alcohol intervention (McCambridge, Platts, Whooley, & Strang, 2004; Strang, McCambridge, Platts, & Groves, 2004). This technique, a brief motivational enhancement intervention based on motivational interviewing, has potential for incorporation into the repertoire of nursing intervention.

Measurement of Outcomes

Multiple measurements such as self-report, behavioral observation, physiological indicators, and qualitative accounts provide rich data for the study of therapeutic listening. Challenges to outcome measurement include the isolation of an independent variable (therapeutic listening as an intervention) from other confounding variables and the complexity of the multifaceted phenomenon of therapeutic listening that may necessitate multivaried study design (Bennett, 1995). Antecedents to interventions (e.g., clients' characteristics) have to be taken into consideration just as the process of interventions (e.g., short- and long-term improvements in nurses' knowledge, skills, attitudes, and behavior after training) and client outcomes need to be evaluated (Harrington et al., 2004; Kruijver et al., 2000).

Positive changes in psychological variables such as anxiety, depression, hostility, or nursing care satisfaction are potential client outcomes of therapeutic listening. It may also be useful to examine physiological measures (heart rate, blood pressure, respiratory rate, temperature, oxygen saturation, EEG) as outcomes of therapeutic interchange. Outcomes may also include clinical variables such as length of stay, response to illness, mood, adherence, disease control, morbidity, and health care cost.

Precautions

Therapeutic listening has at its heart the intent to be helpful, so few precautions seem warranted. However, sensitivity and awareness to cultural variations of communication styles are vital to interventional effectiveness. Cultural differences in meanings of certain words, styles and approaches, or certain nonverbal behaviors such as silence, touch, or smile may adversely affect therapeutic communication. Maintaining professional boundaries during therapeutic listening is important; empathy with clients is to be demonstrated within professional and therapeutic guidelines. Referrals for professional counseling may be indicated when there are psychiatric crises. Ethical dilemmas may result if the principle of respecting clients' autonomy and confidentiality conflicts with the principle of maintaining professional responsibility and integrity (e.g., taking action based on sensitive information shared in the therapeutic exchange).

USES

Listening is an intervention that is applicable to virtually an unlimited number of care situations. Active listening is a vital technique that may be used to elicit patients' perspectives on their illness (Simpson et al., 1991). Practitioners are admonished to continue listening to patients throughout their visits, as patients may disclose vital information in the closing moments of their appointments (White, Levinson, & Roter, 1994). Selected patient population examples describing the use of listening are included in Table 5.2. Managers in the health care field may also reap benefits from active listening (Boyd, 1998; Kubota, Mishima, & Nagata, 2004). Table 5.3 presents web sites of national and international professional organizations where online resources for details of therapeutic listening can be found.

TABLE 5.2   Selected Uses of Listening

Adolescent mental health (Claveirole, 2004; Street & Svanberg, 2003)

Cancer (Harris & Templeton, 2001; Hirose, 1999)

Culturally diverse populations (Davidhizar, 2004)

Day surgery (Foy & Timmins, 2004)

Emergency care (O'Gara & Fairhurst, 2004; O'Hagan, Webb, & Moore, 2004)

Families of critically ill patients (Garcia de Lucio, Garcia Lopez, Marin Lopez, Hesse, & Caamano Vaz, 2000)

Gastrointestinal conditions (Eckes, 1996)

Loss (Gibbons, 1993)

Mentally impaired community-dwelling adults (Sheppard, 1993)

Older adults (Williams, Kemper, & Hummert, 2004)

Pediatric behavioral problems (Herman-Staab, 1994)

Perinatal care (Battersby & Deery, 2001)

Posttraumatic stress (Gidron et al., 2001)

Terminal care (Cherin, Enguidanos, & Brumley, 2001)

Traumatic stress/disasters (Liehr, Mehl, Summers, & Pennebaker, 2004)

TABLE 5.3   Professional Organizations and Online Resources for Therapeutic Listening

---

National

- The National Communication Association http://www.natcom.org
- The Focusing Institute http://www.focusing.org

International

- The International Communication Association http://www.icahdq.org
- The International Listening Association http://www.listen.org
  - International Journal of Listening http://www.listen.org/pages/ijl.htm
- Communication Institute for Online Scholarship http://www.cios.org
  - Electronic Communication Journal http://www.cios.org/www/ejcmain.htm

---

FUTURE RESEARCH

Many questions can be pursued in this area of research. Systematic studies are needed to develop a body of knowledge. Their designs require a new paradigm other than traditional randomization or control because of ethical and feasibility concerns, among other variables. Rather, qualitative studies, case reports, or mixed method designs may be options for understanding the nature and effects of therapeutic listening. Potential questions are as follows:

- Can therapeutic listening via phone or other interactive technology (synchronous and asynchronous) be effective at a distance?

- What are the effects of health care providers' use of listening on patient satisfaction and other outcomes of care?

- Are interventions to improve listening of health care providers cost effective and legitimate areas on which to focus continuous quality improvement (CQI) in order to improve patient safety and quality of care?

- How do multicultural differences manifest in the process and effectiveness of therapeutic listening?

REFERENCES

Arnold, E., & Underman Boggs, K. (1999). *Interpersonal relationships: Professional communication skills for nurses* (3rd ed.). London: Saunders.

Battersby, S., & Deery, R. (2001). Midwifery and research: Comparable skills in listening and the use of language. *Practising Midwife, 4*(9), 24–25.

Bennett, J. A. (1995). Methodological notes on empathy: Further considerations. *Advances in Nursing Science, 18*(1), 36–50.

Boyd, S. D. (1998). Using active listening. *Nursing Management, 29*(7), 55.

Brown, J. B., Boles, M., Mullooly, J. P., & Levinson, W. (1999). Effect of clinician communication skills training on patient satisfaction: A randomized, controlled trial. *Annals of Internal Medicine, 131,* 822–829.

Burnard, P. (1997). *Effective communication skills for health professionals* (2nd ed.). Cheltenham, UK: Nelson Thornes.

Bush, K. (2001). Do you really listen to patients? *RN, 64*(3), 35–37.

Cherin, D., Enguidanos, S., & Brumley, R. (2001). Reflection in action in caring for the dying: Applying organizational learning theory to improve communications in terminal care. *Home Health Care Services Quarterly, 19*(4), 65–78.

Claveirole, A. (2004). Listening to young voices: Challenges of research with adolescent mental health service users. *Journal of Psychiatric & Mental Health Nursing, 11,* 253–260.

Davidhizar, R. (2004). Listening—a nursing strategy to transcend culture. *Journal of Practical Nursing, 54*(2), 22–24.

De Vito, J. A. (1995). *The interpersonal communication book* (7th ed.). New York: HarperCollins.

Eckes, L. M. (1996). Active listening. *Gastroenterology Nursing, 19*(6), 219–220.

Foy, C. R., & Timmins, F. (2004). Improving communication in day surgery settings. *Nursing Standard, 19*(7), 37–42.

Fredriksson, L. (1999). Modes of relating in a caring conversation: A research synthesis on presence, touch and listening. *Journal of Advanced Nursing, 30,* 1167–1176.

Garcia de Lucio, L., Garcia Lopez, F. J., Marin Lopez, M. T., Mas Hesse, B., & Caamano Vaz, M. D. (2000). Training programme in techniques of self-control and communication skills to improve nurses' relationships with relatives of critically ill patients: A randomized controlled study. *Journal of Advanced Nursing, 32,* 425–431.

Gibbons, M. B. (1993). Listening to the lived experience of loss. *Pediatric Nursing, 19,* 597–599.

Gidron, Y., Gal, R., Freedman, S., Twiser, I., Lauden, A., Snir, Y., et al. (2001). Translating research findings to PTSD prevention: Results of a randomized-controlled pilot study. *Journal of Traumatic Stress, 14,* 773–780.

Harrington, J., Noble, L. M., & Newman, S. P. (2004). Improving patients' communication with doctors: A systematic review of intervention studies. *Patient Education and Counseling, 52*(1), 7–16.

Harris, S. R., & Templeton, E. (2001). Who's listening? Experiences of women with breast cancer in communicating with physicians. *Breast Journal, 7,* 444–449.

Herman-Staab, B. (1994). Screening, management, and appropriate referral for pediatric behavior problems. *Nurse Practitioner, 19*(7), 40, 42–43, 46–49.

Hirose, H. (1999). Classifying the empathic understanding of the nurse psychotherapist. *Cancer Nursing, 22,* 204–211.

Kacperek, L. (1997). Non-verbal communication: The importance of listening. *British Journal of Nursing, 6,* 275–279.

Kemper, B. J. (1992). Therapeutic listening: Developing the concept. *Journal of Psychosocial Nursing and Mental Health Services, 30*(7), 21–23.

Kruijver, I. P., Kerkstra, A., Francke, A. L., Bensing, J. M., & van de Wiel, H. B. (2000). Evaluation of communication training programs in nursing care: A review of the literature. *Patient Education and Counseling, 39,* 129–145.

Kubota, S., Mishima, N., & Nagata, S. (2004). A study of the effects of active listening on listening attitudes of middle managers. *Journal of Occupational Health, 46*(1), 60–67.

Lekander, B. J., Lehmann, S., & Lindquist, R. (1993). Therapeutic listening: Key nursing interventions for several nursing diagnoses. *Dimensions of Critical Care Nursing, 12,* 24–30.

Liehr, P., Mehl, M. R., Summers, L. C., & Pennebaker, J. W. (2004). Connecting with others in the midst of stressful upheaval on September 11, 2001. *Applied Nursing Research, 17*(1), 2–9.

McCambridge, J., Platts, S., Whooley, D., & Strang, J. (2004). Encouraging GP alcohol intervention: Pilot study of change-oriented reflective listening (CORL). *Alcohol & Alcoholism, 39*(2), 146–149.

Minamisawa, H., & Mitoh, T. (1997). Relating EEG changes and I–thou feelings during nursing interview. *Journal of Neuroscience Nursing, 29,* 32–38.

Molter, N. C. (2003). Creating a healing environment for critical care. *Critical Care Nursing Clinics of North America, 15,* 295–304.

Myers, S. (2000). Empathic listening: Reports on the experience of being heard. *Journal of Humanistic Psychology, 40*(2), 148–173.

O'Gara, P. E., & Fairhurst, W. (2004). Therapeutic communication: Part 2. Strategies that can enhance the quality of the emergency care consultation. *Accident and Emergency Nursing, 12,* 201–207.

O'Hagan, B., Webb, L., & Moore, K. (2004). Listening and learning from patients. *Emergency Nurse, 12*(7), 12–14.

Olson, J. K., & Hanchett, E. (1997). Nurse-expressed empathy, patient outcomes, and development of a middle-range theory. *Image: Journal of Nursing Scholarship, 29,* 71–76.

Olson, J. K., & Iwasiw, C. L. (1987). Effects of a training model on active listening skills of post-RN students. *Journal of Nursing Education, 26,* 104–107.

Reid-Ponte, P. (1992). Distress in cancer patients and primary nurses' empathy skills. *Cancer Nursing, 15,* 283–292.

Rogers, C. R. (1957). The necessary and sufficient conditions of therapeutic personality change. *Journal of Consulting Psychology, 21,* 95–103.

Rollnick, S., Allison, J., Ballasiotes, S., Barth, T., Butler, C. C., Rose, G. S., et al. (2002). Variations on a theme: Motivational interviewing and its adaptations. In W. R. Miller & S. Rollnick (Eds.), *Motivational interviewing: Preparing people for change* (2nd ed., pp. 270–283). New York: Guilford.

Ryden, M. B., McCarthy, P. R., Lewis, M. L., & Sherman, C. (1991). A behavioral comparison of the helping styles of nursing students, psychotherapists, crisis interveners, and untrained individuals. *Archives of Psychiatric Nursing, 5,* 185–188.

Sandelowski, M. (1994). We are the stories we tell: Narrative knowing in nursing practice. *Journal of Holistic Nursing, 12,* 23–33.

Schlesinger, H. J. (1994). How the analyst listens: The pre-stages of interpretation. *International Journal of Psycho-Analysis, 75,* 31–37.

Sheppard, M. (1993). Client satisfaction, extended intervention, and interpersonal skills in community mental health. *Journal of Advanced Nursing, 18,* 246–259.

Simpson, M., Buckman, R., Stuart, M., Maguire, P., Lipkin, M., Novack, D., et al. (1991). Doctor–patient communication: The Toronto Consensus Statement. Consensus Development Conference. *British Medical Journal, 303*(6814), 1385–1387.

Strang, J., McCambridge, J., Platts, S., & Groves, P. (2004). Engaging the reluctant GP in care of the opiate users. *Family Practice, 21*(2), 150–154.

Street, C., & Svanberg, J. (2003, July–August). Listening to young people. *Mental Health Today,* 28–30.

Sundeen, S. J., Stuart, G. W., Rankin, E. A. D., & Cohen, S. A. (1998). *Nurse–client interaction: Implementing the nursing process* (6th ed.). St. Louis, MO: Mosby.

Vitello-Cicciu, J. M. (2002). Exploring emotional intelligence: Implications for nursing leaders. *Journal of Nursing Administration, 32*(4), 203–210.

Wanzer, M. B., Booth-Butterfield, M., & Gruber, K. (2004). Perceptions of health care providers' communication: Relationships between patient-centered communication and satisfaction. *Health Communication, 16*, 363–384.

Whaley, L., & Wong, D. (1996). *Essentials of pediatric nursing* (5th ed). St. Louis: Mosby.

White, J., Levinson, W., & Roter, D. (1994). "Oh by the way . . . ": The closing moments of the medical visit. *Journal of General Internal Medicine, 9*, 24–28.

Williams, K., Kemper, S., & Hummert, M. L. (2004). Enhancing communication with older adults: Overcoming elderspeak. *Journal of Gerontological Nursing, 30*(10), 17–25.

PART II

Mind–Body Therapies

OVERVIEW

Many complementary therapies can be placed in this category. According to the National Center for Complementary/Alternative Medicine (NCCAM), mind–body therapies encompass those that promote the mind's capacity to have an impact on the functioning of the body. This definition does not mention that the reverse is also true—that therapies that affect the body can have an impact on the mind. Neither does the definition make reference to the spiritual realm that is a part of a holistic perspective. The more encompassing perspective, mind-body-spirit, will be the focus in this book.

Mind–body therapies stand in opposition to the long held, beliefs that underlie Western biomedicine in which the body and mind are examined separately. This separation was based on the philosophy of René Descartes. Nursing care, on the other hand, has been based on a holistic philosophy. Florence Nightingale documented the impact that therapies such as music have on the whole person (Nightingale, 1936). Despite the literature on a holistic philosophy and the emphasis that has been given to holistic assessments, in actuality the biomedical model has often predominated in nursing until recently. Other health professionals are also shifting away from the dichotomy of mind and body and are viewing persons from a holistic perspective.

An emerging body of research provides the basis for the use of mind–body therapies. From Herbert Benson's work in the 1960s on the effect of transcendental meditation on blood pressure to the increasing number of psychoneuroimmunological studies, the interconnectedness of the mind and body is being documented. Measurement of multiple outcomes (physiological, psychological, and spiritual) is needed in which complementary therapies are tested. Such studies pose challenges for identifying and measuring outcomes.

Many of the therapies in this category have been used by nurses. These include imagery, music, prayer, and humor. Many other mind–body therapies such as internal qi gong, soul retrieval, sweat lodges, and body psychotherapy are less familiar to nurses. The therapies chosen for inclusion in part II are ones that nurses frequently use and on which nurses have conducted research. These are imagery, music, humor, yoga, biofeedback, meditations, prayer, storytelling, and animal-assisted therapy.

REFERENCE

Nightingale, F. (1936/1992). *Notes on nursing*. Philadelphia: Lippincott.

CHAPTER 6

Imagery

Janice Post-White and Maura Fitzgerald

Imagery is a mind–body intervention that uses the power of the imagination to effect change in physical, emotional, or spiritual dimensions. Throughout our daily lives we constantly see images, feel sensations, and make impressions. A picture makes us angry or sad, a smell brings us to a past moment, a sound makes the muscles in our neck tighten. A billboard showing a cool glass of lemonade makes our mouths water, and a fondly remembered song on the radio takes us back to carefree feelings of youth. Images evoke physical and emotional responses and help us understand the meaning of events.

Imagery is described as "the world's oldest and greatest healing resource" (Achterberg, 1985, p. 3), and is used in many ancient healing traditions to effect cure, alleviate suffering, and facilitate spiritual transformation. Throughout time, healers and shamans have used imagery to access the patient's subconscious mind and belief system in order to open communication among the body, mind, and spirit. In spiritual life, experiences are images reflecting us back to ourselves (Epstein, 2004).

Imagery is commonly used in modern health care, most often in the form of guided imagery, clinical hypnosis, or self-hypnosis. In the mid-1950s, the American Medical Association and the American Psychiatric Association recognized hypnosis as a therapeutic tool (Lee, 1999). Nurses, physicians, psychologists, and others use it in their practice for treatment of acute and chronic illness, relief of symptoms, and enhancement of wellness. Imagery has become standard therapy to alleviate anxiety and promote relaxation in adults and children, and has been successfully used to relieve both chronic and procedural pain and insomnia, prevent allergic responses, and lower high blood pressure. Imagery is a hallmark of current stress-management programs and is a technique used to promote deep relaxation, gain psychological insight, and progress on a chosen spiritual path.

DEFINITION

Imagery is the formation of a mental representation of an object, a place, an event, or a situation that is perceived through the senses. It is based on the individual's own imagination and cognitive processing and can be practiced as an independent activity (self-hypnosis) or guided by a professional (guided imagery).

Imagery can be active or passive. For adults and adolescents, physical and mental relaxation tends to facilitate imagery. Younger children often do not need to assume a relaxed state. Imagery may be receptive, with the individual perceiving messages from the body, or it may be active, with the individual cognitively evoking thoughts or ideas. Active imagery can be outcome- or end-state–oriented, in which case the individual envisions a goal, such as being healthy and well, or it can be process-oriented, in which case the mechanism of the desired effect is imagined, such as envisioning a strong immune system fighting a viral infection or tumor.

Images employ all the senses—visual, aural, tactile, olfactory, proprioceptive, and kinesthetic. Although imagery is often referred to as "visualization," it includes imagining through any sense and not just being able to "see something" in the mind's eye. While inducing imagery, the individual often imagines seeing, hearing, smelling, tasting, and/or touching something in the image.

SCIENTIFIC BASIS

Imagery is thought to modify disease and reduce symptoms by lowering the stress response, which is mediated by psychoneuroimmune interactions. The stress response is triggered when a situation or event (perceived or real) threatens physical or emotional well-being or when the demands of a situation exceed available resources. One of the goals of imagery is to reframe stressful situations from negative responses of fear and anxiety to positive images of healing and well-being (Dossey, 1995). Imagery also can be used to increase emotional awareness and restructure the meaning of a situation. Emotional responses to situations trigger the limbic system and signal physiologic changes in the peripheral and autonomic nervous systems, resulting in the characteristic fight-or-flight stress response. The right cerebral hemisphere stores images, which can be evoked through memories (Epstein, 2004). Over time, chronic stress results in adrenal and immune suppression and may be the most harmful to cellular immune function, impairing the ability to ward off viruses and tumor cells (Pert, Dreher, & Ruff, 1998). Redefining negative responses to positive images and meaning reduces the physiologic stress response of the body.

Extensive rat model research by Robert Ader and Nicholas Cohen in the 1970s confirmed that the immune system can be conditioned by expectations and beliefs (Ader & Cohen, 1981; Ader, Felten, & Cohen, 1991). Subsequent research in psychoneuroimmunology attempted to explain the mechanisms of how the brain and body communicate through cellular interactions. Receptors for neuropeptides, neurohormones, and cytokines reside on neural and immune cells and induce biochemical changes when activated. Serotonin and dopamine are two neurotransmitters that increase with stress and activate hypothalamic activity through receptor signaling (Black, 1995). There is overlap between the neuronal pathways and brain structures that are activated in imagery and those that are active in the actual use of the sense (Djordjevic, Zatorre, Petrides, Boyle, & Jones-Gotaman, 2005; Gulyas, 2001; Kraemer, Macrae, Green, & Kelley, 2005; Yoo, Lee, & Choi, 2001). As a result, the brain and the body respond to both real and imagined situations in a similar fashion.

A cascade of signaling events in response to perceived or actual stress results in the release of corticotropin-releasing hormone (CRH) from the hypothalamus, adrenocorticotropin-releasing hormone (ACTH) from the pituitary, norepinephrine and epinephrine from the adrenal medulla and peripheral sympathetic nerve terminals, and immunosuppressive cortisol from the adrenal cortex. These interactions are bi-directional and changes in one system will influence the others.

Although immune responses to emotional states are extremely complex, in general, acute stress activates cardiac sympathetic activity and increases plasma catecholamines and natural killer cell activity, whereas chronic stress (or inescapable or unpredictable stress) is associated with suppression of NK cells and interleukin-1 beta (β) and other pro-inflammatory cytokines (Cacioppo et al., 1998; Glaser et al., 2001). These effects appear to be mediated by the influence of stress hormones on T helper 1 (Th1) and T helper 2 (Th2) components (Maes et al., 1998). The degree of response also varies. Cacioppo and colleagues hypothesize that persons who have large physiologic responses to everyday stressors have "high stress reactivity" and are at greater risk for disease susceptibility, even when coping, performance, and perceived stress are comparable. And although genetic factors remain to be studied, baseline levels of neuroendocrine activity are likely to be regulated by genes and may determine the degree of natural resistance to disease, independent of external stimuli and stressors (Bonneau, Mormede, Vogler, McClearn, & Jones, 1998). The amazing heterogeneity in individual responses to stressful situations may determine not only how the individual responds, but also which interventions are more effective for individual adaptation.

INTERVENTION

Techniques

Imagery may be practiced independently, with a coach or teacher, or with a videotape or audiotape. The most effective imagery intervention is one that is specific to individuals' personalities, to their preferences for relaxation and specific settings, their developmental age, and the desired outcomes. An example of the steps of a general imagery session is outlined in Table 6.1.

Imagery sessions for adults and adolescents are usually 10–30 minutes in length, whereas most children tolerate 10–15 minutes. The session typically begins with a relaxation exercise or a focused "centering" situation or event for children. A technique that works well for both children and adults is to focus on slow and expansive breathing, which facilitates relaxation as the breath moves lower into the chest and the diaphragm and abdominal muscles are used more than the upper chest muscles. Other techniques include progressive muscle relaxation or focusing on a word or object. Relaxation helps make the mind more open to new information (Benson, 1993), but is not required for imagery. Some children use active imagery very successfully and may use their bodies to demonstrate or respond to their image.

Once the client is in a relaxed or "altered" state, the practitioner suggests an image of a relaxing, peaceful, or comforting place or introduces a predetermined and agreed-upon image suggested by the client. Scenes commonly used to induce relaxation include watching a sunset or clouds float by, sitting on a warm beach or by a fire on a snowy evening, or floating through water or space. The scene used is often one

TABLE 6.1 General Guided Imagery Technique

1. Achieving a relaxed state
    A. Find a comfortable sitting or reclining position (not lying down).
    B. Uncross any extremities.
    C. Close your eyes or focus on one spot or object in the room.
    D. Focus on breathing with abdominal muscles—with each breath say to yourself "in" and "out." Notice your breath as it moves in and out. With your next breath let the exhalation be just a little longer and notice how the inhalation that follows is deeper. And as you notice that let your body become even more relaxed.
    E. Feel your body becoming heavy and warm—from the top of your head to the tips of your fingers and toes.
    F. If your thoughts roam, bring your mind back to thinking of your breathing and your relaxed body.

2. Specific suggestions for imagery
    A. In your mind, go to a place you enjoy and where you feel good.
    B. What do you see—hear—taste—smell—and feel?
    C. Take a few deep breaths and enjoy being there.
    D. Now imagine yourself the way you want to be . . . (Describe the desired goal specifically).
    E. Imagine what steps you will need to take to be the way you want to be.
    F. Practice these steps now—in this place where you feel good.
    G. What is the first thing you are doing to help you be the way you want to be?
    H. What will you do next?
    I. When you reach your goal of the way you want to be—feel yourself, touch yourself, embrace yourself, listen to the sounds surrounding you.

3. Summarize process and reinforce practice
    A. Remember that you can return to this place, this feeling, this way of being anytime you want.
    B. You can feel this way again by focusing on your breathing, relaxing, and imagining yourself in your special place.
    C. Come back to this place and envision yourself the way you want to be every day.

4. Return to present
    A. When you are ready you may return to the room we are in.
    B. You will feel relaxed and refreshed and be ready to resume your activities.
    C. You may open your eyes and tell me about your experience when you are ready.

that the client has actually experienced previously and found to be relaxing. Children may prefer active images that involve motion, such as flying or playing a sport.

For directed imagery, the practitioner guides the imagery, using positive suggestions to alleviate specific symptoms or conditions (outcome or end-state imagery) or to rehearse or "walk through" an event (process imagery). Images do not need to be anatomically correct or vivid. Symbolic images may be the most powerful healing images because they are drawn from individual beliefs, culture, and meaning. For example, a 54-year-old woman with metastatic breast cancer watched her Alaskan Huskie dogs devour their breakfast and then used imagery to envision them scouring her body for tumor cells.

The ability to use guided imagery for therapeutic purposes is related to the individual's hypnotic ability or the ability to enter an altered state of consciousness and to become involved or absorbed in the imagery (Kwekkeboom, Huseby-Moore, & Ward, 1998). Some individuals have naturally high hypnotic abilities. They recall pictures more accurately, generate more complex images, have higher dream recall frequency in the waking state, and make fewer eye movements in imagery than poor visualizers.

Imagery has been used extensively in children and adolescents as well as with adults. Children as young as age 4 who have language skills that are adequate to understand the suggestions, can benefit from imagery (Olness & Kohen, 1996). Young children often are better at imagery because of their natural active use of their imaginations. It has been found that hypnotizability rises through early childhood, peaking somewhere between ages 7 and 14 and then leveling off into adolescence and adulthood (Olness & Kohen).

When practitioners do imagery with children, techniques must be modified to suit their developmental and cognitive age, as well as their personal preferences. Adjustments may include reducing the length of time and modifying the types of imagery used. Children often do not like to close their eyes. Preschool and school-age children most often imagine in an active state; therefore muscle relaxation is not necessarily a goal. For example, a group of 9- to 12-year-old boys with sickle cell disease were being taught guided imagery as a pain control technique. When asked what special place they would like to go to they requested a trip to a local amusement park and a ride on the roller coaster. During the imagery many of them were physically and vocally active, swaying from side to side and moving their arms up and down. At the end of the visualization they all reported feeling like they had been in the park (absorption) and gave examples of things they felt, saw, heard, or smelled.

Recognizing individual and developmental preferences for settings, situations, and relaxation or stimulation can improve the effectiveness of the imagery and reduce time and frustration with learning it. Practicing imagery oneself is extremely helpful in guiding others.

Measurement of Outcomes

Evaluating and measuring outcomes are important in determining the effectiveness and value of imagery in clinical practice. Clinical outcomes of imagery include physical signs of relaxation, less distress, lower levels of anxiety and depression, a sense of meaning, purpose, competency, and positive changes in attitude or behavior (Post-White & Johnson, 1991). Health services benefits may reduce costs, morbidity, and length of stay, and improve functional performance and quality of life.

The outcomes measured should reflect the client's situation and the conceptual framework providing the rationale for the use of imagery. If imagery is used to facilitate relaxation and progression during the birthing experience, outcomes might include reduced level of pain, decrease in medications taken, perceived helpfulness, and progression of labor. If imagery is used to control symptoms in clients undergoing chemotherapy for cancer, expected outcomes might include reduced nausea, vomiting, and fatigue; enhanced body image; positive mood states; and improved functional abilities. When imagery is used to reduce the stress response and promote relaxation, outcomes may include increased oxygen saturation levels, lower blood pressure and heart rate, warmer extremities, reduced muscle tension, greater alpha waves on EEG, and lower anxiety.

One of the most difficult determinations to make is whether the outcomes are solely the result of imagery or a combination of interventions. Learning and practicing imagery often changes other health-related behaviors, such as getting more sleep, eating a healthier diet, stopping smoking, or exercising regularly. The therapist's presence, attention, and compassion also may be an intervention independent of the imagery process. Because the ability to generate images and become involved in them as if they were real may moderate the effects of imagery on outcomes (Kwekkeboom et al., 1998), it is important to assess the ability to image. Several instruments can be used to measure the effectiveness of the ability to image (Achterberg & Lawlis, 1984; Marks, 1973; Sheehan, 1967; Shor & Orne, 1962) and the level of absorption (Tellegen, 1993).

Precautions

The physical and emotional risks of mind–body techniques are virtually nonexistent as long as they are not used in place of conventional medicine

(Goleman & Gurin, 1993). There are few reports of adverse events and there were no reports of adverse events or side effects reported in a systematic review of guided imagery for cancer (Roffe, Schmidt, & Ernst, 2005). Kwekkeboom and colleagues (1998) reported increased anxiety in 3 of 15 subjects using imagery specifically to reduce anxiety associated with a stressful task. However, the authors also acknowledge that the imagery was perceived as pleasant, despite the inability to relieve anxiety. Some individuals have anecdotally reported airway constriction or difficulty breathing when they focus on breathing techniques. Using another centering method, such as focusing on an object in the room or repeating a mantra, can reduce this distressing response and still induce relaxation.

The expertise and training of the nurse should guide judgment in using imagery to achieve outcomes in practice. Imagery techniques can be easily applied to managing symptoms (pain, nausea, vomiting) and facilitating relaxation, sleep, or anxiety reduction. Advanced techniques such as age regression and management of depression or posttraumatic stress disorder require further training.

USES

Imagery has been used therapeutically in a variety of conditions and populations (Table 6.2). Pain and cancer are two conditions in which imagery has been helpful in both adults and children.

Pain

Whether pain is from cancer, other illness, side effects of treatment, injury, or physical stress on the body, emotional factors contribute to pain perception, and mind–body interventions such as imagery can help make pain more manageable. Stress, anxiety, and fatigue decrease the threshold for pain, making the perceived pain more intense. Imagery can break this cycle of pain-tension-worry-anxiety-pain. Relaxation with imagery decreases pain directly by reducing muscle tension and related spasms and indirectly by lowering anxiety and improving sleep, both of which influence pain perception. Imagery also is a distraction strategy; vivid, detailed images using all senses tend to work best for pain control. In addition, cognitive reappraisal/restructuring used with imagery can increase a sense of control over the ability to reframe the meaning of pain.

Imagery is especially helpful in muscle tension–related pain, such as some headaches and migraines (Baumann, 2002; Ilacqua, 1994). Imagery also eases pain associated with childbirth (Rees, 1995), dental procedures,

TABLE 6.2 Conditions for Which Imagery Has Been Tested in Children and Adults

Clinical Conditions	Selected Sources
Children	
Asthma/COPD	Hackman, Stern, & Gershwin (2000); Louie (2004)
Burn dressing change	Foertsch, O'Hara, Stoddard, & Kealey (1998)
Cancer	Steggles et al. (1997)
Cardiac catheterization	Pederson (1995)
Chronic dyspnea	Anbar (2001a, 2001b)
Emotional and behavioral disorders	Olness & Kohen (1996)
Managing procedural pain	Broome, Rehwaldt, & Fogg (1998); Liossi & Hatira (1999); Stevens et al. (1994); Butler et al. (2005)
Nausea and vomiting	Keller, 1995
Pain	Anbar (2001a); Ball et al. (2003); Baumann (2002); Broome, Rehwaldt, & Fogg (1998); Huth, Broome, & Good (2004); Lambert (1999); Walco et al. (1992)
Adults	
Asthma	Epstein et al. (2004)
Phobias, anxiety	Thompson & Coppens (1994)
Childbirth/postpartum care	Rees (1995); Rossi (1986)
Depression & fatigue in HIV	Eller (1995)
Anxiety and pain medication use following coronary artery bypass surgery	Ashton et al. (1997)
Surgical outcomes	Mandle et al. (1996)
Protective cardiac factors	Mandle et al. (1996)
Psoriasis	Zachariae et al. (1996)
Anxiety during cancer treatment	Baider et al. (1994); Decker & Cline-Elsen (1992); Feldman & Salzberg (1990); Walker (1998)
Nausea and vomiting during cancer treatment	Burish & Jenkins (1992); Troesch et al. (1993)
Five-year survival in lymphoma	Ratcliffe et al. (1995)
Immune response in healthy volunteers	Johnson et al. (1996); Rider et al. (1990); Walker et al. (1993); Zachariae et al. (1994)
Immune response in breast cancer	Anderson (1992); Gruber et al. (1993); Post-White et al. (1996); Richardson et al. (1997); Walker et al. (1996)
Cancer pain	Syrjala et al. (1995); Wallace (1997)
Postoperative pain	Antall & Kresevic (2004)
Comfort during cancer therapy	Kolcaba & Fox (1999)
Sleep	Richardson (2003)

and surgery (Mandle, Jacobs, Arcari, & Domar, 1996; Manyande et al., 1995). Although highly hypnotizable persons benefit more readily than others, practically all patients can learn to better manage their pain and pain-related stresses through simple imagery exercises (Spira & Spiegel, 1992).

Guided imagery has been used extensively with children to alleviate pain and anxiety (Huth, Broome, & Good, 2004; Lambert, 1999; Rusy & Weisman, 2000; Steggles, Damore-Petingola, Maxwell, & Lightfoot, 1997). Imagery is particularly helpful in getting a child through a medical procedure with a safe and effective level of sedation/analgesia and as little movement as possible (Butler, Symons, Henderson, Shortliffe, & Spiegel, 2005). Suggestions to breathe deeply and to relax or be comfortable are combined with vivid images of a favorite place. It is best to introduce the child to breathing techniques and explore favorite places prior to the procedure. In critical or emergency situations, however, imagery has been successfully employed without preliminary work (Kohen, 2000).

Distraction imagery is most useful for dealing with exhausting and severe pain and painful procedures. Suggestions for drawing attention completely from the physical pain include floating or other pleasant sensations, recalling a pleasant past experience or feeling, or distracting oneself from the pain source by rubbing fingers together or squeezing and releasing hands.

Several studies document the effectiveness of imagery to reduce acute procedural pain in children. In one study of chronic pain, imagery and progressive muscle relaxation were effective for reducing chronic recurrent abdominal pain and improving quality of life, social functioning, and school attendance after 10 months of training and practice (Youssef et al., 2004).

In two studies of children with cancer undergoing procedures, relaxation, distraction, and imagery reduced pain during lumbar puncture in a single arm study of 28 children and adolescents (Broome, Rehwaldt, & Fogg, 1998). Clinical hypnosis and cognitive restructuring also reduced pain and anxiety, in comparison to a control condition, in 30 children undergoing bone marrow biopsy (Liossi & Hatira, 1999).

In a study of 26 children undergoing elective surgical procedures, preoperative imagery reduced postoperative pain scores and length of stay in comparison to standard preoperative education, despite the same dose of pain medication (Lambert, 1996). Two other studies measuring the effectiveness of imagery in reducing procedural pain in children found no differences in distress behaviors and pain with cardiac catheterization in comparison to a control group (Pederson, 1995) and during burn dressing changes (Foertsch, O'Hara, Stoddard, & Kealey, 1998).

The focus with moderate pain is to alter the interpretation or perception of pain. Metaphors for pain can be used to dissociate from the pain and gain control (initially over the metaphor used), thereby reducing the intensity of the pain. Another alternative is to identify pleasant sensations with the metaphor. Associations with hot or cold temperature also can be used, with the individual concentrating on raising and lowering the intensity/level and associating pleasant sensations with different temperatures.

Focusing and transferring analgesia is most effective for mild pain. Several techniques can be used, such as imagining the area being injected with anesthetic, being wooden, or being painted a color that numbs the area. It is helpful to numb an unaffected area first, such as a "hand in glove" anesthesia, and then transfer that numbness to the painful area (Levitan, 1992). Although elements of relaxation, vividness, and distraction were important to pain reduction, Zachariae and Bjerring (1994) and De Pascalis and colleagues (2004) found that focused analgesia was the most effective in reducing acute pain, particularly in subjects with high hypnotizable ratings.

Cancer Pain

Imagery interventions in oncology have focused on four areas: efficacy in pain management, influence on surgical outcomes, improvement in quality of life, and changes in immunity (Lee, 1999). Pain specific to cancer and its treatment can be acute or chronic. In a randomized pretest–posttest study of 67 hospitalized patients with cancer pain, imagery combined with progressive muscle relaxation reduced pain sensation, intensity, and severity and lowered non-opioid breakthrough analgesia use (Sloman, 1995). Similarly, in two clinical trials of bone marrow transplant patients, Syrjala and colleagues measured reduced levels of mucositis-related pain in the imagery/hypnosis group (Syrjala, Cummings, & Donaldson, 1992; Syrjala, Donaldson, Davis, Kippes, & Carr, 1995). Twice-weekly imagery sessions included progressive muscle relaxation, deep relaxation, transference of sensations, and individualized imagery.

Despite its use in cancer, there are few randomized controlled studies documenting the effectiveness of imagery for cancer-related pain (Wallace, 1997). However, a National Institutes of Health technology assessment panel concluded that behavioral therapies for chronic cancer pain should be accepted as standard treatment and reimbursed similar to medical treatments (Eastman, 1995). Kwekkeboom (1999) proposed a model to help predict the effectiveness of cognitive-behavioral cancer pain management strategies. In a subsequent pilot study testing the relationships among predictive variables in a path analysis model, imaging ability was the strongest predictor of mean pain intensity, positive affect, and perceived control over the pain (Kwekkeboom, Kneip, & Pearson, 2003). Outcome expectancy was not a predictor of imagery success.

Other factors proposed to influence imagery's success include the dose of imagery. Great variability exists in how frequently imagery is recommended. In an attempt to quantify this effect, Van Kuiken (2004) conducted a meta-analysis of 16 published studies since 1996. Although the final sample of 10 studies was too small for statistical analysis, Van Kuiken concluded that imagery practice up to 18 weeks increases the effectiveness of the intervention. A minimum dose was not determined and further study is needed to explore a dose relationship with outcomes. To help with standardization of imagery interventions and generalizability, other documentation should include a detailed description of the specific interventions used, outcomes affected by the imagery, and factors influencing effectiveness.

Cancer Outcomes

Although several prospective randomized studies found that imagery increased survival in patients with cancer (Fawzy et al., 1993; Grossarth-Maticek & Eysenck, 1989; Spiegel, Bloom, Kraemer, & Gottheil, 1989; Walker, 1998), and reduced time to engraftment in 23 patients undergoing bone marrow transplant (Sahler, Hunter, & Liesveld, 2003), many other factors also influence cancer outcomes. Psychosocial factors such as depression (Walker, 1998) and diagnostic factors such as stage of disease (Ratcliffe, Dawson, & Walker, 1995) are consistent covariates in explaining survival outcomes.

A common explanation for how imagery may improve cancer outcomes is postulated through increasing cellular immune function. Some studies have demonstrated increases in natural killer cytotoxicity (Fawzy et al., 1993; Fawzy et al., 1990; Gruber, Hall, Hersh, & Dubois, 1988; Gruber et al., 1993; Gruzelier, 2002; Walker et al., 1996), NK numbers (Bakke, Purtzer, & Newton, 2002), and T cell responses (Gruber et al., 1988; Gruber et al., 1993), whereas others have found no differences (Post-White et al., 1996; Richardson et al., 1997) or decreases (Zachariae, Hansen, et al., 1994) in natural killer cell numbers and cytotoxicity. Despite inconclusive effects on cancer outcome, imagery interventions have consistently improved coping responses and psychological states in patients with cancer, suggesting that imagery may mediate psychoneuroimmune outcomes in breast and other cancers (Walker, 2004). Further study is needed to determine the clinical significance of immunological effects.

In a systematic review of guided imagery as an adjuvant cancer therapy for symptom distress, Roffe and colleagues (2005) evaluated the evidence from six studies using imagery as a single intervention in cancer. Three studies reported significant effects on anxiety (Sloman, 2002), comfort during radiation therapy (Kolcaba & Fox, 1999), and emotional response to chemotherapy (Troesch et al., 1993). No effects were found on physical symptoms, which may be partially explained by few distressing symptoms in the subjects. The literature search identified 103 articles investigating imagery for cancer. Guided imagery has recently been identified as one of the 10 most frequently recommended integrative therapies for cancer on the Internet (Schmidt & Ernst, 2004). The low methodological quality of the studies suggests that rigorous research in imagery for cancer is not as prevalent as actual use in clinical practice.

FUTURE RESEARCH

Despite documented relationships between the mind and the body, many of the intervention trials testing the effectiveness of guided imagery and other mind–body interventions lack the scientific rigor of randomized controlled clinical trials. Wild and Espie (2004) conclude that there is insufficient evidence for the efficacy of hypnosis to manage procedural pain in pediatric oncology, largely because of the lack of high-quality research studies. Small sample sizes and lack of standardized control groups limit the generalizability of the findings. However, the clinical evidence for effect remains strong, and more scientifically rigorous research testing outcomes are needed.

Key questions that remain to be answered are whether psychoneuroimmune responses to imagery influence clinical outcomes and quality of life and if so, how they work to mediate psychosocial and clinical outcomes. Determining personal preferences for use of imagery and specific types of imagery is important for demonstrating significant clinical effects. Measuring clinical outcomes relevant to quality of life and health/illness states is critical to demonstrating cost effectiveness and efficacy of imagery as an intervention useful in practice. As a low cost, noninvasive intervention, imagery has the potential to be effective in reducing pain and distress across several conditions.

Questions to be pursued include:

1. Is imagery more effective than relaxation alone in producing stress-reducing outcomes?

2. Does the type of imagery (outcome or process) produce different outcomes? Does imaging the immune system in cancer actually influence immune response?

3. Are there certain characteristics of individuals that determine their ability to respond to imagery and produce desired outcomes? Are there certain individuals or conditions for which imagery should not be recommended?

4. What are the long-term effects of imagery? Over time, can imagery reduce stress, improve coping, enhance well-being, create healthier lifestyles, and reduce illness in individuals?

WEB SITES FOR IMAGERY

Academy for Guided Imagery, Inc. (2004). Professional Certification Program. http://www.academyforguidedimagery.com/programinfo.php

American Holistic Nurses Association. (2004). http://www.ahna.org/home/home.html

American Society of Clinical Hypnosis. Undated. http://www.asch.net/. Certification, workshops, resources.

Cancer Imagery (2002–2005). http://cancerimagery.com/index.html. Cancer Imagery research (pain, resources).

Imagination, Mental Imagery, Consciousness, and Cognition: Scientific, Philosophical, and Historical Approaches by Nigel Thomas (November 11, 2004). http://www.calstatela.edu/faculty/nthomas/

InnerVision Studio, Inc. (2000). Research on Guided Imagery, Hypnosis, and Relaxation Techniques. http://www.innervisionstudioinc.com/research.htm

Beyond Ordinary Nursing. (2004). Integrative Imagery Training for Health Professionals. http://www.integrativeimagery.com/index.htm. Certificate program, Continuing education credits for holistic healing, post-graduate classes.

REFERENCES

Achterberg, J. (1985). *Imagery in healing: Shamanism and modern medicine.* Boston: Shambhala.

Achterberg, J., & Lawlis, G. F. (1984). *Imagery and disease: Diagnostic tools?* Champaign, IL: Institute for Personality and Ability Testing.

Ader, R., & Cohen, N. (1981). Conditioned immunopharmacologic responses. In R. Ader (Ed.), *Psychoneuroimmunology* (pp. 281–319). New York: Academic Press.

Ader, R., Felten, D. L., & Cohen, N. (1991). *Psychoneuroimmunology* (2nd ed.). San Diego: Academic Press.

Anbar, R. D. (2001a). Self-hypnosis for the treatment of functional abdominal pain in childhood. *Clinical Pediatrics, 40*(8), 447–451.

Anbar, R. D. (2001b). Self-hypnosis for management of chronic dyspnea in pediatric patients. *Pediatrics, 107*(2):e21 [electronic version].

Anderson, B. L. (1992). Psychological interventions for cancer patients to enhance the quality of life. *Journal of Consulting and Clinical Psychology, 60*, 552–568.

Antall, G. F., & Kresevic, D. (2004). The use of guided imagery to manage pain in an elderly orthopaedic population. *Orthopedic Nursing, 23*(5), 335–340.

Ashton, C., Whitworth, G. C., Seldomridge, J. A., Shapiro, P. A., Weinberg, A. D., Smith, C. R., et al. (1997). Self-hypnosis reduces anxiety following coronary artery bypass surgery: A prospective, randomized trial. *Journal of Cardiovascular Surgery, 38*, 69–75.

Baider, L., Uziely, B., & De-Nour, A. K. (1994). Progressive muscle relaxation and guided imagery in cancer patients. *General Hospital Psychiatry, 16*(5), 340–347.

Bakke, A. C., Purtzer, M. Z., & Newton, P. (2002). The effect of hypnotic-guided imagery on psychological well-being and immune function in patients with prior breast cancer. *Journal of Psychosomatic Research, 53*(6), 1131–1137.

Ball, T. M., Shapiro, D. E., Monheim, C. J., & Wydert, J. A. (2003). A pilot study of the use of guided imagery for the treatment of recurrent abdominal pain in children. *Clinical Pediatrics, 42*(6), 527–532.

Baumann, R. J. (2002). Behavioral treatment of migraine in children and adolescents. *Pediatric Drugs, 4*(9), 555–561.

Benson, H. (1993). The relaxation response. In D. Goleman & J. Gurin (Eds.), *Mind/body medicine* (pp. 233–258). Yonkers, NY: Consumers Union of the United States.

Black, P. H. (1995). Psychoneuroimmunology: Brain and immunity. *Scientific American Science and Medicine, 2*(6), 16–25.

Bonneau, R. H., Mormede, P., Vogler, G. P., McClearn, G. E., & Jones, B. C. (1998). A genetic basis for neuroendocrine-immune interactions. *Brain, Behavior, and Immunity, 12*, 83–89.

Broome, M. E., Rehwaldt, M., & Fogg, L. (1998). Relationships between cognitive behavioral techniques, temperament, observed distress, and pain reports in children and adolescents during lumbar puncture. *Journal of Pediatric Nursing, 13*(1), 48–51.

Burish, T. G., & Jenkins, R. A. (1992). Effectiveness of biofeedback and relaxation training in reducing the side effects of cancer chemotherapy. *Health Psychology, 11*(1), 17–23.

Butler, L. D., Symons, B. K., Henderson, S. L., Shortliffe, L. D., & Spiegel, D. (2005). Hypnosis reduces distress and duration of an invasive medical procedure for children. *Pediatrics, 115*(1), e77–85.

Cacioppo, J. T., Berntson, G. G., Malarkey, W. B., Kiecolt-Glaser, J. K., Sheridan, J. F., Poehlmann, K., et al. (1998). Autonomic, neuroendocrine, and immune responses to psychological stress: The reactivity hypothesis. *Annals of the New York Academy of Sciences, 1*(840), 664–673.

Decker, T. W., & Cline-Elsen, J. (1992). Relaxation therapy as an adjunct in radiation oncology. *Journal of Clinical Psychology, 48*(3), 388–393.

De Pascalis, V., Bellusci, A., Gallo, C., Magurano, M. R., & Chen, A. C. (2004). Pain-reduction strategies in hypnotic context and hypnosis: ERI and SCRs during a secondary auditory task. *International Journal of Clinical and Experimental Hypnotism, 52*(4), 343–363.

Djordjevic J., Zatorre, R. J., Petrides, M., Boyle, J. A., & Jones-Gotaman, M. (2005). Functional neuroimaging of odor imagery. *Neuroimage, 24*(3), 791–801.

Dossey, B. (1995). Complementary Modalities Part 3: Using imagery to help your patient heal. *American Journal of Nursing, 96*(6), 41–47.

Eastman, P. (1995). Panel endorses behavioral therapy for cancer pain (news). *Journal of the National Cancer Institute, 87*(22), 1666–1667.

Eller, L. S. (1995). Effects of two cognitive-behavioral interventions on immunity and symptoms in persons with HIV. *The Society of Behavioral Medicine, 17*(4), 339–348.

Epstein, G. (2004). Mental imagery: The language of spirit. *Advances, 20*(3), 4–10.

Epstein, G. N., Halper, J. P., Barrett, E. A., Birdsal, C., McGee, M., Baron, K. P., et al. (2004). A pilot study of mind–body changes in adults with asthma who practice mental imagery. *Alternative Therapies, 10*(4), 66–71.

Fawzy, F. I., Fawzy, N. W., Hyun, C. S., Elashoff, R., Guthrie, D, Fahey, J. L., et al. (1993). Malignant melanoma: Effects of an early structured psychiatric intervention, coping and affective state on recurrence and survival 6 years later. *Archives of General Psychiatry, 50,* 681–689.

Fawzy, F. I., Kemeny, M. E., Fawzy, N. W., Elashoff, R., Morton, D., Cousins, N., & Fahey, J. L. (1990). A structured psychiatric intervention for cancer patients II. Changes over time in immunological measures. *Archives of General Psychiatry, 47,* 729–735.

Feldman, C. S., & Salzberg, H. C. (1990). The role of imagery in the hypnotic treatment of adverse reactions to cancer therapy. *Journal of the South Carolina Medical Association, 86*(5), 303–306.

Foertsch, C. E., O'Hara, M. W., Stoddard, F. J., & Kealey, G. P. (1998) Treatment-resistant pain and distress during pediatric burn-dressing changes. *Journal of Burn Care and Rehabilitation, 19,* 219–224.

Gil, K. M. (2001). Daily coping practice predicts treatment effects in children with sickle cell disease. *Journal of Pediatric Psychology, 26*(3), 163–173.

Glaser, R., MacCallum, R. C., Laskowski, B. F., Malarkey, W. B., Sheridan, J. F., & Kiecolt-Glaser, J. K. (2001). Evidence for a shift in the Th-1 to Th-2 cytokine response associated with chronic stress and aging. *Journal of Gerontology A: Biological Science and Medical Science, 56*(8), M477–M482.

Goleman, D., & Gurin, J. (Eds.). (1993). *Mind/body medicine.* Yonkers, NY: Consumer Report Books.

Grossarth-Maticek, R., & Eysenck, H. J. (1989). Length of survival and lymphocyte percentage in women with mammary cancer as a function of psychotherapy. *Psychological Reports, 65,* 315–321.

Gruber, B. L., Hall, N. R., Hersh, S. P., & Dubois, P. (1988). Immune system and psychologic changes in metastatic cancer patients while using ritualized relaxation and guided imagery: A pilot study. *Scandinavian Journal of Behavioral Therapy, 17,* 25–46.

Gruber, B. L., Hersh, S. P., Hall, N. R., Waletzky, L. R., Kunz, J. F., Carpenter, J. K., et al. (1993). Immunological responses of breast cancer patients to behavioral interventions. *Biofeedback and Self Regulation, 18*(1), 1–22.

Gruzelier, J. H. (2002). A review of the impact of hypnosis, relaxation, guided imagery and individual differences on aspects of immunity and health. *Stress, 5*(2), 147–163.

Gulyas, B. (2001). Neural networks for internal reading and visual imagery of reading: A PET study. *Brain Research Bulletin, 54*(3), 319–328.

Hackman, R. M., Stern, J. S., & Gershwin, M. E. (2000). Hypnosis and asthma: A critical review. *Journal of Asthma, 37*(1), 1–15.

Huth, M. M., Broome, M. E., & Good, M. (2004). Imagery reduces children's postoperative pain. *Pain, 110*(1–2), 439–448.

Ilacqua, G. E. (1994). Migraine headaches: Coping efficacy of guided imagery training. *Headache, 34*(2), 99–102.

Johnson, V. C., Walker, L. G., Whiting, P., Heys, S. D., & Eremin, O. (1996). Can relaxation training and hypnotherapy modify the immune response to acute stress, and is hypnotisability relevant? *Contemporary Hypnosis, 13,* 100–108.

Keller, V. (1995). Management of nausea and vomiting in children. *Journal of Pediatric Nursing, 10*(5), 280–286.

Kohen, D. (2000, June). Integrating hypnosis into practice. *Introductory Workshop in Clinical Hypnosis.* St. Paul, MN: University of Minnesota and the Minnesota Society of Clinical Hypnosis.

Kolcaba, K., & Fox, C. (1999). The effects of guided imagery on comfort of women with early stage breast cancer undergoing radiation therapy. *Oncology Nursing Forum, 26*(1), 67–72.

Kraemer, D. J., Macrae, C. N., Green, A. E., & Kelley, W. M. (2005). Musical imagery: Sound of silence activates auditory cortex. *Nature, 434*(7030), 158.

Kwekkeboom, K. (1999). A model for cognitive-behavioral interventions in cancer pain management. *Image: Journal of Nursing Scholarship, 31,* 151–156.

Kwekkeboom, K., Huseby-Moore, K., & Ward, S. (1998). Imaging ability and effective use of guided imagery. *Research in Nursing and Health, 21,* 189–198.

Kwekkeboom, K., Kneip, J., & Pearson, L. (2003). A pilot study to predict success with guided imagery for cancer pain. *Pain Management Nursing, 4*(3), 112–123.

Lambert, S. (1996). The effects of hypnosis/guided imagery on the postoperative course of children. *Developmental and Behavioral Pediatrics, 17*(5), 307–310.

Lambert, S. (1999). Distraction, imagery, and hypnosis: Techniques for management of children's pain. *Journal of Child and Family Nursing, 2*(1), 5–15.

Lee, R. (1999). Guided imagery as supportive therapy in cancer treatment. *Alternative Medicine Alert, 2*(6), 61–64.

Levitan, A. A. (1992). The use of hypnosis with cancer patients. *Psychiatric Medicine, 10*(1), 119–131.

Liossi, C., & Hatira, P. (1999). Clinical hypnosis versus cognitive behavioral training for pain management with pediatric cancer patients undergoing bone marrow aspirations. *The International Journal of Clinical Hypnosis, 47*(2), 104–116.

Louie, S. W. (2004). The effects of guided imagery relaxation in people with COPD. *Occupational Therapy International, 11*(3), 145–159.

Maes, M., Song, C., Lin, A., De Jongh, R., Van Gastel, A., Kenis, G., et al. (1998). The effects of psychological stress on humans: Increased production of pro-inflammatory cytokines and a Th1-like response in stress-induced anxiety. *Cytokine, 10*(4), 313–318.

Mandle, C. L., Jacobs, S. G., Arcari, P. M., & Domar, A. D. (1996). The efficacy of relaxation response interventions with adult patients: A review of the literature. *Journal of Cardiovascular Nursing, 10*(3), 4–26.

Manyande, A., Berg, S., Gettins, D., Stanford, S. C., Mazhero, S., Marks, D. F., et al. (1995). Preoperative rehearsal of active coping imagery influences subjective and hormonal responses to abdominal surgery. *Psychosomatic Medicine, 57*(2), 177–182.

Marks, D. F. (1973). Visual imagery differences in the recall of pictures. *British Journal of Psychology, 64*, 17–24.

Olness, K., & Kohen, D. (1996). *Hypnosis and hypnotherapy with children* (3rd ed.). New York: Guilford.

Pederson, C. (1995). Effect of imagery on children's pain and anxiety during cardiac catheterization. *Journal of Pediatric Nursing, 10*(6), 365–374.

Pert, C. B., Dreher, H. E., & Ruff, M. R. (1998). The psychosomatic network: Foundations of mind–body medicine. *Alternative Therapies, 4*(4), 30–41.

Post-White, J., & Johnson, M. K. (1991). Complementary nursing therapies in clinical oncology practice: Relaxation and imagery. *Dimensions in Oncology Nursing, 5*(2), 15–20.

Post-White, J., Schroeder, L., Hannahan, A., Johnston, M. K., Salscheider, N., & Grandt, N. (1996). Response to imagery/support in breast cancer survivors. *Oncology Nursing Forum, 23*(2), 355.

Ratcliffe, M. A., Dawson, A. A., & Walker, L. G. (1995). Personality inventory L-scores in patients with Hodgkin's disease and non-Hodgkin's lymphoma. *Psycho-Oncology, 4*, 39–45.

Rees, B. L. (1995). Effect of relaxation with guided imagery on anxiety, depression, and self-esteem in primaparas. *Journal of Holistic Nursing, 13*(3), 255–267.

Richardson, M. A., Post-White, J., Grimm, E. A., Moye, L. A., Singletary, S. E., & Justice, B. (1997). Coping, life attitudes, and immune responses to imagery and group support after breast cancer. *Alternative Therapies in Health and Medicine, 3*(5), 62–70.

Richardson, R. (2003). Effects of relaxation and imagery on the sleep of critically ill adults. *Dimensions of Critical Care Nursing, 22*(4), 182–190.

Rider, M., Achterberg, J., Lawlis, F. G., Goven, A., Toledo, R., & Butler, J. R. (1990). Effect of immune system imagery on secretory IgA. *Biofeedback and Self-Regulation, 15*(4), 317–333.

Roffe, L., Schmidt, K., & Ernst, E. (2005). A systematic review of guided imagery as an adjuvant cancer therapy. *Psycho-oncology.* (in press). Electronic version published online January 13, 2005.

Rossi, E. L. (1986). *The psychobiology of mind-body healing: New concepts of therapeutic hypnosis.* New York: Norton.

Rusy, L. M., & Weisman, S. J. (2000). Complementary therapies for acute pediatric pain management. *Pediatric Clinics of North America, 47*(3), 589–599.

Sahler, O. L., Hunter, B. C., & Liesveld, J. L. (2003). The effect of using music therapy with relaxation imagery in the management of patients undergoing bone marrow transplantation: A pilot feasibility study. *Alternative Therapies in Health & Medicine, 9*(6), 70–74.

Schmidt, K., & Ernst, E. (2004). Assessing websites on complementary and alternative medicine for cancer. *Annals of Oncology, 15,* 733–742 [electronic version].

Sheehan, P. W. (1967). A shortened form of Betts questionnaire upon mental imagery. *Journal of Clinical Psychology, 23,* 386–389.

Shor, R. E., & Orne, E. C. (1962). Norms on the Harvard Group Scale of Hypnotic Susceptibility. *International Journal of Clinical and Experimental Hypnosis, 11,* 39–47.

Sloman, R. (1995). Relaxation and the relief of cancer pain. *Nursing Clinics of North America, 30*(4), 697–709.

Sloman, R. (2002). Relaxation and imagery for anxiety and depression control in community patients with advanced cancer. *Cancer Nursing, 25*(6), 432–435.

Spiegel, D., Bloom, J. R., Kraemer, H. C., & Gottheil, E. (1989). Effect of psychosocial treatment on survival of patients with metastatic breast cancer. *Lancet, 2*(8668), 888–891.

Spira, J. L., & Spiegel, D. (1992). Hypnosis and related techniques in pain management. *Hospice Journal, 8*(1–2), 89–119.

Steggles, S., Damore-Petingola, S., Maxwell, J., & Lightfoot, N. (1997). Hypnosis for children and adolescents with cancer: An annotated bibliography 1985–1995. *Journal of Pediatric Oncology Nursing, 14*(1), 27–32.

Stevens, M. M., Pozza, L. D., Cavelletto, B., Cooper, M. G., & Kilham, H. A. (1994). Pain and symptom control in paediatric palliative care. *Cancer Surveys, 21,* 211–231.

Syrjala, K. L., Cummings, C., & Donaldson, G. W. (1992). Hypnosis or cognitive behavioral training for the reduction of pain and nausea during cancer treatment: A controlled clinical trial. *Pain, 48,* 137–146.

Syrjala, K. L., Donaldson, G. W., Davis, M. W., Kippes, M. E., & Carr, J. E. (1995). Relaxation and imagery and cognitive-behavioral training reduce pain during cancer treatment: A controlled clinical trial. *Pain, 63,* 189–198.

Tellegen, A. (1993). *Multidimensional Personality Questionnaire manual.* Minneapolis: University of Minnesota Press.

Thompson, M. B., & Coppens, N. M. (1994). The effects of guided imagery on anxiety levels and movement of clients undergoing magnetic resonance imaging. *Holistic Nursing Practice, 8*(2), 59–69.

Troesch, L. M., Rodehaver, C. B., Delaney, E. A., & Yanes, B. (1993). The influence of guided imagery on chemotherapy-related nausea and vomiting. *Oncology Nursing Forum, 20*(8), 1179–1185.

Van Kuiken, D. (2004). A meta-analysis of the effect of guided imagery practice on outcomes. *Journal of Holistic Nursing, 22*(2), 164–179.

Walco, G. A., Varni, J. W., & Ilowite, N. T. (1992). Cognitive-behavioral pain management in children with juvenile rheumatoid arthritis. *Pediatrics, 89*(6), 1075–1079.

Walker, L. G. (1998). Hypnosis and cancer: Host defences, quality of life and survival. *Contemporary Hypnosis, 15*(1), 34–38.

Walker, L. G. (2004). Hypnotherapeutic insights and interventions: A cancer odyssey. *Contemporary Hypnosis, 21*(1), 35–45.

Walker, L. G., Johnson, V. C., & Eremin, O. (1993). Modulation of the immune response to stress by hypnosis and relaxation training in normals: A critical review. *Contemporary Hypnosis, 10*, 19–27.

Walker, L. G., Miller, I., Walker, M. B., Simpson, E., Ogston, K., Segar, A., et al. (1996). Immunological effects of relaxation training and guided imagery in women with locally advanced breast cancer. *Psycho-Oncology, 5*(3), Suppl. 16.

Wallace, K. (1997). Analysis of recent literature concerning relaxation and imagery interventions for cancer pain. *Cancer Nursing, 20*(2), 79–87.

Wild, M. R., & Espie, C. A. (2004). The efficacy of hypnosis in the reduction of procedural pain and distress in pediatric oncology: A systematic review. *Developmental and Behavioral Pediatrics, 25*(3), 207–213.

Yoo, S. S., Lee, C. U., & Choi, B. G. (2001). Human brain mapping of auditory imagery: Event-related functional MRI study. *Neuroreport, 12*(14), 3045–3049.

Youssef, N. N., Rosh, J. R., Loughran, M., Schuckalo, S. G., Cotter, A. N., Verga, B. G., et al. (2004). Treatment of functional abdominal pain in childhood with cognitive behavioral strategies. *Journal of Pediatric and Gastroenterological Nutrition, 39*(2), 192–196.

Zachariae, R., & Bjerring, P. (1994). Laser-induced pain-related brain potentials and sensory pain ratings in high and low hypnotizable subjects during hypnotic suggestions of relaxation, dissociated imagery, focused analgesia, and placebo. *The International Journal of Clinical and Experimental Hypnosis, XLII* (1), 56–80.

Zachariae, R., Hansen, J. B., Andersen, M., Jinquan, T., Petersen, K. S., Simonsen, C., et al. (1994). Changes in cellular immune function after immune specific guided imagery and relaxation in high and low hypnotizable healthy subjects. *Psychotherapy and Psychosomatics, 61*(1–2), 74–92.

Zachariae, R., Oster, H., Bjerring, P., & Kragballe, K. (1996). Effects of psychologic intervention on psoriasis: A preliminary report. *Journal of the American Academy of Dermatology, 34*(6), 1008–1015.

CHAPTER 7

Music Intervention

Linda Chlan

Music has been used throughout history as a treatment modality. From the time of the ancient Egyptians, the power of music to affect health has been noted. Nursing's pioneering leader Florence Nightingale recognized the healing power of music (1860). Today nurses can use music in a variety of settings to benefit patients and clients.

DEFINITIONS

The *American Heritage Dictionary® of the English Language* defines music as "the art of arranging sounds in time so as to provide a continuous, unified and evocative composition, as through melody, harmony, rhythm, and timbre" (2000). Alvin (1975) delineated five main elements of music. The character of a piece of music and its effects depend on the qualities of these elements and their relationships to one another:

- Frequency or pitch is produced by the number of vibrations of a sound—the highness or lowness of a musical tone noted by the letters A, B, C, D, E, F, G. Rapid vibrations tend to act as a stimulant, whereas slow vibrations bring about relaxation.

- Intensity creates the volume of the sound, related to the amplitude of the vibrations. A person's like or dislike of certain music partially depends on intensity, which can be used to produce intimacy (soft music) or power (loud music).

- Tone color or timbre is a nonrhythmical, subjective property that results from harmony. Psychological significance results from the timbre of music because of associations with past events or feelings.

- Interval is the distance between two notes related to pitch, which creates melody and harmony. Melody results from how musical pitches are sequenced and the interval between them. Harmony results from the way pitches are sounded together, described by the listener as consonant (conveying the feeling of restfulness) or dissonant (conveying the feeling of tension). Cultural norms determine what a listener deems enjoyable and pleasant.

- Duration creates rhythm and tempo. Duration refers to the length of sounds, and rhythm is a time pattern fitted into a certain speed. Rhythm is what influences one to move with music in a certain manner and can convey peace and security, whereas repetitive rhythms can elicit feelings of depression. Continuous sounds that are repeated at a slow pace and become gradually slower produce decreased levels of responsiveness. Strong rhythms can awaken feelings of power and control.

From a nursing perspective, music intervention is the use of music for therapeutic purposes to promote patient/client health and well-being. Music therapists are employed in many health care facilities, and countless situations exist in which nurses can implement music intervention in a patient's plan of care. In order not to confuse the practice of music therapy with the use of music from a nursing perspective, the term *music intervention* will be used in this chapter.

SCIENTIFIC BASIS

Music is complex and affects the physiological, psychological, and spiritual aspects of human beings. Individual responses to music can be influenced by personal preferences, the environment, education, and cultural factors.

Entrainment, a physics principle, is a process whereby two objects vibrating at similar frequencies will tend to cause mutual sympathetic resonance, resulting in their vibrating at the same frequency (Maranto, 1993). Music and physiological processes (heartbeat, blood pressure, body temperature, adrenal hormones) are composed on vibrations that occur in a regular, periodic manner and consist of oscillations (Saperston, 1995). Rhythm and tempo of music can be used to synchronize or entrain body rhythms (e.g., heart rate, respiratory pattern) with resultant changes in physiological states. Certain properties of music (less than 80 beats per minute with fluid, regular rhythm) can be used to promote relaxation by causing body rhythms to slow down or "entrain" with the slower beat and regular, repetitive rhythm of selected music (Robb, Nichols, Rutan, Bishop, & Parker, 1995).

Likewise, music can decrease anxiety by occupying attention channels in the brain with meaningful, distractive auditory stimuli (Bauldoff, Hoffman, Zullo, & Sciurba, 2002). Music intervention provides a patient/client with a familiar, comforting stimulus that can evoke pleasurable sensations while refocusing the individual's attention onto the music instead of on stressful thoughts or other environmental stimuli.

INTERVENTION

Determination of a person's music preferences through assessment is essential; among the tools developed for use by nurses is one by Chlan and Tracy (1999). This assessment instrument elicits information on how frequently music is listened to, the type of preferred musical selections, and the reason a person listens to music. For some people the purpose of listening to music may be to relax whereas others may prefer music that stimulates and invigorates. After assessment data have been gathered, appropriate techniques with specific music can then be implemented.

Techniques

The use of music can take many forms, from listening to selected tapes or compact discs (CDs) to singing or drumming. A number of factors should be kept in mind when considering the specific technique: the type of music and personal preferences, active versus passive involvement, on an individual basis or use in a group, length of time to use music, and desired outcomes. Two of the more commonly used music intervention techniques will be discussed here: individual listening and group work.

Individual Music Listening

Providing the means for patients to listen to music is the intervention technique most frequently implemented by nurses. Cassette tapes and

CDs make it easy to provide music intervention for patients/clients in all types of settings. Tape or CD players are relatively inexpensive; they are small and can be used even in the most crowded confines such as critical care units. Auto-reverse capabilities of tape players allow patients to listen to music for any length of time without having to turn the tape over. CD players have superior sound clarity and track-seeking that allows immediate selection of a desired piece. Comfortable headphones allow patients private listening that does not disturb others. Equipment selected for music intervention should be easy for patients to use with minimal effort.

With only a very modest outlay of money, a nursing unit can establish a tape or CD library containing a wide variety of selections to meet various music preferences. The Public Radio Music Source (www.prms.org) offers a great variety of music for purchase. It is also easy to individualize tapes or CDs to meet the preferences of each patient. (Attention to copyright laws is necessary when reproducing tapes or downloading music from Internet sites.)

Although various music genres are available on the radio, commercial messages and talking are deterrents to using them for music intervention. Likewise, one cannot control the quality of the radio signal reception or the specific music selections.

Group Music Making

Music can be used for patient groups as a powerful integrating force. Music creates interrelationships among the members and between the listener and the music. One method of group music making is drumming, a form of rhythmic auditory stimulation. Drumming circles induce relaxation by entraining theta and alpha brain waves, leading to altered states of consciousness by activation of the limbic brain region with the lower brain (Winkelman, 2003). Drumming circles have been used effectively to reduce burnout and improve mood in nursing students (Bittman et al., 2004) and to enhance recovery from a variety of chemical addictions (Winkelman, 2003).

Nurses should consult with experts in drumming prior to implementing this type of group music making. The American Music Therapy Association web site (www.musictherapy.org) can provide assistance in locating a music therapist. Further, diversity in the preferences, interests, and abilities of individuals in a group or securing an appropriate site for a group session may necessitate implementing music on an individual basis; groups also require more planning than do individual sessions.

Types of Music for Intervention

Careful attention to the selection of the music contributes to its therapeutic effect. For example, music to induce relaxation has a regular rhythm, less than 80 beats per minute, no extreme pitch or dynamics, and a melodic sound that is smooth and flowing (Robb et al., 1995). Past experiences can influence one's response to music as well. Specific selections may be associated with happy or sad occasions and events, and cultural influences will also impact one's musical preferences. Across five pain intervention studies Caucasian persons preferred orchestra music, African American persons jazz, and Taiwanese persons harp music (Good et al., 2000). However, other investigators have found that minority elders tend to prefer music that is familiar to their own cultural background, rather than Western music (Lai, 2004). These disparate findings highlight the need for careful music preference assessment prior to intervention.

Older persons may prefer patriotic and popular songs from an earlier era or hymns with slower tempos played with familiar instruments (Moore, Staum, & Brotons, 1992). Religious music may be welcomed by persons unable to attend religious services.

Classical music is thought to evoke greater enjoyment and interest with repeated listening, whereas popular music declines in effectiveness with repetition (Bonny, 1986). Bonny believes that patients in a weakened state respond less to popular music and are more receptive to the stimulus of classical music that has endured over time. In any event, providing a choice and considering a person's musical preferences are imperative.

New Age, synthesized, or nontraditional music has become very popular. This type of music differs from traditional music, which is characterized by tension and release (Guzzetta, 1995). However, some experts think that this type of synthesized music is not appropriate for relaxation due to the novelty of the stimulus and the absence of the usual forms found in more traditional and American music (Bonny, 1986; Hanser, 1988). Music perceived as unfamiliar will cause an orienting response that may undermine goals for intervention (Maranto, 1993).

Guidelines

Music intervention for the purpose of relaxation utilizes music as a pleasant stimulus to block out sensations of anxiety, fear, and tension and to divert attention from unpleasant thoughts (Thaut, 1990). A minimum of 20 minutes is necessary to induce relaxation along with some form of relaxation exercise, such as deep breathing, prior to initiating music intervention (Guzzetta, 1995).

Although the definition of relaxing music may vary by individual, factors affecting response include musical preferences, familiar selections, and cultural background. Relaxing music should have a tempo at or below a resting heart rate (less than 80 beats); predictable dynamics; fluid melodic movement; pleasing harmonies; regular rhythm without sudden changes; and tonal qualities that include strings, flute, piano, or specially synthesized music (Robb et al., 1995). One of the most widely used classical music selections for relaxation is Pachelbel's Canon in D Major, which is frequently included in commercially available relaxation tapes. Table 7.1 outlines the basic steps for implementing music intervention for promoting relaxation.

Measurement of Outcomes

The outcome indices for evaluating the effectiveness of music vary, depending on the purpose for which music is implemented. Outcomes may be physiological or psychological alterations and include a decrease in anxiety or stress arousal, promotion of relaxation, increase in social

TABLE 7.1   Guidelines for Music Intervention for Relaxation

1. Ascertain that patient has adequate hearing.
2. Ascertain patient's like/dislike for music.
3. Assess music preferences and previous experience with music for relaxation.
4. Provide a choice of relaxing selections; assist with tape/CD selections as needed.
5. Determine agreed-upon goals for music intervention with patient.
6. Complete all nursing cares prior to intervention; allow for a minimum of 20 minutes of uninterrupted listening time.
7. Gather equipment (CD or cassette tape-player, cassettes/CDs, headphones, batteries) and ensure all are in good working order.
8. Assist patient to a comfortable position as needed; ensure call-light is within easy reach and assist patient with equipment as needed.
9. Enhance environment as needed (draw blinds, close door, turn off lights, etc.).
10. Post a Do Not Disturb sign to minimize unnecessary interruptions.
11. Encourage and provide patient with opportunities to "practice" relaxation with music.
12. Document patient responses to music intervention.
13. Revise intervention plan and goal(s) as needed.

interaction, reduction in the need for medications, and increase in overall well-being. The nurse should carefully consider the goals of intervention and select outcome measurements accordingly.

Precautions

Adaptation occurs if the auditory system is continually exposed to the same type of stimulus (Farber, 1982). Neural adaptation can occur after 3 minutes of continuous exposure, with the result that music is no longer the stimulant and may not have the intended calming influence. Use of stimulation such as music in phase I following head injury may increase intracranial pressure. Music of a stimulating quality should be delayed until the autonomic nervous system has stabilized. Quiet music may be used to induce relaxation and block irritating sounds from the environment; however, the patient's individual response to music should be monitored.

Careful control of volume is essential. Permanent ear damage results from exposure to high frequencies and volumes. Decibels higher than 90 dBSL cause discomfort (Idzoriek, 1982), and fatigue occurs more frequently when stimulation is at higher frequencies (Farber, 1982).

Initiating music intervention without first assessing a person's likes and dislikes may produce deleterious effects. Because of music's effect on the limbic system, it can bring about intense emotional responses. Use of portable players with headphones may be inappropriate for patients in psychiatric settings who may use the equipment cords for self-harm.

USES

Music has been tested as a therapeutic intervention with many different patient populations, with a majority of the nursing literature focusing on individualized music listening. Table 7.2 shows those patient populations and the numerous purposes for which music has been implemented. Two frequent uses will be highlighted here.

Decreasing Anxiety and Stress

One of the strongest effects of music is anxiety reduction (Standley, 1986). Music can enhance the immediate environment, provide a diversion, and lessen the impact of potentially disturbing sounds for pediatric patients (Barrera, Rykov, & Doyle, 2002; Klein & Winkelstein, 1996), for patients

TABLE 7.2   Uses of Music Intervention

Orientation/minimizing disruptive behaviors

Elders (Clark, Lipe, & Bilbrey, 1998; Gerdner, 1997; Janelli, Kanski, Jones, & Kennedy, 1995; Sambandham & Schirm, 1995)

Restrained patients (Janelli & Kanski, 1998)

Decreasing anxiety

Pediatrics (Barrera et al., 2002; Klein & Winkelstein, 1996)

Surgical (Augustin & Hains, 1996; Yung, Chui-Kam, French, & Chan, 2002)

Cardiac patients (Hamel, 2001; White, 1992, 1999)

Flexible sigmoidoscopy (Chlan, Evans, Greenleaf, & Walker, 2000)

Ventilator-dependent ICU patients (Chlan, 1998; Wong, Lopez-Nahas, & Molassiotis, 2001)

Pain management

Acute pain (Good, 1995; Good et al., 1999; Good et al., 2001; Laurion & Fetzer, 2003; Shertzer & Keck, 2001)

Chronic pain (Schorr, 1993)

Invasive procedures/pediatrics (Berlin, 1998)

Stress reduction and relaxation

Elderly patients undergoing ophthalmic surgery (Golden & Izzo, 2001)

NICU patients (Burke, Walsh, Oehler, & Gingras, 1995; Kemper, Martin, Block, Shoaf, & Woods, 2004)

Nursing students (Bittman et al., 2004)

Stimulation

Depression in older adults (Hanser & Thompson, 1994)

Sleep disturbances in older adults (Mornhinweg & Voignier, 1995)

Increasing children's sociability (Aasgaard, 2001)

Head injury (Formisano et al., 2001; Jones, Hux, Morton-Anderson, & Knepper, 1994)

Distraction

Adjunct to spinal or general anesthesia (Lepage, Drolet, Girard, Grenier, & DeGagne, 2001; Nilsson, Rawal, Unesthahl, Zetterberg, & Unosson, 2001)

Burn care (Fratianne et al., 2001; Prensner, Yowler, Smith, Steele, & Fratianne, 2001)

Cardiac patients on bedrest (Cadigan et al., 2001)

High-dose chemotherapy (Ezzone, Baker, Rosselet, & Terepka, 1998)

Cardiac laboratory environmental enhancement (Thorgaard, Henriksen, Pedersbaek, & Thomsen, 2003)

---

experiencing a variety of surgical procedures (Augustin & Hains, 1996; Yung et al., 2002), coronary care unit patients (Hamel, 2001; White, 1992, 1999), and ventilator-dependent ICU patients (Chlan, 1998; Wong et al., 2001). Music can be an effective intervention for enhancing the newborn ICU (NICU) environment and reducing stress (Kemper et al., 2004) with such improvements as enhanced oxygenation during suctioning (Chou, Wang, Chen, & Pai, 2003) and increased feeding rates (Standley, 2003).

Distraction

Music is an effective intervention for distraction, particularly for procedures that induce untoward symptoms and distress. It can reduce noise annoyance in the ICU for cardiac surgery patients (Byers & Smyth, 1997). It has been found to be an effective diversional adjunct in the care of persons with burns (Fratianne et al., 2001; Prensner et al., 2001), management of nausea and vomiting induced by chemotherapy (Ezzone et al., 1998), and nausea and pain intensity after bone marrow transplantation (Sahler, Hunter, & Liesveld, 2003), for distress in children undergoing immunizations (Megel, Houser, & Gleaves, 1998), or can reduce the amount of sedation required for adults during colonoscopy (Lee et al., 2002; Smolen, Topp, & Singer, 2002).

FUTURE RESEARCH

Although the evidence base is increasing, the following are areas in which research is needed to further build the science of music intervention:

1. Recent meta-analyses have been published on the strong, consistent effects of music intervention for premature infants (Standley, 2002) and for children and adolescents with autism (Whipple, 2004). A large body of work is available on music intervention for symptom management, such as anxiety, nausea, and vomiting. An up-to-date meta-analysis articulating effect sizes for these symptoms that nurses typically manage would make a significant contribution to the scientific base of music intervention.

2. Cost and cost savings are significant issues in health care today. Little is known about the potential cost savings that could be realized with music intervention. Research is needed to determine

if music is a cost-effective or cost-neutral intervention and, if cost effective, in which patient-care settings.

3. Much of the nursing research focuses on immediate or short-term effects of music intervention. It is not known if music can be effective for managing symptoms and distress in persons with chronic conditions or improving their quality of life.

4. There is a paucity of investigations as to the appropriate or optimal timing for delivery of music intervention to enhance effectiveness and for which specific patient populations or symptoms.

5. Many published studies have used convenience samples limited to single centers. Randomized, multisite clinical trials are needed to determine if music indeed is effective in natural settings that are not as highly controlled by the investigator and under what conditions.

Although intervention research itself is labor intensive, there is a need for additional research on music intervention. The knowledge base of music intervention to promote patient/client health and well-being can be expanded through high-quality research and by dissemination of those findings in a timely manner.

REFERENCES

Aasgaard, T. (2001). An ecology of love: Aspects of music therapy in the pediatric oncology environment. *Journal of Palliative Care, 17*(3), 177–181.

Alvin, J. (1975). *Music therapy.* New York: Basic Books.

American Heritage® Dictionary of the English Language (4th ed.). (2000). Boston, MA: Houghton Mifflin.

American Music Therapy Association. Retrieved from www.musictherapy.org

Augustin, P., & Hains, A. (1996). Effect of music on ambulatory surgery patients' preoperative anxiety. *AORN Journal, 63*(4), 750–758.

Barrera, M., Rykov, M., & Doyle, S. (2002). The effects of interactive music therapy on hospitalized children with cancer: A pilot study. *Psycho-Oncology, 11*(5), 379–388.

Bauldoff, G., Hoffman, L., Zullo, T., & Sciurba, I. (2002). Exercise maintenance following pulmonary rehabilitation: Effect of distractive stimuli. *Chest, 122*(3), 948–954.

Berlin, B. (1998). Music therapy with children during invasive procedures: Our emergency department's experience. *Journal of Emergency Nursing, 24*(6), 607–608.

Bittman, B., Snyder, C., Liebfreid, F., Stevens, C., Westengard, J., & Umbach, P. (2004, July 9). Recreational music-making: An integrative group intervention for reducing burnout and improving mood states in first-year associate degree nursing students: Insights and economic impact. *International Journal of Nursing Education Scholarship, 1*. Retrieved from www.bepress.com/ijnes/vol1/iss1.

Bonny, H. (1986). Music and healing. *Music Therapy, 6*(1), 3–12.

Burke, M., Walsh, J., Oehler, J., & Gingras, J. (1995). Music therapy following suctioning. *Neonatal Network, 14*(7), 41–49.

Byers, J., & Smyth, K. (1997). Effect of music intervention on noise annoyance, heart rate, and blood pressure in cardiac surgery patients. *American Journal of Critical Care, 6*(3), 183–191.

Cadigan, M., Caruso, N., Haldeman, S., McNamara, M., Noyes, D., Spadafora, M., et al. (2001). The effects of music on cardiac patients on bedrest. *Progress in Cardiovascular Nursing, 16*(1), 5–13.

Chlan, L. (1998). Effectiveness of a music therapy intervention on relaxation and anxiety for patients receiving ventilatory assistance. *Heart & Lung, 27*(3), 169–176.

Chlan, L., Evans, D., Greenleaf, M., & Walker, J. (2000). Effects of a single music therapy intervention on anxiety, discomfort, satisfaction, and compliance with screening guidelines in outpatients undergoing screening flexible sigmoidoscopy. *Gastroenterology Nursing, 23*(4), 148–156.

Chlan, L., & Tracy, M. (1999). Music therapy in critical care: Indications and guidelines for intervention. *Critical Care Nurse, 19*(3), 35–41.

Chou, L., Wang, R., Chen, S., & Pai, L. (2003). Effects of music therapy on oxygen saturation in premature infants receiving endotracheal suctioning. *Journal of Nursing Research, 11*(3), 209–215.

Clark, M., Lipe, A., & Bilbrey, M. (1998). Use of music to decrease aggressive behavior in people with dementia. *Journal of Gerontological Nursing, 24*(7), 10–17.

Ezzone, S., Baker, C., Rosselet, R., & Terepka, E. (1998). Music as an adjunct to antiemetic therapy. *Oncology Nursing Forum, 25*(9), 1551–1556.

Farber, S. (1982). *Neurorehabilitation.* Philadelphia: Saunders.

Formisano, R., Vinicola, V., Penta, F., Matteis, M., Brunelli, S., & Weckel, J. (2001). Active music therapy in the rehabilitation of severe brain injured patients during coma recovery. *Annali Dell Insituto Superiore di Sanita, 37*(4), 627–630.

Fratianne, R., Prensner, J., Huston, M., Super, D., Yowler, C., & Standley, J. (2001). The effect of music-based imagery and musical alternate engagement on the burn debridement process. *Journal of Burn Care & Rehabilitation, 22*(1), 47–53.

Gerdner, L. (1997). An individualized music intervention for agitation. *Journal of the American Psychiatric Nurses Association, 3*(6), 177–184.

Golden, A., & Izzo, J. (2001). Normalization of hypertensive responses during ambulatory surgical stress by perioperative music. *Psychosomatic Medicine, 63*(3), 487–492.

Good, M. (1995). A comparison of the effects of jaw relaxation and music on postoperative pain. *Nursing Research, 44*(1), 52–57.

Good, M., Picot, B., Salem, S., Chin, C., Picot, S., & Lane, D. (2000). Cultural differences in music chosen for pain relief. *Journal of Holistic Nursing, 18*(3), 245–260.

Good, M., Stanton-Hicks, M., Grass, J., Anderson, G., Choi, C., Schoolmeesters, L., et al. (1999). Relief of postoperative pain with jaw relaxation, music and their combination. *Pain, 81*(1, 2), 163–172.

Good, M., Stanton-Hicks, M., Grass, J., Anderson, G., Lai, H., Roykulcahroen, V., et al. (2001). Relaxation and music to reduce postsurgical pain. *Journal of Advanced Nursing, 33*(2), 208–215.

Guzzetta, C. (1995). Music therapy: Hearing the melody of the soul. In B. Dossey, L. Keegan, C. Guzzetta, & L. Kolkmeier (Eds.), *Holistic nursing* (pp. 670–698). Gaithersburg, MD: Aspen.

Hamel, W. (2001). The effects of music intervention on anxiety in the patient waiting for cardiac catheterization. *Intensive and Critical Care Nursing, 17*(2), 279–285.

Hanser, S. (1988). Controversy in music listening/stress reduction research. *The Arts in Psychotherapy, 15*(2), 211–217.

Hanser, S., & Thompson, L. (1994). Effects of a music therapy strategy on depressed older adults. *Journal of Gerontology, 49*(6), 265–269.

Idzoriek, P. (1982). Comparison of auditory and strong tactile stimuli on responsiveness. Unpublished Plan B Project. University of Minnesota, School of Nursing, Minneapolis.

Janelli, L., & Kanski, G. (1998). Music for untying restrained patients. *Journal of the New York State Nurses Association, 29*(1), 13–15.

Janelli, L., Kanski, G., Jones, H., & Kennedy, M. (1995). Exploring music intervention with restrained patients. *Nursing Forum, 30*(4), 12–18.

Jones, R., Hux, C., Morton-Anderson, A., & Knepper, L. (1994). Auditory stimulation effect on a comatose survivor of traumatic brain injury. *Archives of Physical Medicine and Rehabilitation, 75*(1), 164–171.

Kemper, K., Martin, K., Block, S., Shoaf, R., & Woods, C. (2004). Attitudes and expectations about music therapy for premature infants among staff in the neonatal intensive care unit. *Alternative Therapies in Health & Medicine, 10*(2), 50–54.

Klein, S., & Winkelstein, M. (1996). Enhancing pediatric health care with music. *Pediatric Health Care, 10*(1), 74–81.

Lai, H. L. (2004). Music preference and relaxation in Taiwanese elderly people. *Geriatric Nursing, 25*(5), 286–291.

Laurion, S., & Fetzer, S. J. (2003). The effect of two nursing interventions on the postoperative outcomes of gynecologic laparoscopic patients. *Journal of Perianesthesia Nursing, 18*(4), 254–261.

Lee, D., Chan, K., Poon, C., Ko, C., Cha, K., Sin, K., et al. (2002). Relaxation music decreases the dose of patient-controlled sedation during colonoscopy: A prospective randomized controlled trial. *Gastrointestinal Endoscopy, 55*(1), 33–36.

Lepage, C., Drolet, P., Girard, M., Grenier, Y., & DeGagne, R. (2001). Music decreases sedative requirements during spinal anesthesia. *Anesthesia and Analgesia, 93*, 912–916.

Maranto, C. (1993). Applications of music in medicine. In M. Heal & T. Wigram (Eds.), *Music therapy in health and education* (pp. 153–174). London: Jessica Kingsley.

Megel, M., Houser, C., & Gleaves, L. (1998). Children's responses to immunization: Lullabies as a distraction. *Issues in Comprehensive Pediatric Nursing, 21*(3), 129–145.

Moore, R., Staum, M., & Brotons, M. (1992). Music preferences of the elderly: Repertoire, vocal ranges, tempos, and accompaniments for singing. *Journal of Music Therapy, 29*(4), 236–252.

Mornhinweg, G., & Voignier, R. (1995). Music for sleep disturbance in the elderly. *Journal of Holistic Nursing, 13*(3), 248–254.

Nightingale, F. (1860/1969). *Notes on nursing*. New York: Dover.

Nilsson, U., Rawal, N., Unesthahl, L., Zetterberg, C., & Unosson, M. (2001). Improved recovery after music and therapeutic suggestions during general anesthesia: A double-blind randomized controlled trial. *Acta Anesthesiologica Scandinavica, 45*, 812–817.

Prensner, J., Yowler, C., Smith, L., Steele, A., & Fratianne, R. (2001). Music therapy for assistance with pain and anxiety management in burn treatment. *Journal of Burn Care & Rehabilitation, 22*(1), 83–88.

Public Radio Music Source. Retrieved from www.prms.org

Robb, S., Nichols, R., Rutan, R., Bishop, B., & Parker, J. (1995). The effects of music-assisted relaxation on preoperative anxiety. *Journal of Music Therapy, 32*(1), 3–12.

Sahler, O., Hunter, B., & Liesveld, J. (2003). The effect of using music therapy with relaxation imagery in the management of patients undergoing bone marrow transplantation: A pilot feasibility study. *Alternative Therapies in Health & Medicine, 9*(6), 70–74.

Sambandham, M., & Schirm, V. (1995). Music as a nursing intervention for residents with Alzheimer's disease in long-term care. *Geriatric Nursing, 16*(2), 79–83.

Saperston, B. (1995). The effects of consistent tempi and physiologically interactive tempi on heart rate and EMG responses. In T. Wigram, B. Saperston, & M. West (Eds.), *The art and science of music therapy: A handbook* (pp. 58–79). Newark, NJ: Harwood Academic Publishers.

Schorr, J. (1993). Music and pattern change in chronic pain. *Advances in Nursing Science, 15*(4), 27–36.

Shertzer, K., & Keck, J. (2001). Music and the PACU environment. *Journal of PeriAnesthesia Nursing, 16*(2), 90–102.

Smolen, D., Topp, R., & Singer, L. (2002). The effect of self-selected music during colonoscopy on anxiety, heart rate and blood pressure. *Applied Nursing Research, 16*(2), 126–130.

Standley, J. (1986). Music research in medical/dental treatment: Meta-analysis and clinical applications. *Journal of Music Therapy, 23*(2), 56–122.

Standley, J. (2002). A meta-analysis of music therapy for premature infants. *Journal of Pediatric Nursing, 17*(2), 107–113.

Standley, J. (2003). The effect of music-reinforced sucking on feeding rate of premature infants. *Journal of Pediatric Nursing, 18*(3), 169–173.

Thaut, M. (1990). Physiological and motor responses to music stimuli. In R. Unkefer (Ed.), *Music therapy in the treatment of adults with mental disorders: Theoretical bases and clinical interventions* (pp. 33–49). New York: Schirmer Books.

Thorgaard, B., Henriksen, B., Pedersbaek, G., & Thomsen, I. (2003). Specially selected music in the cardiac laboratory—an important tool for improvement of the well-being of patients. *European Journal of Cardiovascular Nursing, 3*(1), 21–26.

Whipple, J. (2004). Music in intervention for children and adolescents with autism: A meta-analysis. *Journal of Music Therapy, 41*(2), 90–106.

White, J. (1992). Music therapy: An intervention to reduce anxiety in the myocardial infarction patient. *Clinical Nurse Specialist, 6*(2), 58–63.

White, J. (1999). Effects of relaxing music on cardiac autonomic balance and anxiety after acute myocardial infarction. *American Journal of Critical Care, 8*(4), 220–230.

Winkelman, M. (2003). Complementary therapy for addiction: "Drumming out Drugs." *American Journal of Public Health, 93*(4), 647–651.

Wong, H., Lopez-Nahas, V., & Molassiotis, A. (2001). Effects of music therapy on anxiety in ventilator-dependent patients. *Heart & Lung, 30*(5), 376–387.

Woolf, H. (Ed.). (1979). *Merriam-Webster's collegiate dictionary* (9th ed.). Springfield, MA: Merriam-Webster.

Yung, P., Chui-Kam, S., French, P., & Chan, T. (2002). A controlled trial of music and pre-operative anxiety in Chinese men undergoing transurethral resection of the prostate. *Journal of Advanced Nursing, 39*(4), 352–359.

CHAPTER 8

Humor

Kevin Smith

A merry heart doeth good like a medicine, but a broken spirit
drieth the bones.
—Proverbs 17:22

Throughout history, human beings have accorded a beneficial effect to
joy and mirth. Greek philosophers including Plato and Aristotle wrote
treatises on humor (McGhee, 1979). The German philosopher Immanuel
Kant, in 1790, set forth similar physical effects of humor and characterized it as a talent that enabled one to look at things from a different
perspective (Haig, 1988). In medieval physiology, humor referred to the
four principal fluids of the body: blood, phlegm, choler (yellow bile),
and melancholy (black bile). A proper balance of the four was called
good humor, and a preponderance of any one constituted ill humor
(Robinson, 1991).

That humor and laughter can improve our ability to cope with
difficulties and to stay healthy is a popular notion. Interest in this area
has increased since Norman Cousins's account of the role of laughter in
his recovery from a painful collagen disorder (1979). The belief that
humor and laughter positively influence health, and the scientific evidence
will be reviewed to provide a basis for the use of humor by nurses and
others providing health care.

Nursing journal articles continue to address many facets of humor, such as laughter and stress management (Paquet, 1993; Smith, 2003; Woodhouse, 1993), humor as a nursing intervention (Hunt, 1993; Mornhinweg & Voignier, 1995), humor and the older adult (Herth, 1993), humor and healing (Macaluso, 1993), and the positive physiologic effects of humor (Lambert & Lambert, 1995). Humor organizations and publications are increasing, humor workshops are being offered to nurses and other health care providers, and many continuing education offerings are incorporating humorous presentations or activities.

Humor can be used as a specific therapy or with other therapies as a parallel intervention. The goals in using humor as an intervention are to enhance the well-being of the client, to enhance the therapeutic relationship between the nurse and the client, and to bring hope and joy to the situation. Humor creates an outlet for stress for both client and nurse. It can be used to foster trust and a comfortable environment for the client. In addition to incorporating humor into the health care setting with patients, the use of humor in daily and work life is a significant self-care practice for health care professionals. Virtually anyone can develop the requisite skills needed to use humor as an intervention.

DEFINITIONS

> Humor is the good-natured side of truth.
> —Mark Twain

The Association for Applied and Therapeutic Humor (2005) defines therapeutic humor as follows:

> Any intervention that promotes health and wellness by stimulating a playful discovery, expression, or appreciation of the absurdity or incongruity of life's situations. This intervention may enhance work performance, support learning, improve health, or be used as a complementary treatment of illness to facilitate healing or coping, whether physical, emotional, cognitive, social, or spiritual. (www.aath.org)

Nurse and humor expert Vera Robinson (1978) described the phenomenon of humor as "any communication which is perceived by any of the interacting parties as humorous and leads to laughing, smiling or a feeling of amusement" (p. 193). The dictionary defines it as "the quality of being laughable or comical," and "the ability to perceive, enjoy, or express what is comical or funny." Humor can be the process of either producing or perceiving the comical. What is personally defined or perceived as funny and its physical manifestations vary among individuals. However, there are predictable stimuli for laughter and usual responses.

Why Do We Laugh?

There are many different reasons that we laugh. Sometimes the response is simply for the fun of it; sometimes it is for more important reasons. Here we will discuss four basic theories for the laughter response: surprise, superiority, incongruity, and release.

1. *Surprise:* Good humor or a good joke may catch one off guard. The surprise in itself causes a person to laugh. Another type of surprise humor is shock humor. This could be a startling or loud punch line or something taboo or vulgar. Shock humor is not recommended in clinical or therapeutic settings.

2. *Superiority:* The theory of superiority laughter (Robinson, 1991) involves situations in which laughter occurs when one feels superior to an individual or a group. One's laughter is in response to the inferiority, stupidity, or misfortunes of others. In its most simple form this is slapstick humor; a more sophisticated form is political satire. It has been suggested that the essential effect of humor is derived from a sense of mastery or ego strength (Lefcourt & Martin, 1986).

3. *Incongruity:* Schaefner (1981) concisely describes this theory as laughter occurring because of "a perception of an incongruity in a ludicrous context." For example, a man walks into a psychiatrist's office with a duck on his head. The duck says, "Doc, you got to help me get this guy off my tail." Two ideas are juxtaposed in an impossible or absurd situation. The incongruity theory advanced by Kant and other philosophers like Schopenhauer and Spencer emphasized the importance of a sudden surprise, shock, conflict of ideas, or incongruity as a trigger for laughter (Liechty, 1987). Asimov (1992) argues that incongruities put the listener, for a brief moment, in a fantasy world. This suspension of reality readies the listener for the crowning bit of fantasy or the punch line that results in laughter.

4. *Release:* The basic premise of the release theory, as a laughter stimulus, is that humor and laughter help to release tensions and anxieties. Freud (1905) viewed humor as a coping tool that

allows individuals to reduce tension by expressing hostile or obscene impulses in a socially acceptable manner. Morreal (1983) called this the relief theory and notes that humor that produces laughter is a method for venting nervous energy. This release type of laughter is often enhanced in group situations where many share the same anxiety.

Humor Styles

Most of the humor employed on a daily basis with staff and patients is of the spontaneous type: situational humor that arises out of the normal absurdities of the day's activities. This type of humor is also a very effective communication tool when used to break the ice with patients or co-workers. An attempt is made to lighten the situation; this is a sign of caring and allows for a free exchange of thoughts and emotions. Formal humor, or premeditated acts of humor (Smith, 1995), include the sharing of jokes, cartoons, humorous articles or stories; novelty toys or gag gifts; and practical jokes. Formal humor, like most kinds of humor, is usually effective only when it is relevant to the situation in which it is presented. Other more specific humor styles include self-deprecating humor, puns and plays on words, ethnic humor, sarcastic humor, and gallows humor.

Self-deprecating humor may be the most effective and powerful humor tool that nurses can develop and use. To show that one is able to laugh at oneself demonstrates that one is a normal human being with weaknesses who at the same time displays confidence, self-awareness, and self-esteem. Ronald Reagan used this type of humor effectively when critics made derogatory comments about his age during his second run for the presidency. He quipped, "Andrew Jackson was seventy-five years old and still vigorous when he left the White House. I know because he told me" (Klein, 1989, p. 10). Paulsen (1989) stated that gently poking fun at oneself acts as a social lubricant. It shows that a person is at ease with the situation. People are often suspicious or afraid of those without a sense of humor.

Puns and plays on words are simple and straightforward humor styles. Some consider puns to be the lowest form of humor, but pun enthusiasts include Asimov and Freud. Puns typically produce groans rather than laughter. For example, "With friends like you, who needs enemas?"

Ethnic humor is often regional. Using one's own ethnicity or profession as the target of the joke is the most acceptable approach. Sarcastic humor is somewhat risky; overheard sarcasm can make a patient or others think they are the target of the sarcastic comments. Freud (1905) developed a theory about why people laugh at tragedy and death, which he called gallows humor. Such grim humor is typically seen when people are faced with considerable stress. He theorized that jokes allow people to express unconscious aggressive or sexual impulses. Obrldik (1942) asserted that the phenomenon of gallows humor has a definite social purpose. It provides a psychological escape and strengthens the morale of the group and in some situations undermines the morale of the oppressors. Gallows humor is frequently used in situations where individuals are under significant stress, such as emergency rooms, intensive care units, operating rooms, and morgues.

SCIENTIFIC BASIS

Many of the positive physiological effects of humor and laughter have been studied. Humor is the stimulus and laughter the response. Laughter creates a cascade of physiological changes in the body. Fry (1971) studied the effects of mirthful laughter on heart rate and on the oxygen saturation level of peripheral blood and respiratory phenomena. He found that both the arousal and cathartic effects are paralleled in the physiological. Laughter involves extensive physical activity. It increases respiratory activity and oxygen exchange, increases muscular activity and heart rate, and stimulates the cardiovascular system, the sympathetic nervous system, and the production of catecholamines. The arousal state is followed by the relaxation state in which respiration rate, heart rate, and muscle tension return to normal. Although the oxygen saturation of peripheral blood is not affected during this relaxation state, blood pressure is reduced and a state exists similar to the impact of hearty exercise. Fry and Savin (1988) investigated the effects of humor on arterial blood pressure using direct arterial cannulization. Findings showed increases in systolic and diastolic blood pressure that were directly related to the intensity and length of laughter. Blood pressure decreased immediately after the laughter to below the pre-laughter baseline.

Many studies have found that humor and laughter increase levels of salivary immunoglobulin A (S-IgA), a vital immune system protein that is the body's first line of defense against respiratory illnesses. In a controlled study, Dillon, Minchoff, and Baker (1985) demonstrated increased levels of S-IgA in college students who viewed a humorous video. Martin and Dobbin (1988) measured subjects' sense of humor, stress levels, and S-IgA levels and demonstrated that subjects with low scores on the humor scales showed a greater negative relationship between stress and S-IgA than did subjects with high humor scores. Stone, Valdimarsdottir, Jandorf, Cox, and Neale (1987) found that the S-IgA response level was lower on days of negative mood and higher on days of positive mood. Lambert and Lambert (1995) produced similar findings with S-IgA levels in healthy fifth-grade students.

Berk, Tan, and Fry (1989) studied the effects of laughter on the neuroendocrine stress hormones and immune parameters (Berk, Tan, Napier, & Eby, 1989). They found a complex autonomic response with each catecholamine, suggesting that laughter may be an antagonist to the classical stress response. They demonstrated that laughter lowered serum cortisol levels, increased the amount of activated T-lymphocytes, and increased the number and activity of natural killer cells. Laughter stimulated the immune system, counteracting the immunosuppressive effects of stress. Berk, Felten, Tan, Bittman, and Westengard (2001) proposed that interventions of mirthful laughter may be capable of modulating neuroendocrine and neuroimmune parameters and may be an adjunct to other therapies.

Friedman and Ulmer (1984) assigned hundreds of heart attack survivors to one of two groups. The control group received standard advice regarding medications, diet, and exercise. The treatment group received additional counseling on relaxation, smiling, laughing at themselves, admitting mistakes, taking time to enjoy life, and renewing their religious faith. Over 3 years, the treatment group experienced half as many repeat heart attacks as the control group.

In the pediatric oncology setting, Dowling, Hockenberry, and Gregory (2003) found a direct relationship between a high sense of humor and psychological adjustment to cancer as well as fewer incidences of infection among children with high coping humor scores. Yet Schofield and colleagues (2004) found no evidence that a high level of optimism prior to treatment improved survival in patients with non-small-cell lung carcinoma.

Psychological Perspectives

Humor has been considered an adaptive coping mechanism. Freud (1905) regarded humor and laughter as two of the few socially acceptable means for releasing pent-up frustrations and anger, a cathartic mechanism for preserving psychic or emotional energy. Humor and laughter alter our perspective in various situations. Laughter can counteract negative emotions; it allows people to transcend predicaments, overcome painful circumstances, and cope with difficulties. By focusing energy elsewhere, humor can diffuse the stress of difficult events (Klein, 1989). The use of humor has been shown to reduce threat-induced anxiety (Yovetich, Dale, & Hudak, 1990).

INTERVENTION

There are many approaches, techniques, and tools that can be used for utilizing humor as an intervention. A first step in deciding how and when to use humor is to complete a humor assessment, first of yourself, then of your patient.

Assessment

A humor interview guide was developed to explore older adults' perceptions of humor (Herth, 1993; see Table 8.1). This assessment could be adapted for use in clinical settings or used in research. The assessment is completed by the provider and then by the client.

When completing an assessment of one's own sense of humor, one should consider what type of humor seems most natural. Consider preferences for spontaneity versus formal humor. Like all skills, you can always work on improving your sense of humor. Strickland (1993) says that the first and biggest barrier to using humor is the fear of appearing foolish or of losing control over one's self-image.

Part of the humor assessment of a patient is determining what type of humor is appropriate to use for the patient and the particular situation. Humor that is divisive in any way should be avoided. Investigate the patient's and family's prior use of humor and whether they currently appreciate and value humor and laughter (Davidhizar & Bowen, 1992).

TABLE 8.1   Humor Assessment Interview Guide

---

1. When you think of humor, what kinds of images or thoughts come to mind?
2. Was humor a part of your life when you were younger?
3. Is humor still a part of your life?
4. How has humor been helpful or not helpful at this time in your life?
5. If humor is helpful, what do you do to maintain humor in your life?
6. Are there certain times when you appreciate humor more than other times?
7. When has humor been a negative experience?
8. What types of activities do you find amusing or enjoyable?

Note: From "Humor and the Older Adult," by K. A. Herth, 1993, *Applied Nursing Research*, 64, pp. 146–153. Copyright 1993, Philadelphia, PA: W. B. Saunders Company. Used with permission.

Spontaneous humorous comments on a neutral topic such as the weather, equipment, or yourself can help you to see if the individual is open to humor, though readiness for humor may not always be apparent.

Techniques

Table 8.2 shows a variety of approaches to intervention. Ackerman, Henry, Graham, and Coffey (1994) developed a model for incorporating humor into the health care setting and described the steps to create a humor program. Humorous materials were made available to patients through a "chuckle wagon" cart that was taken to their rooms. A humor resource center was developed to assist nurses in incorporating humor into their patient care, and a patient satisfaction evaluation tool was developed to assess the patients' response to the humor cart. Table 8.3

TABLE 8.2   Selected Techniques and Activities to Provide and Support Humor Interventions

1. Assemble/collect humor resources (create humor rooms, humor carts, humorous videos).
2. Invite guest performers (comedians, magicians, clowns).
3. Wear a humorous item, silly button, necktie, etc.
4. Display humorous photos of staff.
5. Have a cartoon bulletin board with favorites from staff and patients displayed each week.
6. Play music that encourages playful movement.
7. Support and applaud the efforts of staff and patients to use humor.

TABLE 8.3   Selected Online Humor Resources

1. Association for Applied and Therapeutic Humor: www.aath.org
2. The Joyful Noiseletter: www.joyfulnoiseletter.com
3. The Humor Project: www.humorproject.com
4. International Society for Humor Studies (ISHS): http://www.hnu.edu/ishs/
5. World Laughter Tour: http://worldlaughtertour.com/
6. Hospital Clown Newsletter: http://hospitalclown.com/
7. Comedy Cures Foundation: www.comedycures.org
8. The Humor Collection: http://www.thehumorcollection.org/
9. Dr. Thorson's Humor Scale: http://spiritualityhealth.com/newsh/items/self-test/item_8508.html

provides several humor web sites that contain material for humor interventions.

Measurement of Effectiveness

Although physical laughter is not an essential outcome of humor, physical responses to a humor intervention are obvious indicators of effectiveness. According to Black (1984), the multiple physical manifestations of the laughter response cover a range from smiling to belly laughing. Other positive responses may be the relief of symptoms, facial expression, degree of involvement in activities, and strengthening of the relationship between caregiver and client.

Lefcourt and Martin (1986) developed the Situational Humor Response Questionnaire (SHRQ) for determining an individual's response to particular types of humor. It has been used in numerous studies and has been validated as effectively measuring humor. Diverse elements, such as developmental or cultural factors, may also influence an individual's response to humor. It is important to be alert to the variations and subtleties of a patient's response.

Precautions

There are a variety of factors that practitioners should consider when using humor. The timing of the use of humor in the clinical setting is crucial to its success. Leiber (1986) cautioned that one must assess the patient's receptiveness to humor. Crane (1987) states that there are times when humor is contraindicated. What may be funny to patients when they are feeling well may not seem funny during an illness episode. Humor and laughter have no place at the height of a crisis, although they can be useful to allay tension as the crisis subsides. Inside jokes among health care professionals can seem offensive or callous to outsiders who may overhear them. Laughing at others negates confidence and destroys teamwork, whereas laughing *with* others builds confidence, brings people together, and pokes fun at our common dilemmas (Goodman, 1992). Patients may use inappropriate or sexually aggressive remarks under the pretext of joking, in which case further assessment may be indicated to determine the underlying reason for the aggressive verbal behavior.

USES

Humor may be effectively used in highly stressful situations to overcome tensions and to facilitate patient catharsis or expression of fear and anxiety. Ziv (1984) described the use of humor as a defense mechanism for dealing with anxieties. As a provider of patient care, one must be sensitive to the fact that the patient's use of humor could be an attempt to avoid facing more serious issues or feelings. Humorous distraction may be used to reduce preoperative anxiety (Gaberson, 1991). Humor has also been used as an adjunct for enhancing postoperative recall of the exercise routines that were taught preoperatively (Parfitt, 1990). It may be used effectively for problems associated with communication, anxiety, grieving, powerlessness, or social isolation (Hunt, 1993).

The psychological impact of humor and laughter has been studied as an adjunct in the management of psychiatric patients (Saper, 1988, 1990) and may be an effective intervention as part of psychotherapy (Rosenheim & Golan, 1986). Moody (1978) studied and has incorporated the use of positive emotions and humor in dealing with the fear, anxiety, and pain that go along with cancer and other chronic conditions. In the oncology setting, humor provides benefits related to *psychological* aspects of patients, such as using humor as a defense mechanism; *communication,* by creating a more relaxed mood between patients and providers; and *social situations,* using humor to establish relationships with the many individuals involved in their care (Joshua, Cotroneo, & Clarke, 2005). In a group of men with testicular cancer, humor was found to ease difficult interactions, but health care providers should take cues from their patients to determine whether the use of humor is appropriate (Chapple & Ziebland, 2004). Humor has also been advocated as an intervention for elderly clients (Hulse, 1994).

Berger, Coulehan, and Belling (2004) describe potential risks and benefits of using humor in the clinical encounter. The recipient may find some aspect of the humor inappropriate and the health professional may risk embarrassment, which could harm the therapeutic relationship. The provider can start the encounter with low-risk humor, such as the self-deprecating kind, which can enhance communication without being offensive.

Humor may be used to increase comfort or raise the pain threshold. Cogan, Cogan, Waltz, and McCue (1987) studied the effects of laughter and relaxation on discomfort thresholds. In a group of volunteers, tolerance levels of physical discomfort were measured after members of the group either listened to a laughter-inducing narrative, an uninteresting narrative tape, or had no intervention. Patient discomfort thresholds increased (patients could handle more pain) in the laughter-inducing scenario.

The use of humor is particularly appropriate in situations involving short-term pain such as some nursing treatments (e.g., injections) and recovery from procedures or surgery.

FUTURE RESEARCH

The therapeutic use of humor by nurses has been and will continue to be an important aspect of providing patient care. Awareness of the importance of humor is increasing, as demonstrated by the plethora of articles published in support of humor as an intervention, numerous scientific studies regarding its use, and an increase in the number of educational offerings. A greater understanding is needed of how humor, laughter, and positive emotions benefit the physiology and potential healing capacity of individuals. Nurses can use this same information to incorporate humor into their lives to make their work and personal lives more enjoyable and to become more effective providers of care. Research questions to be addressed include:

1. What are the physiological effects of humor on patients who are critically ill?
2. How can the use of humor be taught and the effectiveness of its use be measured?
3. Can the systematic use of humor speed healing or enhance outcomes of acute illness?
4. Can humor be utilized in care environments to reduce stress and enhance nurse satisfaction and retention?

REFERENCES

Ackerman, M., Henry, M., Graham, K., & Coffey, N. (1994). Humor won, humor too: A model to incorporate humor into the health care setting (revised). *Nursing Forum, 29*(2), 15–21.

Asimov, I. (1992). *Asimov laughs again*. New York: HarperCollins.

Association for Applied and Therapeutic Humor. (2000). Retrieved from www.aath.org

Berger J., Coulehan, J., & Belling, C. (2004). Humor in the physician–patient encounter. *Archives of Internal Medicine, 164*(8), 825–830.

Berk, L., Felten, D., Tan, S., Bittman, B., & Westengard, J. (2001). Modulation of neuroimmune parameters during the eustress of humor-associated mirthful laughter. *Alternative Therapies in Health and Medicine, 7*(2), 62–76.

Berk, L., Tan, S., & Fry, W. (1989). Neuroendocrine and stress hormone changes during mirthful laughter. *American Journal of Medical Sciences, 298*(6), 390–396.

Berk, L., Tan, S., Napier, B., & Eby, W. (1989). Eustress of mirthful laughter modifies natural killer cell activity. *Clinical Research, 37*(1), 115A.

Black, D. (1984). Laughter. *Journal of the American Medical Association, 25*(21), 2995–2998.

Chapple, A., & Ziebland, Z. (2004). The role of humor for men with testicular cancer. *Qualitative Health Research, 14*(8), 1123–1139.

Cogan, R., Cogan, D., Waltz, W., & McCue, M. (1987). Effects of laughter and relaxation on discomfort thresholds. *Journal of Behavioral Medicine, 10,* 139–144.

Cousins, N. (1979). *Anatomy of an illness.* New York: Norton.

Crane, A. L. (1987). Why sickness can be a laughing matter. *RN, 50,* 41–42.

Davidhizar, R., & Bowen, M. (1992). The dynamics of laughter. *Archives of Psychiatric Nursing, 6*(2), 132–137.

Dillon, K., Minchoff, B., & Baker, K. (1985). Positive emotional states and enhancement of the immune system. *International Journal of Psychiatry in Medicine, 15*(1), 3–17.

Dowling, J. S., Hockenberry, M., & Gregory, R. L. (2003). Sense of humor, childhood cancer stressors, and outcomes of psychosocial adjustment, immune function, and infection. *Journal of Pediatric Oncology Nursing, 20*(6), 271–292.

Freud, S. (1905). *Jokes and their relation to the unconscious.* New York: Norton. (Originally: Der Witz und seine Beziehung zum Unbewussten. Leipzig and Vienna: Durtricke, 1960.)

Friedman, M., & Ulmer, D. (1984). *Treating type A behavior—and your heart.* New York: Knopf.

Fry, W. (1971). Mirth and oxygen saturation of peripheral blood. *Psychotherapy and Psychosomatics, 19,* 76–84.

Fry, W. F., & Savin, M. (1988). Mirthful laughter and blood pressure. *Humor, 1,* 49–62.

Gaberson, K. (1991). The effect of humorous distraction on preoperative anxiety. *AORN Journal, 54*(6), 1258–1264.

Goodman, J. (1992). Laughing matters: Taking your job seriously and yourself lightly. *Journal of the American Medical Association, 267*(13), 1858.

Haig, R. A. (1988). *The anatomy of humor: Biopsychosocial and therapeutic perspectives.* Springfield, IL: Charles C Thomas.

Herth, K. A. (1993). Humor and the older adult. *Applied Nursing Research, 6*(4), 146–153.

Hulse, J. (1994). Humor: A nursing intervention for the elderly. *Geriatric Nursing, 15*(2), 88–90.

Hunt, A. H. (1993). Humor as a nursing intervention. *Cancer Nursing, 16*(1), 34–39.

Joshua, A., Cotroneo, A., & Clarke, S. (2005). Humor and oncology. *Journal of Clinical Oncology, 23*(3), 645–648.

Klein, A. (1989). *The healing power of humor.* Los Angeles: Jeremy P. Tarcher.

Lambert, R., & Lambert, N. K. (1995). The effects of humor on secretory immuno-globulin-A levels in school-aged children. *Pediatric Nursing, 21*(1), 16–19.

Lefcourt, H. M., & Martin, R. A. (1986). *Humor and life stress: Antidote to adversity.* New York: Springer Verlag.

Leiber, D. B. (1986). Laughter and humor in critical care. *Dimensions in Critical Care Nursing, 5*(3), 162–170.

Liechty, R. D. (1987). Humor and the surgeon. *Archives of Surgery, 122,* 519–522.

Macaluso, M. C. (1993). Humor, health and healing. *American Nephrology Nurses Association Journal, 20*(1), 14–16.

Martin, R., & Dobbin, J. (1988). Sense of humor, hassles, and immunoglobulin evidence for a stress-moderating effect of humor. *International Journal of Psychiatry in Medicine, 18*(2), 93–105.

McGhee, P. (1979). *Humor: Its origin and development.* San Francisco: Freeman.

Moody, R. A. (1978). *Laugh after laugh.* Jacksonville, FL: Headwaters.

Mornhinweg, G., & Voignier, R. (1995). Holistic nursing interventions. *Orthopedic Nursing, 14*(4), 20–24.

Morreal, J. (1983). *Taking laughter seriously.* Albany: State University of New York Press.

Obrldik, A. (1942). Gallows humor: A sociological phenomenon. *American Journal of Sociology, 47,* 709–716.

Paquet, J. (1993, November/December). Laughter and stress management. *Today's OR Nurse,* 13–17.

Parfitt, J. M. (1990). Humorous preoperative teaching: Effect of recall of postoperative exercise routines. *AORN Journal, 52*(1), 114–120.

Paulsen, T. (1989). *Making humor work: Take your job seriously and yourself lightly.* Los Altos, CA: Crisp.

Robinson, V. (1978). Humor in nursing. In C. Carlson & B. Blackwell (Eds.), *Behavioral concepts and nursing interventions* (pp. 129–152). Philadelphia: Lippincott.

Robinson, V. M. (1991). *Humor and the health professions* (2nd ed.). Thorofare, NJ: Slack.

Rosenheim, E., & Golan, G. (1986). Patients' reactions to humorous interventions in psychotherapy. *American Journal of Psychotherapy, 40*(1), 110–124.

Saper, B. (1988). Humor in psychiatric healing. *Psychiatric Quarterly, 59*(4), 306–319.

Saper, B. (1990). The therapeutic use of humor for psychiatric disturbances in adolescents and adults. *Psychiatric Quarterly, 61*(4), 261–272.

Schaefner, N. (1981). *The art of laughter.* New York: Columbia University Press.

Schofield, P., Ball, D., Smith, J., Borland, R., O'Brien, P., Davis, S., et al. (2004). Optimism and survival. *Cancer, 100*(6), 1276–1282.

Simon, J. M. (1989). Humor techniques for oncology nurses. *Oncology Nursing Forum, 16*(5), 667–670.

Smith, K. L. (1995). *Medicinal mirth: The art and science of therapeutic humor.* Presentation to North Memorial Hospice and Home Care, Minneapolis.

Smith, K. (2003). Clinical wit and wisdom. *Advances for Nurse Practitioners, 11*(12), 83.

Stone, A., Valdimarsdottir, H., Jandorf, L., Cox, D., & Neale, J. (1987). Evidence that IgA antibody is associated with daily mood. *Journal of Personality and Social Psychology, 52,* 988–993.

Strickland, D. (1993, November/December). Seriously, laughter matters. *Today's OR Nurse, 19*–24.

Woodhouse, D. K. (1993). The aspects of humor in dealing with stress. *Nursing Administration Quarterly, 18*(1), 80–89.

Yovetich, N. A., Dale, A., & Hudak, M. (1990). Benefits of humor in reduction of threat induced anxiety. *Psychological Reports, 66,* 51–58.

Ziv, A. (1984). *Personality and sense of humor.* New York: Springer Verlag.

CHAPTER 9

Yoga

Miriam E. Cameron

Anyone, regardless of health or beliefs, can benefit from yoga. The regular practice of yoga heals and strengthens the body, sharpens the mind, and calms the spirit. Yoga's do-it-yourself prescription for stress management and optimal health has no side effects and does not require medications or expensive equipment and treatments (Kabat-Zinn, 2005). Nurses do yoga themselves and use it as a complementary, alternative, and primary therapy. Currently, millions of people around the world practice yoga, primarily for physical fitness and relaxation (Feuerstein, 2003). However, it offers much more than physical poses, breathing techniques, and relaxation (Cameron & Parker, 2004).

Yoga consists of a systematic ethical and spiritual path of consciousness transformation, as yogis in India and Tibet have advocated for centuries and Western researchers are now discovering (Frawley, 1999). Doing yoga brings the body, mind, and spirit into harmony with each other and the universe. As practitioners let go of ego, which underlies suffering and most illnesses, they recognize that they are linked to every being, the environment, and larger forces of the universe. Developing gratefulness for this vast interconnectedness, they do their best to relieve suffering for all beings (Arya, 1998). They sift out the unreal from the real and allow their true nature to shine forth. Then their inner wisdom flows spontaneously through all the cells of the body, promoting optimal health, inner freedom, creativity, peace, and joy (Feuerstein, 2003; Hartranft, 2003).

DEFINITION

Yoga, an ancient Indian art and science, means union or joining together of the individual and universal spirit. Two millennia ago, the Indian sage Patanjali systemized yoga into the *Yoga Sutra*, a treatise consisting of 196 compact observations. This unique blend of theoretical knowledge and practical application is a primary text for yoga (Bharati, 2001). In the *Yoga Sutra*, Patanjali analyzed how we know what we know and why we suffer. He described a meditative program through which to fulfill the primary purpose of consciousness: to see things as they really are and achieve freedom from suffering (Hartranft, 2003). Through yoga, he explained, we can rein in our tendency to gravitate toward external things, to identify with them, and to try to find happiness through them. Systematic practice of yoga teaches us how to turn inward and become aware of our true nature. Only then, he wrote, can we understand how to develop happiness and wisdom. By becoming still, we can abide in this deep, absorptive knowing (Feuerstein, 2003).

Patanjali described yoga as consisting of eight interconnected limbs, or aspects of the whole. If they are practiced simultaneously, they lead progressively to higher stages of ethics, spirituality, health, and awareness. The first five limbs still the mind and body in preparation for the last three limbs. The eight limbs and their Sanskrit names are as follows:

1. Ethical behavior (yama): nonviolence, truthfulness, nonstealing, chastity, and noncovetousness. Practitioners avoid causing any harm or getting involved in harmful activities and relationships. They become gentle, loving, free from anger, and helpful.

2. Personal behavior (niyama): purity, commitment, contentment, self-study, and surrender to the infinite. Practitioners make wise lifestyle choices in order to develop a healthy body, mind, and spirit that can fully practice all eight limbs.

3. Posture (asana): carefully designed physical poses to methodically stretch, condition, and massage the body. Practitioners perform these postures deliberately without strain or competition to bring the body into harmony with consciousness.

4. Breath control (pranayama): regulation and refinement of inhalation and exhalation of the breath to expand prana (life-force).

Practitioners learn how the breath, consisting of air and prana, affects well-being and the length and quality of life.

5. Sensory inhibition (pratyahara): right management of the senses and ability to go beyond them. Practitioners temporarily withdraw the senses from the external world into the interior self, such as by closing the eyes and looking inward.

6. Concentration (dharana): focusing steadily and without interruption on an object or field, such as the breath or a mantra. Practitioners give all their mental energy to whatever they are examining in order to develop and extend their powers of attention.

7. Meditation (dhyana): the capacity to sustain attention without distraction, leading to a profound state of quiet and relaxation. As practitioners develop awareness of the inner self and universal spirit, they perceive the truth of things.

8. Ecstasy (samadhi): a transcendent state of oneness, truth, wisdom, joy, and peace. Practitioners experience integration with the universal spirit and understanding of ultimate reality (Bharati, 2001; Cameron, 2002; Frawley, 1999; Hartranft, 2003).

SCIENTIFIC BASIS

Yoga is based on ancient observations, principles, and theories of the mind-body-spirit connection. Qualified teachers have passed down this precise knowledge to their students from one generation to the next. For centuries, these teachers have made health claims, many of which are now being validated by Western scientists. Researchers have found that the systematic practice of yoga treats symptoms and prevents both onset and recurrence of symptoms. Poor body alignment and breathing are major factors in health problems. Yoga improves body alignment and the use of extremities, as well as strengthens cardiorespiratory responses (Sinha, Ray, Pathak, & Selvamurthy, 2004). The vital organs and endocrine glands become rehabilitated and more efficient. The autonomic nervous system stabilizes (Harinath et al., 2004).

Research indicates that yoga enhances self-regulation, healing, and well-being (Telles & Naveen, 2004). It has promoted mindfulness, concentration, circulation, oxygen uptake, flexibility, and strength (Sinha et al., 2004). Yoga practitioners have developed resilience to stress, which has reduced their risk for cardiorespiratory diseases and other health problems (West, Otte, Geher, Johnson, & Mohr, 2004). Elderly women have decreased breathing frequency and increased breathing amplitude (de Barros et al., 2003). In children, yoga has improved depth perception (Raghuraj & Telles, 2003) and mental health (Bhushan, 2003).

INTERVENTION

Each of Patanjali's eight limbs is a potential nursing intervention. Nurses can teach ethical behavior (1st limb) and personal behavior (2nd limb). Table 9.1 describes "Corpse Pose," a posture that any conscious person can do; thousands of other poses condition all parts of the body (3rd limb). Table 9.2 explains Alternate Nostril Breathing, one of many breathing techniques that nurses can integrate into care (4th limb). Table 9.3 describes one kind of meditation that incorporates the 5th through 8th limbs.

The best way to learn yoga is to do it. Books, classes, and audiovisual aids describe beginning to advanced levels. Qualified teachers can assist nurses to do yoga and to use it as a nursing intervention. Yoga Alliance (www.yogaalliance.org) and International Association of Yoga Therapists (www.iayt.org) are currently developing standards.

Measurement of Outcomes

Nurses can measure outcomes by asking individuals how they feel after doing yoga. Most health problems develop over time, and yoga may not

TABLE 9.1   Corpse Pose (Savasana)

1. Lie flat on your back with arms relaxed near your sides, palms turned up, and head, trunk, and legs in a straight line. If you feel uncomfortable, put a small pillow or blanket under your head and a pillow or rolled blanket under your knees.
2. Close your eyes, keep your eyes still, relax your face, and allow your body to sink.
3. Focus on breathing slowly and evenly through your nose and from your abdomen.
4. When you are ready, open your eyes, bend your knees, turn to your right, and get up.

Nurses can use Corpse Pose to encourage deep relaxation and to treat hypertension, anxiety, insomnia, chronic fatigue, and other health problems.

Note: Adapted from "The Corpse," by L. Payne & R. Usatine, 2002, *Yoga Rx: A Step-By-Step Program to Promote Health, Wellness, and Healing for Common Ailments.* New York: Broadway Books, p. 70.

TABLE 9.2 Alternate Nostril Breathing (ANB)

1. Lie in Corpse Pose or sit comfortably with a straight back in a chair or on the floor.
2. Place your right thumb on the side of your right nostril, and your ring and little fingers on the side of your left nostril.
3. Use your thumb to close the right nostril and inhale deeply and slowly through the left nostril.
4. Use your ring and little fingers to close the left nostril and exhale deeply and slowly through the right nostril.
5. Reverse the process: Inhale through the right nostril while blocking the left nostril, and exhale through the left nostril while blocking the right nostril.
6. Over time, as you continue to practice, gradually increase the length of your breath and sessions until you reach your comfortable maximum.

Nurses can use ANB to create balance and harmony by allowing each nostril equal time and to strengthen the breath of the nostril that is chronically weaker.

Note: Adapted from "Alternate Nostril Breathing," by L. Payne & R. Usatine, 2002, *Yoga Rx: A Step-By-Step Program to Promote Health, Wellness, and Healing for Common Ailments*. New York: Broadway Books, p. 45.

TABLE 9.3 Meditation

1. Lie in Corpse Pose or sit comfortably with a straight back in a chair or on a meditation cushion. Close your eyes, relax completely, and look inward.
2. Focus on your breath. As you inhale through the nose, silently count "One." Exhale. On the next in-breath, count, "Two," and so on. When your mind wanders away, go back to one again. If you reach 10, go back to one again.
3. When you are deeply relaxed, open up to your own inner experience. Simply observe and let go of whatever arises, without attachment, judgment, or direction.
4. Over time, as you systematically meditate, you will be able to hang on to this open-ended awareness for longer periods without distraction.

Nurses can use meditation as an intervention to enhance the immune system, promote a profound state of quiet and relaxation, and develop harmony and wisdom.

Note: Adapted from "Meditation" by M. E. Cameron, 2002, *Karma & Happiness: A Tibetan Odyssey in Ethics, Spirituality, and Healing*, Minneapolis, MN: Fairview Press, pp. 226–228.

alleviate them right away. Minor difficulties often respond quickly, but serious problems require sustained, patient practice. Yoga advocates gradual change. Optimal benefits occur from regular practice. Short-term outcomes are notable, however, for they include a more relaxed attitude, decreased anxiety, improved balance, and increased musculoskeletal flexibility. Faithful practice produces long-term outcomes of better physical, spiritual, and mental health.

Precautions

Complications may result from doing yoga in a harmful manner, such as straining to do yoga poses and breathing (Johnson, Tierney, & Sadighi, 2004). Some reports have described psychotic symptoms for the first time after meditation, and precipitation of acute psychotic episodes after meditation in persons with a history of psychosis (Naveen & Telles, 2003). Yoga discourages anything unnatural or hurtful. Practitioners can avoid adverse effects by doing yoga gently and in moderation and by developing an attitude of noncompetition and relaxation. Although yoga teachers and other aids can be invaluable, individuals must seek their own inner wisdom (Kabat-Zinn, 2005).

USES

Nurses use yoga as a separate intervention and as part of an integrated health program in all areas of nursing practice. Table 9.4 lists current research findings about the benefits of yoga for persons with specific health problems. Yoga can help nurses reduce their own health problems and become a healing presence. By doing yoga themselves and using it as an intervention, nurses promote nonreactivity of the mind and inner calmness that embraces, rather than denies, difficult circumstances in a healing manner (Ott, 2004).

FUTURE RESEARCH

Additional research is needed to understand yoga's scientific basis and how to use it as a nursing intervention. Research findings are difficult to compare and apply because the various studies use different parts of yoga. Yoga therapists adapt the practice to the needs of people with specific or persistent health problems not usually addressed in a group class (Payne & Usatine, 2002), but research is needed to validate this

TABLE 9.4 Recent Research Findings: The Benefits of Yoga for Specific Health Problems

- *Asthma:* may improve symptoms and reduce bronchodilator use (Cooper et al., 2003).
- *Attention Deficit Hyperactivity Disorder (ADHD) in boys:* reduced symptoms (Jensen & Kenny, 2004).
- *Cancer:* enhanced quality of life, decreased stress, improved endocrine function (Carlson, Speca, Patel, & Goodey, 2004; Rosenbaum et al., 2004); improved sleep-related functions (Cohen, Warneke, Fouladi, Rodriguez, & Chaoul-Reich, 2004).
- *Carpal Tunnel Syndrome:* significant benefit (Muller et al., 2004); may be effective (Goodyear-Smith & Arroll, 2004).
- *Chronic Low Back Pain:* may be beneficial (Galantino et al., 2004).
- *Dementia Caregiver Stress:* improved physical, emotional functioning (Waelde, Thompson, & Gallagher-Thompson, 2004).
- *Depression:* improved mood (Woolery, Myers, Sternlieb, & Zeltzer, 2004).
- *Diabetes:* promoted management (Elder, 2004).
- *Hypertension:* reduced heart rate, systolic pressure, and diastolic pressure (Vijayalakshmi, Bhavanani, Patil, & Babu, 2004).
- *Irritable Bowel Syndrome:* decreased bowel symptoms and anxiety, enhanced parasympathetic response (Taneja et al., 2004).
- *Mental Illness:* decreased symptoms of obsessive-compulsive disorder (OCD), phobias, anxiety disorders, and anger (Shannahoff-Khalsa, 2004).
- *Multiple Sclerosis:* decreased fatigue (Oken et al., 2004).
- *Osteoarthritis:* may benefit knees (Grober & Thethi, 2003).
- *Pulmonary Tuberculosis:* reduced symptoms (Viswcswaraiah & Telles, 2004).
- *Substance Abuse:* decreased symptoms (Shannahoff-Khalsa, 2004).
- *Stroke:* improved balance and movement (Bastille & Gill-Body, 2004).

work. Because most research was conducted for brief time periods, longitudinal studies are needed to shed light on yoga's long-term effects. New qualitative methodologies may be required to examine the holistic nature of yoga. Some research questions are:

1. Which specific yoga techniques are therapeutic for particular health problems?

2. What characterizes individuals who systematically practice yoga?

3. How can individuals be encouraged to do yoga regularly?

4. What are effective strategies for teaching nurses to do yoga themselves?

REFERENCES

Arya, P. U. (1998). *Philosophy of hatha yoga*. Honesdale, PA: The Himalayan International Institute.

Bastille, J. V., & Gill-Body, K. M. (2004). A yoga-based exercise program for people with chronic poststroke hemiparesis. *Physical Therapy, 84*, 33–48.

Bharati, S. V. (2001). *Yoga sutras of Patanjali with the exposition of Vyasa: A translation and commentary* (Vol. II). Delhi, India: Motile Banarsidass.

Bhushan, L. I. (2003). Yoga for promoting mental health of children. *Journal of Indian Psychology, 21*, 45–53.

Cameron, M. E. (2002). *Karma & happiness: A Tibetan odyssey in ethics, spirituality, and healing*. Minneapolis, MN: Fairview.

Cameron, M. E., & Parker, S. A. (2004). The ethical foundation of yoga. *Journal of Professional Nursing, 5*, 275–276.

Carlson, L. E., Speca, M., Patel, K. D., & Goodey, E. (2004). Mindfulness-based stress reduction in relation to quality of life, mood, symptoms of stress and levels of cortisol, dehydroepiandrosterone sulfate (DHEAS) and melatonin in breast and prostate cancer outpatients. *Psychoneuroendocrinology, 29*, 448–474.

Cohen, L., Warneke, C., Fouladi, R. T., Rodriguez, M. A., & Chaoul-Reich, A. (2004). Psychological adjustment and sleep quality in a randomized trial of the effects of a Tibetan yoga intervention in patients with lymphoma. *Cancer, 100*, 2253–2260.

Cooper, S., Osborne, J., Newton, S., Harrison, V., Thompson, C. J., Lewis, S., et al. (2003). Effect of two breathing exercises (buteyko and pranayama) in asthma: A randomised controlled trial. *Thorax, 58*, 674–679.

de Barros, R. M., Leite, M. R., Brenzikofer, L. R., Filho, E. C., Figueroa, P. J., & Iwanowicz, J. B. (2003). Respiratory pattern changes in elderly yoga practitioners. *Journal of Human Movement Studies, 44*, 387–400.

Elder, C. (2004). Ayurveda for diabetes mellitus: A review of the biomedical literature. *Alternative Therapies in Health & Medicine, 10*, 44–50.

Feuerstein, G. (2003). *The deeper dimension of yoga: Theory and practice*. Boston: Shambhala.

Frawley, D. (1999). *Yoga and ayurveda: Self-healing and self-realization*. Twin Lakes, WI: Lotus.

Galantino, M. L., Bzdewka, T. M., Eissler-Russo, J. L., Holbrook, M. L., Mogck, E. P., Geigle, P., et al. (2004). The impact of modified hatha yoga on chronic low back pain: A pilot study. *Alternative Therapies in Health & Medicine, 10*, 56–59.

Goodyear-Smith, F., & Arroll, B. (2004). What can family physicians offer patients with carpal tunnel syndrome other than surgery? A systematic review of nonsurgical management. *Annals of Family Medicine, 2*, 267–273.

Grober, J. S., & Thethi, A. K. (2003). Osteoarthritis: When are alternative therapies a good alternative? *Consultant, 43*, 197–200.

Harinath, K., Malhotra, A. S., Pal, K., Prasad, R., Kumar, R., Kain, T. C., et al. (2004). Effects of hatha yoga and meditation on cardiorespiratory performance, psychologic profile, and melatonin secretion. *Journal of Alternative Complementary Medicine, 10,* 261–268.

Hartranft, C. (2003). *The Yoga-Sutra of Patanjali: A new translation with commentary.* Boston: Shambhala.

Jensen, P. S., & Kenny, D. T. (2004). The effects of yoga on the attention and behavior of boys with attention-deficit/hyperactivity disorder (ADHD). *Journal of Attention Disorders, 7,* 205–216.

Johnson, D. B., Tierney, M. J., & Sadighi, P. J. (2004). Kapalabhati pranayama: Breath of fire or cause of pneumothorax? A case report. *Chest, 125,* 1951–1952.

Kabat-Zinn, J. (2005). *Coming to our senses: Healing ourselves and the world through mindfulness.* New York: Hyperion.

Muller, M., Tsui, D., Schnurr, R., Biddulph-Deisroth, L., Hard, J., & MacDermid, J. C. (2004). Effectiveness of hand therapy interventions in primary management of carpal tunnel syndrome: A systematic review. *Journal of Hand Therapy, 17,* 210–228.

Naveen, K. V., & Telles, S. (2003). Yoga and psychosis: Risks and therapeutic potential. *Journal of Indian Psychology, 21,* 34–37.

Oken, B. S., Kishiyama, S., Zajdel, D., Bourdette, D., Carlsen, J., Haas, M., et al. (2004). Randomized controlled trial of yoga and exercise in multiple sclerosis. *Neurology, 62,* 2058–2064.

Ott, M. J. (2004). Mindfulness meditation: A path of transformation & healing. *Journal of Psychosocial Nursing and Mental Health Services, 42*(7), 22–29, 54–55.

Payne, L., & Usatine, R. (2002). *Yoga Rx: A step-by step program to promote health, wellness, and healing for common ailments.* New York: Broadway Books.

Raghuraj, P., & Telles, S. (2003). A randomized trial comparing the effects of yoga and physical activity programs on depth perception in school children. *Journal of Indian Psychology, 21,* 54–60.

Rosenbaum, E., Gautier, H., Fobair, P., Neri, E., Festa, B., Hawn, M., et al. (2004). Cancer supportive care, improving the quality of life for cancer patients. A program evaluation report. *Supportive Care in Cancer, 12,* 293–301.

Shannahoff-Khalsa, D. S. (2004). An introduction to Kundalini yoga meditation techniques that are specific for the treatment of psychiatric disorders. *Journal of Alternative Complementary Medicine, 10,* 91–101.

Sinha, B., Ray, U. S., Pathak, A., & Selvamurthy, W. (2004). Energy cost and cardiorespiratory changes during the practice of Surya Namaskar. *Indian Journal of Physiology & Pharmacology, 48,* 184–190.

Taneja, I., Deepak, K. K., Poojary, G., Acharya, I. N., Pandey, R. M., & Sharma, M. P. (2004). Yogic versus conventional treatment in diarrhea-predominant irritable bowel syndrome: A randomized control study. *Applied Psychophysiology & Biofeedback, 29,* 19–33.

Telles, S., & Naveen, K. V. (2004). Changes in middle latency auditory evoked potentials during meditation. *Psychological Reports, 94,* 398–400.

Vijayalakshmi, P., Bhavanani, A. B., Patil, A., & Babu, K. (2004). Modulation of stress induced by isometric handgrip test in hypertensive patients following yogic relaxation training. *Indian Journal of Physiology & Pharmacology, 48,* 59–64.

Visweswaraiah, N. K., & Telles, S. (2004). Randomized trial of yoga as a complementary therapy for pulmonary tuberculosis. *Respirology, 9,* 96–101.

Waelde, L. C., Thompson, L., & Gallagher-Thompson, D. (2004). A pilot study of a yoga and meditation intervention for dementia caregiver stress. *Journal of Clinical Psychology, 60,* 677–687.

West, J., Otte, C., Geher, K., Johnson, J., & Mohr, D. C. (2004). Effects of Hatha yoga and African dance on perceived stress, affect, and salivary cortisol. *Annals of Behavioral Medicine, 28,* 114–118.

Woolery, A., Myers, H., Sternlieb, B., & Zeltzer, L. (2004). A yoga intervention for young adults with elevated symptoms of depression. *Alternative Therapies in Health & Medicine, 10,* 60–63.

CHAPTER 10

Biofeedback

Marion Good

This chapter provides an overview of biofeedback, its scientific basis, health conditions in which it is useful, and a technique that can be used by nurses trained in its practice.

DEFINITION

Biofeedback is based on a holistic perspective in which the mind and body are not separated. Its goal is increased control over one's functioning. Biofeedback is defined by Williams, Nigl, and Savine (1981) as

> The technique of using equipment (usually electronic) to reveal to human beings some of their internal physiological events, normal and abnormal, in the form of visual and auditory signals in order to teach them to manipulate these otherwise involuntary or unfelt events by manipulating the displayed signals. This technique inserts a person's volition into the gap of an open feedback loop, hence the artificial name of biofeedback. (p. 22)

The holistic philosophy behind biofeedback and its focus on helping persons gain more control over their functioning make the intervention an appropriate one for nurses to use. Biofeedback has been used to control

117

functions related to all areas of the body including muscle strengthening or relaxation, the brain activity, and somatic and autonomic nervous system (ANS) responses. Responses to control efforts are monitored and feedback is provided to the patient concerning the degree of control achieved so that the person can eventually control the response without feedback.

SCIENTIFIC BASIS

The following provide the basis for the use of biofeedback:

- Biofeedback originated from research in the fields of psychophysiology, learning theory, and behavioral theory. For centuries it was believed that responses such as heart rate were beyond the individual's control.

- In the 1960s scientists found that the autonomic nervous system (ANS) had an afferent as well as a motor system, and control of its functions was possible with instrumentation and conditioning.

- The basis for biofeedback is a skills acquisition model in which persons determine the relationship between ANS functioning and their voluntary muscle or cognitive/affective activities. They learn skills to control these activities, which are then reinforced by a visual and/or auditory display on the biofeedback instrument. The display informs the person whether control has been achieved, reinforcing learning.

- Behavioral strategies, such as relaxation, modify physiological activity and are often part of biofeedback treatment.

- Biofeedback can also be used with relaxation strategies to control autonomic responses that affect brain waves, peripheral vascular activity, heart rate, blood glucose, and skin conductance.

- Biofeedback combined with exercise can strengthen muscles weakened by conditions such as chronic pulmonary disease, knee surgery, or age, and can recruit auxiliary motor nerves in hemiplegia.

- Combined with positioning and biomechanics, biofeedback can reduce injury from repetitive activities like typing (Barthel, Miller, Deardorff, & Portenier, 1998).

INTERVENTION

Nurses are ideal professionals to provide biofeedback because of their knowledge of physiology, psychology, and health and illness states. However, they need to acquire special information and skills in order to use it. It is recommended that information be gained from classes and workshops available in many locations and that nurses using biofeedback become certified by the Biofeedback Certification Institute of America, www.bcia.org. The Association for Applied Psychophysiology and Biofeedback (AAPB) is an excellent resource for information and can be contacted at 10200 W. 44th Avenue, Wheat Ridge, CO 80033 (303-422-8436). Although nursing practice acts differ across states, the nurses' network of AAPB is working toward nationwide acceptance of autonomous nursing biofeedback practice and inclusion of its principles in basic nursing education programs (Smart, 1990).

Technique

A biofeedback unit consists of a sensor that monitors the patient's physiological activity and a transducer that converts what is measured into an electronic visual or auditory display to the patient. Frequently measured physiological parameters include muscle depolarization, which is monitored by electromyogram (EMG), and peripheral temperature.

Biofeedback provides information about changes in a physiological parameter when behavioral treatments such as relaxation or strengthening exercises are used for a health problem. For example, a relaxation tape helps persons relax muscles to reduce blood pressure while the EMG biofeedback instrument informs the learner of progress (i.e, reduced tension in the muscle). Temperature feedback is also used with relaxation. As muscles relax, circulation improves and the fingers and toes become warmer. When exercises are used to strengthen perineal muscles in preventing urinary incontinence, success in contracting the correct muscles may be monitored by a pressure sensor inserted into the vagina. In health conditions exacerbated by stress, biofeedback is often combined with stress-management counseling.

Biofeedback is most frequently used in an office or clinic setting in seven to twelve 30-minute training sessions (Brown, 1977). Prior to beginning training at the initial session, the therapist and patient should decide upon the number of sessions. If the patient has not achieved mastery or control of a function at the end of the agreed-upon number of sessions, the reasons and the need for further sessions should be discussed.

The first session is devoted to assessing the patient, choosing the appropriate mode of feedback, discussing the roles of the nurse and patient, and obtaining baseline measurements. Measuring several parameters helps in getting valid baseline data. Because success will be determined by changes from baseline, it is essential that these be accurate and reflect the true status of the parameter being used. The first session will be longer than subsequent ones, perhaps lasting 1 to 2 hours. Behavioral exercises are provided. It is important that patients understand the content of this session so they can use the equipment.

The therapist plays a key role in the success of biofeedback. It is helpful for the nurse to have advanced training in relaxation, imagery, and stress-management counseling. Because practice of the behavioral techniques is vital, the nurse who succeeds in motivating patients to practice at home will have patients who achieve their goals.

The final sessions focus on integration of the learning into the person's life. The patient is connected to the machine but does not receive feedback while practicing the technique; the nurse monitors the degree of control achieved. Descriptions of stressful situations are provided, and the person is asked to practice the procedure as if in those situations. Final measurements are taken. Follow-up sessions at 1 month and 6 months are advocated.

Guideline for Biofeedback-Assisted Relaxation

A protocol for using biofeedback with cognitive-behavioral interventions for relaxation and stress management is found in Table 10.1. This technique could be used for hypertension, anxiety, asthma, irritable bowel syndrome, headache, or chronic pain because muscle relaxation improves these conditions. The protocol should be tailored to the patient, condition, and type of feedback.

Various types of relaxation exercises such as autogenic phrases or systematic relaxation may be used. To increase patient awareness of the relaxed state versus tension, progressive muscle relaxation with alternate contraction and relaxation may be helpful. Imagery may relax patients by distracting the mind and reducing negative or stressful thoughts. Hypnosis and self-hypnosis also produce an alternative state of mind. Music relaxes and distracts and may be used with relaxation or imagery.

It is important to keep the requirements for home practice simple, interesting, and meaningful. Boredom with the same relaxation tape, failure to find a convenient time to practice, and lack of noticeable improvements may decrease adherence to home practice. Changing to a new relaxation technique can revive interest. To integrate new skills

TABLE 10.1 Biofeedback Protocol

1. Before first session:

    - Determine health problem for which biofeedback treatment is sought.
    - Ask for physician's name so care can be coordinated. Give information on location, time commitment, and cost.
    - Request a 2-week patient log with medications and the frequency and severity of the health problem (e.g., number, intensity, and time of headaches).
    - Answer questions.

2. First session:

    - Interview patient for a health history; include the specific health condition.
    - Assess abilities for carrying out current medical regimen and behavioral intervention. Assess cultural preferences for behavioral treatments.
    - Discuss rationale for using biofeedback, type of feedback, and behavioral intervention.
    - Explain that the role of the nurse is to provide ten 50-minute sessions once a week, using the biofeedback instrument to supply physiological information.
    - Explain that the patient is the major factor in the successful use of biofeedback and that it is important to continue to keep a log of the health problem, including home practice sessions. The patient should consult the physician if health problems occur.
    - Explain the procedure. If using frontal muscle tension feedback, apply 3 sensors to the forehead after cleaning the skin with soap and water and applying gel. Set the biofeedback machine and operate according to instructions.
    - Obtain baseline EMG readings of frontal muscle tension for 5 minutes while the patient sits quietly with closed eyes.
    - Instruct the patient to practice taped relaxation instructions for 20 minutes while the EMG sensors are on the forehead. Ask the patient to watch the biofeedback display for information on the decreasing level of muscle tension.
    - Review the 2-week record of the health problem and set mutually determined goals.
    - Give a tape and instructions for practicing relaxation at home. Provide a log to record practice and responses. Discuss timing, frequency, length, and setting for practice.
    - Discuss self-care for any possible side effects to the behavioral intervention.

(continued)

TABLE 10.1   *(continued)*

3. Subsequent sessions:

- Open the session with a 20-minute review of the health-problem log, stressors, and ways used for coping in the past week; provide counseling for adaptive coping.
- Apply sensors and earphones and let the patient practice relaxation for 20 minutes while watching the display. Quietly leave the room after the patient masters the technique.
- Vary relaxation techniques to maintain interest and increase skill.
- Give instructions for incremental integration of relaxation into daily life. For example, add 30-second mini-relaxation exercises for busy times of the day.

4. Final session:

- Conduct the session as above; obtain final EMG readings.
- Discuss a plan for ongoing practice and management of stress after treatment ends.

into daily life, patients can progress to mini-relaxation and use of cues (thoughts, positions, or activities) to signal relaxation. Other intervention protocols are found in the literature for children (Olness & Kohen, 1996), and adults (Coxe, 1994; King, 1992; Schwartz & Associates, 1995).

Although some patients have multiple symptoms requiring treatment, training should only address one symptom at a time. Other symptoms can be treated sequentially after mastery of the first one is attained. The patient decides which symptom will be treated first.

Measurement of Outcomes

Feedback parameters that reflect mastery of the behavioral intervention or control of the health problem are found in Table 10.2. Frequently used parameters include heart rate, muscle tension, peripheral temperature, blood pressure, and EEG neurofeedback. EMG monitoring demonstrates changes more quickly than temperature or galvanic skin response, but the choice may depend on its appropriateness to the health condition. Temperature feedback is used in peripheral vascular problems, but health care outcomes may be fewer episodes of painful vasoconstriction. EMG feedback and temperature feedback are used in persons with diabetes mellitus, tension headache, and chronic pain. Outcomes may include

TABLE 10.2 Parameters Used for Feedback to Patients

Airway resistance	Forced expiratory	Peripheral skin
Blood pressure	volume	temperature
Blood volume	Galvanic skin response	Tidal volume
Bowel sounds	Gastric pH	Tracheal noise
EEG neurofeedback	Heart rate	Vagal nerve stimulation
EMG muscle feedback	Heart rate variability	Vaginal pressure
		Visual

decreased glycoslated hemoglobin, headaches, urinary incontinence, or pain.

Precautions

Biofeedback should be used cautiously, if at all, in persons with depression psychosis, seizures, and hyperactive conditions. Those with rigid personalities may be unwilling to change their mode of functioning (Williams et al., 1981). However, negative reactions may be related to relaxation rather than to biofeedback, and may be avoided by means of patient education and the type of relaxation used (Schwartz & Schwartz, 1995).

Biofeedback-assisted relaxation is expected to lower blood pressure and heart and respiratory rates. Excessive decreases should be avoided in patients with cardiac conditions, hemodynamic instability, or multiple illnesses.

Use of relaxation therapies may also reduce the amount of medication needed to control diabetes mellitus, hypertension, and asthma. This should be discussed with patients and physicians; responses should be carefully monitored. For example, in persons with diabetes there is also the potential for hypoglycemic reactions to occur if patient education and adjustments in insulin or diet are not made. Patients should be taught to manage hypoglycemia and blood glucose. The nurse should keep simple carbohydrates, glucagon, and a blood glucose monitor in the office and have the expertise to administer them. Home practice can be timed to avoid low blood glucose (McGrady & Bailey, 1995).

Electric shock is a potential hazard when any electrical equipment is used. Dangerous levels of current flow may arise from equipment malfunction or operator error. The AAPB publishes a list of companies whose products have met their safety code.

Although biofeedback is noninvasive, cost effective, and very promising in the treatment of many conditions, it is not a miracle intervention.

It requires that the therapist be knowledgeable about the health problem, intervention, and medication effects, with a sincere interest in patient outcome. Patient time, attention, and motivation are also necessary for success. To control the condition, ongoing use of the behavioral technique may be needed after biofeedback sessions end. This should be made very clear before training is initiated.

USES

Biofeedback has been used in the treatment of many medical and psychological problems. The AAPB web site lists 34 conditions in which biofeedback has been studied in research and has an efficacy rating of 3 (probably efficacious) out of a possible 5 (efficacious and specific). Biofeedback has been shown to be efficacious in multiple observational, clinical, and wait list controlled studies, including replications. The visitor to the web site can click on the health condition of interest and obtain information on the level of evidence, the reason biofeedback would help this condition, and the supporting evidence.

Yucha and Gilbert (2004) review the efficacy ratings for most of the disorders that have been treated with biofeedback. Two examples of health conditions for which the best evidence is available at 5 (*efficacious and specific*) are elimination disorders and migraine and tension headache in adults and children. Biofeedback treatment of hypertension in adults, anxiety in adults and children, and attention deficit disorder in children are at 4 (efficacious). Other conditions and populations treated with biofeedback are described in Table 10.3.

Tension Headache

Controlled clinical and follow-up studies have shown that biofeedback reduces tension headaches in adults and children. Tension headaches are caused by prolonged tension in the face, jaws, neck, and shoulders. Muscle tension feedback is used to teach patients to recognized the amount of tension and relax the muscles using relaxation therapy. Yucha and Gilbert (2004) and Sherman (2004) found rigorous studies showing that biofeedback is as good as or better than any medication. The effects last for most people as long as they continue to practice the behavioral techniques they learned. For example Bussone, Grazzi, D'Amico, Leone, and Andrasik (1998) found that juvenile tension-type headache sufferers treated with biofeedback-assisted relaxation continued to improve and were superior to the control condition (86% vs. 50%) at 6- and 12-month follow-

TABLE 10.3 Biofeedback Is "Probably Efficacious" for These Conditions and Populations

Alcoholism	Insomnia
Anxiety	Irritable bowel syndrome
Arthritis	Jaw area pain
Asthma	Knee pain
Attention deficit disorder/ hyperactivity disorder	Low back pain
	Non-cardiac chest pain
Breathing problems	Pain
Chest pain	Phantom limb pain
Chronic pain	Posture related pain
Constipation	Raynaud's syndrome
Drug addiction	Stump pain
Epilepsy/seizure disorders	Subluxication of the patella
Fecal elimination disorder	Substance abuse
Headaches (migraine, tension, menstrual, pediatric)	Temporomandibular disorders
	Traumatic brain injury
Hypertension	Urinary elimination disorders
Hyperventilation	Vulvar vestibulitis
Incontinence (urinary, fecal)	

(Association for Applied Psychophysiology and Biofeedback)

up. Similarly, others found that children and adolescents with episodic tension-type headache had measurably improved symptoms immediately following treatment, with further gains over three years (Grazzi et al., 2001).

Children and Adolescents

Olness and Kohen (1996) describe many conditions in children and adolescents, such as migraine, hypertension, and fecal incontinence, in which biofeedback, combined with hypnotherapy, teaches them to change their thoughts in order to bring about changes in their bodies. The authors describe special biofeedback equipment, age-appropriate explanations and inductions, and many imaginative techniques that appeal to children. The techniques for children include a "Mind Over Body" machine, and software with games or traffic lights as feedback signals. The behavioral intervention that they use is hypnotherapy, including teaching the child self-hypnosis. They have taught parents and child health care professionals, including nurses, to facilitate and reinforce what the children have been taught. For example, researchers found that a computer game to give pelvic floor biofeedback was well accepted in 15 children with chronic voiding dysfunction (Pfister et al., 1999).

Differences in Use Across Cultures

Cultural differences in use of biofeedback therapies have not been found, and biofeedback studies have been reported from other countries, indicating that the idea and the equipment do cross cultures, but comparisons across countries are lacking. In addition, evidence of use in primarily Hispanic or black clinics in the United States was missing in the literature. Health insurance coverage varies widely among plans (Association for Applied Psychophysiology and Biofeedback, 2005), and because cultural background is often linked to economic issues, it is possible that lower income families lack the resources to pay for biofeedback treatment and/ or it may not be available in their clinics.

Cultural differences are likely to exist in some of the health conditions treated by biofeedback. Some biofeedback researchers have stratified their experimental and control groups on race and a few have examined differential effects. McGrady and Roberts (1992) found that Whites but not Blacks had significantly decreased systolic blood pressure and increased finger temperature with biofeedback, perhaps due to greater peripheral resistance in blacks with hypertension. More studies of cultural differences are needed.

FUTURE RESEARCH

There continues to be great need for controlled clinical trials to determine the effectiveness, acceptability, and durability of biofeedback in treating physiological and psychological conditions in children, adults, and minorities. Nurses employing biofeedback can address the following questions:

1. What is the acceptance of biofeedback treatment by persons in minority groups as compared to acceptance by Caucasians?
2. Are there differences in immediate and long-term effects when culturally appropriate behavioral treatments are given along with biofeedback?
3. While controlling for acceptance and culturally appropriate behavioral treatments, are there differences in effects on health conditions between Caucasian and minority patients?

4. Do children who reduce their headaches with biofeedback-relaxation continue to practice at home and maintain lower levels when the sessions are completed?

5. Does biofeedback-assisted relaxation reduce anxiety and respiratory rate when a patient is weaned from a ventilator?

REFERENCES

Association for Applied Psychophysiology and Biofeedback (AAPB). Retrieved March 1, 2005, from http://www.aapb.org

Barthel, H. R., Miller, L. S., Deardorff, W. W., & Portenier, R. (1998). Presentation and response of patients with upper extremity repetitive use syndrome to a multidisciplinary rehabilitation program: A retrospective review of 24 cases. *Journal of Hand Therapy, 11*(3), 191–199.

Biofeedback Certification Institute of America. Retrieved March 1, 2005, from www.bcia.org

Brown, B. (1977). *Stress and the art of biofeedback.* New York: Bantam.

Bussone, G., Grazzi, L., D'Amico, D., Leone, M., & Andrasik, F. (1998). Biofeedback-assisted relaxation training for young adolescents with tension-type headache: A controlled study. *Cephalalgia, 18*(7), 463–467.

Campinha-Bacote, J., Campinha-Bacote, D., & Allbright, J. (1992). C.A.R.E. (Culturally-specific Africentric Relaxation Exercise). *Transcultural C.A.R.E.* Associates, 11108 Huntwicke Place, Cincinnati OH, 241.

Coxe, J. (1994). Assessment for biofeedback and behavioral therapy for urinary incontinence. *Urologic Nursing, 14*, 82–84.

Good, M., Picot, B. L., Salem, S. G., Chin, C. C., Picot, S. F., & Lane, D. (2000). Cultural differences in music chosen for pain relief. *Journal of Holistic Nursing, 18*(3), 245–260.

Grazzi, L., Andrasik, F., D'Amico, D., Leone, M., Moschiano, F., & Bussone, G. (2001). Electromyographic biofeedback-assisted relaxation training in juvenile episodic tension-type headache: Clinical outcome at three-year follow-up. *Cephalalgia, 21*(8), 798–803.

King, T. I. (1992). The use of electromyographic biofeedback in treating a client with tension headaches. *The American Journal of Occupational Therapy, 46*, 839–842.

McGrady, A. (1994). Effects of group relaxation training and thermal biofeedback on blood pressure and related physiological and psychological variables in essential hypertension. *Biofeedback and Self-Regulation, 19*, 51–66.

McGrady, A., & Bailey, B. K. (1995). Biofeedback-assisted relaxation and diabetes mellitus. In M. S. Schwartz and Associates (Eds.), *Biofeedback: A practitioner's guide* (2nd ed., pp. 471–489). New York: Guilford Press.

McGrady, A., Bailey, B. K., & Good, M. (1992). Biofeedback-assisted relaxation in insulin dependent diabetes mellitus: A controlled study. *Diabetes Care, 14*, 160–165.

McGrady, A., Graham, G., & Bailey, B. (1996). Biofeedback-assisted relaxation in insulin-dependent diabetes: A replication and extension study. *Annals of Behavioral Medicine, 18,* 185–189.

McGrady, A., & Roberts, G. (1992). Racial differences in the relaxation response of hypertensives. *Psychosomatic Medicine, 54*(1), 71–78.

Olness, K., & Kohen, D. P. (1996). *Hypnosis and hypnotherapy with children* (3rd ed.). New York: Guilford.

Pfister, C., Dacher, J. N., Gaucher, S., Liard-Zmuda, A., Grise, P., & Mitrofanoff, P. (1999). The usefulness of a minimal urodynamic evaluation and pelvic floor biofeedback in children with chronic voiding dysfunction. *British Journal of Urology International, 84*(9), 1054–1057.

Schwartz, M. S., & Associates. (1995). *Biofeedback: A practitioner's guide* (2nd ed.). New York: Guilford.

Schwartz, M. S., & Schwartz, N. M. (1995). Problems with relaxation and biofeedback: Assisted relaxation and guidelines for management. In M. S. Schwartz & Associates (Eds.), *Biofeedback: A practitioner's guide* (2nd ed., pp. 288–300). New York: Guilford Press.

Sherman R. (2004). *Pain assessment and intervention from a psychophysiological perspective.* Wheat Ridge CO: Association for Applied Psychophysiology.

Smart, S. (1990). Empowering patients through biofeedback. *California Nurse, 86*(7), 13.

Williams, M., Nigl, A., & Savine, D. (1981). *A textbook of biological feedback.* New York: Human Science Press.

Yucha, C., & Gilbert, C. (2004). *Evidence-based practice in biofeedback and neurofeedback.* Colorado Springs, CO: Association for Applied Psychophysiology and Biofeedback.

CHAPTER 11

Meditation

Mary Jo Kreitzer

Meditation is a self-directed practice for relaxing the body and calming the mind that has been used by people in many cultures since ancient times. It is frequently viewed as a religious practice, although its health benefits have been long recognized. It is a recommended intervention for stress reduction, anxiety and anxiety-related disorders, insomnia, expanding awareness, and overall improvement in well-being. Whereas earlier research studies focused on behavioral outcomes associated with meditation (self-reported changes in anxiety, depression, insomnia, and quality of life), more recent research has documented immunological and neurological changes.

The resurgence in interest in meditation has drawn largely from Eastern religious practices, particularly those of India, China, and Japan. Records substantiate the use of meditation by Hindus in India as early as 1500 BC. Taoists in China and Buddhists in India and China included meditation as an integral part of their religious life. Zen Buddhists in China and Japan reaffirmed the centrality of meditation and practiced a sitting meditation in which a quiet panoramic awareness of whatever is happening at the time is maintained.

Meditation has also been an important aspect of the Western world and the Judeo-Christian tradition. Christian monks and hermits went to the desert to meditate and meditation remains a key element of monastic life. Contemplation, centering prayer, and praying the rosary or repeating the Hail Mary are forms of meditation. West (1979) noted the use of meditation in the American Indian culture, the Kung Zhu/twasi of Africa, and the Native Americans of Alaska of North America. In the United States, the most common forms of meditation are sedentary, although there is an increasing interest in many moving meditations such as the Chinese martial art tai chi, the Japanese martial art of aikido, and walking meditation in Zen Buddhism. Although specific meditative practices vary considerably, the outcomes are similar for all techniques.

DEFINITIONS

Many definitions of meditation can be identified in the literature. West (1979) defined it as an exercise in which the individual focuses attention or awareness in order to dwell upon a single object. Welwood's definition (1979) is broader, describing meditation as a technique that allows individuals to investigate the process of their consciousness and experiences and to discover the more basic underlying qualities of their existence as an animate reality. Intense concentration blocks other stimuli, allowing the person to become more aware of self.

Everly and Rosenfeld (1981) divided meditation techniques into four forms: mental repetition, physical repetition, problem concentration, and visual concentration. In mental repetition the person concentrates on a word or phrase, commonly called a *mantra*. Concentration on breathing is frequently the focus in physical repetition techniques; however, dance or other body movements can be the object of concentration. Jogging, for example, allows for concentrating on a physical activity, repetitive breathing, and the sound of one's feet hitting the ground. In samatha Buddhist meditation, the person watches or concentrates on the breath entering and flowing from the tip of the nostrils. In problem-contemplation techniques, an attempt is made to solve a problem that contains paradoxical components, which Zen terms the *koan*. Visual concentration techniques are akin to imagery.

Borysenko (1988) defines meditation simply as any activity that keeps the attention pleasantly anchored in the present moment. It is the way we learn to access the relaxation response. Kabat-Zinn, Wheeler, and colleagues (1998) note that meditation is fundamentally different from relaxation techniques in both methods and objectives. A common but erroneous assumption is that the goal of meditation is to achieve a specific, highly pleasant meditative state akin to deep relaxation. According to these authors, there is no single meditative state and the overall orientation is one of non-striving and non-doing. Kabat-Zinn (2005) emphasizes that meditation is best thought of as a way of being rather than a collection of techniques. Mindfulness expands our capacity for awareness and for self-knowing. When a mindful state is cultivated, it frees people from routinized thought patterns, senses, and relationships and the destructive mind states and emotions that accompany them. When people are able to escape from highly conditioned, reactive, and habitual thinking, they are able to respond in more effective and authentic ways.

SCIENTIFIC BASIS

An understanding of the scientific basis for meditation is emerging. In 1979, West noted that there were few theoretical explanations for meditation's effectiveness, though various explanations had been proposed, including adaptive regression (Shafii, 1973) and desensitization, as meditating allows the person to deal with unfinished psychic material (Tart, 1971). Everly and Rosenfeld (1981) suggested that the role of the focal device used in meditation is to allow the intuitive, non–ego-centered mode of thought processing to dominate consciousness in place of the normally dominant analytic, ego-centered style. When the left (rational, analytic) hemisphere of the brain is silenced, the intuitive mode produces extraordinary awareness. A positive mood, an experience of unity, an alteration in time-space relationships, an enhanced sense of reality and meaning, and an acceptance of things that seem paradoxical are experienced in this superconscious state. A serious meditator may progress through a continuum from beginning meditation to this superconscious state.

In a report to the National Institutes of Health (1992) on alternative medical systems and practices in the United States, research on meditation was summarized as one of several mind–body interventions. In describing how and why meditation may work, Kenneth Walton, director of the neurochemistry laboratory at Maharishi International University in Fairfield, Iowa, cited the link among chronic stress, serotonin metabolism, and the hippocampal regulation of the hypothalamic-pituitary-adrenocortical (HPA) axis.

Brain imaging techniques such as PET and functional magnetic resonance imaging (fMRI) have emerged over the past 10 years and have enabled scientists to study the human brain in action. Neuroplasticity refers to the structural and functional changes in the brain that result from training and experience. Research on neuroplasticity has confirmed that the brain is not a static organ; rather, it is designed to respond to changing experiences. Neuroplasticity research, Schwartz (Schwartz & Begley, 2002) writes, has documented the ability of neurons to literally forge new connections, to blaze new paths through the cortex and even assume new roles. Research on mental training through meditation published by Lutz and colleagues (Lutz, Greischar, Rawlings, Richard, & Davidson, 2004) has provided the most compelling scientific data thus far on what happens in the brain when people meditate. In a study comparing Tibetan monks with student volunteers, this team of researchers found that meditation is associated with brain changes that allow people to achieve different levels of awareness. Longtime practitioners of meditation were found to have unusually powerful gamma waves and the movement of these waves through the brain was better organized and coordinated than in the students.

INTERVENTION

There is a wide variety of meditation approaches described in the literature; however, the following four techniques will be described: mindfulness meditation, transcendental meditation (TM), centering prayer, and relaxation response.

Techniques

Mindfulness Meditation

Mindfulness, awareness and insight meditation are Western terms used interchangeably to describe the Buddhist practice of vipassana meditation. The goal of this meditative practice is to increase insight by becoming a detached observer of the stream of changing thoughts, feelings, drives, and visions until their nature and origin are recognized. The process includes eliciting the relaxation response, centering on breath, and then focusing attention freely from one perception to the next. In this form of meditation, no thoughts or sensations are considered intrusions. When they drift into consciousness, they become the focus of attention (Kutz et al., 1985).

An extension of the practice of mindfulness meditation is what Borysenko (1988) calls "meditation in action" (p. 91). It involves a "be here now" approach that allows life to unfold without the limitation of prejudgment. Mindfulness exercises are carried out during normal, daily activities using this approach. It requires being open to an awareness of the moment as it is and to what the moment could hold. It produces a relaxed state of attentiveness to both the inner world of thoughts and feelings and the outer world of actions and perceptions. Borysenko notes that mindfulness requires a change in attitude: joy is not sought in finishing an activity, but rather in doing it.

Mindfulness-based stress reduction programs (MBSR) originated with the Stress Reduction Clinic at the University of Massachusetts Medical Center and are currently used in more than 80 clinics, hospitals, and HMOs in the United States and abroad (Kabat-Zinn et al., 1998). It is generally understood that in MBSR instruction, participants receive training in three formal meditation techniques: a body scan meditation, a sitting meditation, and mindful hatha yoga, which involves simple stretches and postures.

Transcendental Meditation

A much-publicized technique, transcendental meditation was developed and introduced into the United States in the early 1960s by the Indian leader Maharishi Mahesh Yogi. It is estimated that there are now well over 2 million practitioners. The concept of TM is relatively simple. Students are given a mantra (a word or sound) to repeat silently over and over again while sitting in a comfortable position. The mantra is selected not for its meaning but strictly for its sound. It is the understanding that this sound alone attracts the mind and leads it effortlessly and naturally to a slightly subtler level of the thinking process. If thoughts other than the mantra come to mind, the student is asked to notice them and return to the mantra. It is suggested that practitioners meditate for 20 minutes in the morning and again in the evening. TM is easily learned and is practiced by people of every age, education, culture, and religion. It is not a philosophy and does not require specific beliefs or changes in behavior or lifestyle (Russel, 1976).

Centering Prayer

Though similar to TM in several respects, centering prayer is based in Christianity and is designed to reduce the obstacles to contemplative prayer and union with God. Thomas Keating (1995), the founder of the centering prayer movement, describes centering prayer as a discipline designed to withdraw our attention from the ordinary flow of thoughts. The understanding is that people tend to identify with their thoughts—the debris that floats along the surface of the river—rather than being in touch with the river itself—the source from which these mental objects are emerging. Keating suggests that like boats or floating debris, our thoughts and feelings must be resting on something. They are resting, he asserts, on the inner stream of consciousness, which is our participation in God's being. In centering prayer, as with TM, people are encouraged to find a comfortable position, to close their eyes, and, to focus on a sacred word. Keating notes that 20 to 30 minutes is the minimum amount of time necessary for most people to establish interior silence and to get beyond their superficial thoughts.

Relaxation Response

This response incorporates four elements that are common in many of the other relaxation techniques: a quiet environment, a mental device, a passive attitude, and a comfortable position.

A quiet environment, which is an element of Benson's technique (1975), eliminates outside stimuli and allows the person to concentrate on the mental device. Some people prefer a church or chapel for meditating, but such a place may not be readily accessible. Playing music while meditating is not advocated because it may draw the person's attention away from the internal processes. People should select the place they wish to use for meditation and continue to use that place. This eliminates adjusting to new surroundings and stimuli each time a person meditates.

Use of a mental device helps shift the mind from logical, externally oriented thought to inner rumination. The purpose of the mental device is to preoccupy oneself with an emotionally neutral, repetitive, and monotonous stimulus. Unlike TM, in which the teacher gives the student a mantra, Benson's technique requires the person to select the mental device that will be used whenever the person meditates. It may be a sound, word, or phrase that is repeated silently or aloud, a phrase or portion of a religious prayer or psalm. Fixation on an object is also sometimes used as the mental device.

Guidelines

Borysenko (1988) describes a simple, step-by-step process incorporating many of the concepts previously described that can be used to teach meditation to patients:

1. Choose a quiet place where you will not be disturbed by other people or by the telephone.
2. Sit in a comfortable position with back straight and arms and legs uncrossed, unless you choose to sit cross-legged on the floor.

3. Close your eyes.

4. Relax your muscles sequentially from head to feet.

5. Focus on your breathing, noticing how the breath goes in and out, without trying to control it in any way.

6. Repeat your focus word silently in time with your breathing.

Borysenko advises meditators to not worry about how they are doing. It is helpful to maintain a passive attitude and allow relaxation to occur at its own pace. When distracting thoughts intrude, meditators are encouraged to ignore them by not dwelling on them and return to repeating the chosen word. Successful meditation usually takes practice—at least once a day for 10 to 20 minutes.

Benson (1975) suggests that people wait for 2 hours after any meal before meditating, as the digestive processes seem to interfere with the elicitation of the relaxation response. He also emphasizes the importance of fitting the technique to the individual and making modifications as necessary. Therefore, before any teaching is initiated, an assessment of the individual is needed to determine what might be the most appropriate technique. This requires that nurses have knowledge about various approaches to meditation.

Measurement of Outcomes

Whereas earlier studies of meditation focused on self-report measures and easy-to-obtain physiologic data (changes in blood pressure, respiratory rate, etc.), there is increased interest in neurobiologic and immune system changes. Lutz and colleagues (2004) documented changes in brain structure and function as a result of prolonged meditation. Robinson, Matthews, and Witek-Janusek (2003), in their study of HIV/AIDS patients, found natural killer cell activity and number increased significantly in the mindfulness-based stress reduction group compared to a control group. It is likely that future meditation research will continue to attempt to elucidate the mechanism of action as well as outcomes associated with meditation.

To document the efficacy of meditation in a clinical setting, nurses can use blood pressure readings, heart rate, and respiratory rate as indicators of its effectiveness. Measures should not only be taken before and immediately after practicing meditation, but also at other times during the day, and records should be kept to determine if changes occur over time. Because the person is resting while meditating, it would be expected that the readings would be lower after practice. It is also important that continued follow-up be done to determine if the effect persists over time.

Precautions

Meditation is not a benign intervention. The nurse must be aware of side effects of the intervention, persons for whom it should not be used, and assessments to be made as the person practices meditation. Careful monitoring of reactions to medications is necessary, as doses may need to be altered. Everly and Rosenfeld (1981) noted problems of overdosage with insulin, sedatives, and cardiovascular medications in people who meditated. Because of the effect meditation can have on the cardiovascular system, blood pressure should be checked before meditation begins. If the systolic pressure is below 90 mm Hg, meditation should not be practiced. Patients should be instructed not to meditate if there is light-headedness or dizziness. Also, individuals should not stand immediately after meditating because a hypotensive state is frequently present.

Benson (1975) notes that hallucinations can occur if the person meditates for several hours at a time. Loss of contact with reality is a possibility, and continued assessment is needed to determine if this is occurring. Lazarus (1976) reported cases of attempted suicide, schizophrenia, and severe depression after the continued practice of meditation. Meditation should not be prescribed for some people; however, the characteristics of people who would be harmed by it are as yet unclear.

USES

There is a substantial body of research supporting the use of meditation for a wide variety of conditions. Table 11.1 lists conditions for which it has been used. Use of meditation for patients with chronic pain, hypertension, and anxiety and generalized stress will be discussed.

In addition to being a low-cost intervention with demonstrated efficacy, there are some data that suggest meditative practices may also impact overall use of health care services. In a study comparing 2,000 people who meditated with a group of non-meditators of comparable age, gender, and profession, it was found that over a 5-year period, use of medical services (visits to the doctor and hospitalizations) by the group that meditated was 30% to 87% less than the group of non-meditators (Orme-Johnson, 1987). The difference was greatest for individuals over 40 years of age.

Conditions/Populations

Chronic Pain

Use of meditation for patients experiencing chronic pain has been well documented experientially and empirically. Early studies of mindfulness-

TABLE 11.1 Conditions for Which Meditation Has Been Used

Anxiety (Kabat-Zinn, Massion, et al., 1992; Miller, Fletcher, & Kabat-Zinn, 1995)

Asthma (Wilson, Honsberger, Chin, & Novey, 1975)

Cancer (Carlson, Speca, Patel, & Goodey, 2004; Speca, Carlson, Goodey, & Angen, 2000)

Carotid atherosclerosis (Castillo-Richmond et al., 2000)

Chronic pain (Kabat-Zinn, Lipworth, & Burney, 1985; Kabat-Zinn et al., 1992)

Coronary artery disease (Zamarra, Schneider, Besseghini, Robinson, & Salerno, 1996)

Coronary care units (Guzzetta, 1989)

Depression (Teasdale et al., 2000)

Diagnostic procedures (Frenn, Fehring, & Kartes, 1986)

Drug abuse (Shafii, 1973)

Fibromyalgia (Astin et al., 2003)

Headache (Benson, Klemchuk, & Graham, 1974)

HIV/AIDS (Robinson et al., 2003)

Hypertension (Schneider, Staggers, Alexander, & Sheppard, 1996)

Irritable bowel syndrome (Keefer & Blanchard, 2002)

Organ transplantation (Gross et al., 2004; Kreitzer, Gross, Ye, Russas, & Treesak, 2005)

Psoriasis (Kabat-Zinn et al., 1998)

Psychotherapy (Bogart, 1991)

based stress reduction examined the impact of MBSR on patients with chronic pain. In a study of 51 patients with chronic pain who had been unsuccessfully treated by conventional methods, Kabat-Zinn (1982) reported significant decreases in pain and in the number of medical symptoms reported by patients enrolled in a 10-week training program. Significant reductions in mood disturbances and psychiatric symptomatology were also noted. One methodological limitation of this study was the lack of a comparison or control group.

A larger clinical trial by Kabat-Zinn et al. (1985) examined the impact of mindfulness meditation on 90 chronic pain patients. Statistically significant reductions were reported in present-moment pain, negative body image, inhibition of activity by pain, symptoms, mood disturbance, and psychological symptomatology including anxiety and depression. A comparison group of chronic pain patients did not show significant improvement on these measures. Improvements reported by the patients who received the 10-week mindfulness meditation training were maintained up to 15 months post-meditation training for all measures except present-moment pain.

A 4-year follow-up of 225 chronic pain patients (Kabat-Zinn, Lip-worth, Burney, & Sellers, 1987) enrolled in an 8-week mindfulness meditation training program documented that improvements in physical and psychological status were maintained: 93% of patients reported the present use of at least one of the three meditation practices taught in the initial training.

In a randomized controlled clinical trial of patients with fibromyalgia (Astin et al., 2003), an 8-week mindfulness-based meditation intervention was compared with an education support group. Pain was one of the primary outcome measures. Comparison of outcomes at baseline with those at 8, 16, and 24 weeks indicated that both groups demonstrated statistically significant improvements across time. However, there was no difference between the mind–body training group and the education support group control. In a 1-year follow-up of relaxation response meditation in patients with irritable bowel syndrome (Keefer & Blanchard, 2002), statistically significant reductions in abdominal pain were found post-course, and these changes were maintained over the long-term.

Hypertension

Because of the decreases in blood pressure experienced by persons who had practiced TM, Benson (1975) explored the effectiveness of the relaxation response in persons with hypertension. Statistically significant changes between the experimental and control groups were found in his initial study. Mean systolic pressures decreased from 146 to 137 mm Hg, and mean diastolic pressures from 93.5 to 88.9 mm Hg in subjects who were taught and who practiced Benson's technique. Blood pressure was not measured immediately after meditation, but readings were taken at random times throughout the day instead. It is hypothesized that meditation counteracts the sympathetic responses of the fight-or-flight reaction to stressors.

A study of hypertensive African Americans (Castillo-Richmond et al., 2000) was designed to measure the impact of a TM program on carotid atherosclerosis. In a randomized controlled trial comparing a TM program with a health education program, groups were matched for teaching format, instructional time, home practice, and expectations of health outcomes. Preliminary findings revealed that the TM program was associated with reduced carotid atherosclerosis. This study is encouraging, given the high incidence of hypertension and cardiovascular disease in the African-American population.

Anxiety and Generalized Stress

Two studies have examined the effect of a group mindfulness-based meditation program on patients with anxiety disorders. In a study of 22 patients diagnosed with generalized anxiety disorder or panic disorder with or without agoraphobia, Kabat-Zinn and colleagues (1992) reported significant reductions in anxiety and depression. These improvements were maintained at a 3-month follow-up. Another follow-up study of this same patient population at 3 years (Miller, Fletcher, & Kabat-Zinn, 1995) revealed maintenance of the gains reported in the original study on the following measures: anxiety, depression, number and severity of panic attacks, mobility, and fear.

Astin (1997) conducted a study of the effect of an 8-week mindfulness-based stress reduction program on 28 medical students who were randomized to an experimental group or a nonintervention control group. Participants in the mindfulness meditation training evidenced significant reductions in overall psychological symptomatology (depression and anxiety), increases in a perceived sense of control, and higher scores on a measure of spiritual experiences. Astin concluded that mindfulness meditation might serve as a powerful cognitive-behavioral coping strategy for transforming the ways in which people respond to life events.

The impact of a mindfulness-based stress reduction program on English- and Spanish-speaking patients cared for in a bilingual inner-city primary care clinic was studied by Roth and Creaser (1997). Data revealed that patients who completed the 8-week training program reported statistically significant decreases in medical and psychological symptoms and improvement in self-esteem. Anecdotal reports of the 79 patients who completed the training program indicated that many experienced changes far more profound than the documented reduction in physical and psychological symptoms. Changes reported included greater peace of mind; more patience; less anger and fewer temper outbursts; better interpersonal communication; more harmonious relationships with family members; improved parenting skills; more restful sleep; decreased use of medications for pain, sleep, and anxiety; decrease or cessation of smoking; weight loss; greater acceptance of aspects of life over which they have no control; greater self-knowledge; and a marked improvement in the overall sense of well-being.

FUTURE RESEARCH

Although nurses are increasingly using meditation in their practice, the research base for its use in nursing is sparse. Much of the current research is being conducted by interdisciplinary teams. Because meditation holds great promise as a therapeutic nursing intervention, nurses should be encouraged to contribute to whatever research is being done. Questions and areas that merit further investigation include:

1. What are the characteristics of people who benefit from meditation? Do people who continue to practice it differ significantly
   from those who abandon it?

2. How easily generalized are the effects of meditation? Does its
   use affect areas of the person's life other than those for which
   it was taught? If the person is taught meditation as a means of
   decreasing hypertension, is there also an improvement in sleep
   or other areas?

3. How does meditation differ in process and outcome from other
   forms of self-regulation such as hypnosis, relaxation, and
   guided imagery?

4. What are biologic and behavioral outcomes associated with
   meditation?

WEB SITES

Mind and Life Institute: www.mindandlife.org
Center for Spirituality and Healing, University of Minnesota: www.csh.umn.
edu/modpub/

REFERENCES

Astin, J. (1997). Stress reduction through mindfulness meditation: Effects of
psychological symptomatology, sense of control, and spiritual experiences.
Psychotherapy and Psychosomatics, 66, 97–106.

Astin, J., Berman, B., Bausell, B., Lee, W., Hochberg, M., & Forys, K. (2003).
The efficacy of mindfulness meditation plus Qigong movement therapy in the
treatment of fibromyalgia: A randomized controlled trial. *Journal of Rheumatology, 30*, 2257–2262.

Benson, H. (1975). *The relaxation response.* New York: Avon.

Benson, H., Klemchuk, H., & Graham, J. (1974). The usefulness of the relaxation
response in the therapy of headache. *Headache, 14*, 49–52.

Bogart, G. (1991). Meditation and psychology: A review of the literature. *American Journal of Psychotherapy, 45*, 383–412.

Borysenko, J. (1988). *Minding the body, mending the mind.* New York: Bantam.

Carlson, L., Speca, M., Patel, K., & Goodey, E. (2004). Mindfulness-based stress
reduction in relation to quality of life, mood, symptoms of stress and levels
of cortisol, dehydroepinandrosterone sulfate (DHEAS) and melatonin in breast
and prostate cancer. *Psychoneuroimmunology, 29*, 448–474.

Castillo-Richmond, A., Schneider, R., Alexander, C., Cook, R., Myers, H., Nidich,
S., et al. (2000). Effects of stress reduction on carotid atherosclerosis in hypertensive African Americans. *Stroke, 31*(3), 568–573.

Everly, G., & Rosenfeld, R. (1981). *The nature and treatment of the stress responses.* New York: Plenum.

Frenn, M., Fehring, R., & Kartes, S. (1986). Reducing stress of cardiac catheterization by teaching relaxation. *Dimensions of Critical Care Nursing, 5,* 108–116.

Gross, C. R., Kreitzer, M. J., Russas, V., Treesak, C., Frazier, P. A., & Hertz, M. I. (2004). Mindfulness meditation to reduce symptoms after organ transplant: A pilot study. *Advances in Mind–Body Medicine, 20*(2), 20–29.

Guzzetta, C. E. (1989). Effects of relaxation and music therapy on patients in a coronary care unit with presumptive acute myocardial infarction. *Heart & Lung, 18,* 609–618.

Kabat-Zinn, J. (1982). An outpatient program in behavioral medicine for chronic pain based on the practice of mindfulness meditation. *General Hospital Psychiatry, 4,* 33–47.

Kabat-Zinn, J. (2005). *Coming to our senses: Healing ourselves and the world through mindfulness.* New York: Hyperion.

Kabat-Zinn, J., Lipworth, L., & Burney, R. (1985). The clinical use of mindfulness meditation for the self-regulation of chronic pain. *Journal of Behavioral Medicine, 8*(2), 163–190.

Kabat-Zinn, J., Lipworth, L., Burney, R., & Sellers, W. (1987). Four-year follow-up of a meditation program for the self-regulation of chronic pain: Treatment outcomes and compliance. *Clinical Journal of Pain, 2,* 159–173.

Kabat-Zinn, J., Massion, A. O., Kristeller, J., Peterson, L. G., Fletcher, K. E., Pbert, L., et al. (1992). The effectiveness of a meditation-based stress reduction program in the treatment of anxiety disorders. *American Journal of Psychiatry, 149,* 936–943.

Kabat-Zinn, J., Wheeler, E., Light, T., Skillings, A., Scharf, M. J., Cropley, T. G., et al. (1998). Influence of a mindfulness meditation–based stress reduction intervention on rates of skin clearing in patients with moderate to severe psoriasis undergoing phototherapy (UVB) and photochemo-therapy (PUVA). *Psychosomatic Medicine, 60,* 625–632.

Keating, T. (1995). *Open mind, open heart.* New York: Continuum.

Keefer, L., & Blanchard, E. (2002). A one year follow-up of relaxation response meditation as a treatment for irritable bowel syndrome. *Behavior Research & Therapy, 40,* 541–546.

Kreitzer, M. J., Gross, C. R, Ye, X., Russas, V., & Treesak, C. (2005) Longitudinal impact of mindfulness meditation on illness burden in solid organ transplant recipients: Results of a pilot study. *Progress in Transplantation, 15*(2), 166–172.

Kutz, I., Leserman, J., Dorrington, C., Morrison, C., Borysenko, J., & Benson, H. (1985). Meditation as an adjunct to psychotherapy. *Psychotherapy and Psychosomatics, 43*(4), 209–218.

Lazarus, A. A. (1976). Psychiatric problems precipitated by transcendental meditation. *Psychological Reports, 39,* 601–602.

Lutz, A., Greischar, L., Rawlings, N., Richard, M., & Davidson, R. (2004). Long-term meditators self-induce high amplitude gamma synchrony during mental practice. *Proceedings of the National Academy of Sciences, 101,* 16,369–16,373.

Miller, J. J., Fletcher, K., & Kabat-Zinn, J. (1995). Three-year follow-up and clinical implications of a mindfulness meditation–based stress reduction intervention in the treatment of anxiety disorders. *General Hospital Psychiatry, 17,* 192–200.

National Institutes of Health. (1992). *Alternative medicine: Expanding medical horizons.* Washington, DC: U.S. Government Printing Office.

Orme-Johnson, D. W. (1987). Medical care litigation and the transcendental meditation program. *Psychosomatic Medicine, 49,* 493–507.

Robinson, F., Matthews, H., & Witek-Janusek, L. (2003). Psycho-endocrine-immune response to mindfulness-based stress reduction in individuals infected with the human immunodeficiency virus: A quasiexperimental study. *Journal of Alternative and Complementary Medicine, 9,* 683–694.

Roth, B., & Creaser, T. (1997). MBSR: Experience with a bilingual inner-city program. *The Nurse Practitioner, 20,* 150–176.

Russel, P. (1976). *The TM technique.* Boston: Routledge and Kegan Paul.

Schneider, R. H., Staggers, F., Alexander, C. N., & Sheppard, W. (1996). A randomized controlled trial of stress reduction for hypertension in older African-Americans. *Hypertension, 2,* 820–827.

Schwartz, J., & Begley, S. (2002). *The mind and the brain.* New York: Regan Books.

Shafii, M. (1973). Adaptive and therapeutic aspects of meditation. *International Journal of Psychoanalysis and Psychotherapy, 2,* 431–443.

Speca, M., Carlson, L., Goodey, E., & Angen, M., (2000). A randomized, wait-list controlled clinical trial: The effect of a mindfulness meditation–based stress reduction program on mood and symptoms of stress in cancer outpatients. *Psychosomatic Medicine, 62,* 613–622.

Tart, C. (1971). A psychologist's experiences with transcendental meditation. *Journal of Transpersonal Psychology, 3,* 135–143.

Teasdale, J., Segal, S., Williams, J., Ridgeway, V., Soulsby, J., & Lau, M. (2000). Prevention of relapse/recurrence in major depression by mindfulness-based cognitive therapy. *Journal of Consulting and Clinical Psychology, 68,* 615–625.

Welwood, J. (1979). *The meeting of the ways: Explorations in east/west psychology.* New York: Schocken.

West, M. (1979). The psychosomatics of meditation. *Journal of Psychosomatic Medicine, 24,* 265–273.

Wilson, A. F., Honsberger, R. W., Chin, R. T., & Novey, H. S. (1975). Transcendental meditation and asthma. *Respiration, 32,* 74–78.

Zamarra, J. W., Schneider, R. H., Besseghini, I., Robinson, D. K., & Salerno, J. W. (1996). Usefulness of the TM program in the treatment of patients with coronary artery disease. *American Journal of Cardiology, 77,* 867–870.

CHAPTER 12

Prayer

Mariah Snyder

Prayer has been identified as a complementary therapy by the National Center for Complementary/Alternative Medicine (2005). Prayer is ubiquitous, having been used by persons of all cultures throughout time. McCaffrey, Eisenberg, Legedza, Davis, and Phillips (2004) reported that 35% of respondents in a national survey used prayer for their own health concerns and of these persons 75% used prayer for their own wellness. Only within recent years have studies on the efficacy of prayer in promoting health been conducted. Some contend (Dusek, Astin, Hibberd, & Krucoff, 2003) that prayer, given its philosophical basis, cannot be studied using randomized clinical trials.

People often equate prayer with religion. Yet prayer, like spirituality, transcends religion. Prayer and spirituality acknowledge the existence of a Greater or Higher Being and that we as humans have a connectedness with this Being. Cultural and religious groups have different names for this Higher Being: God, Supreme Being, Mother Earth, Master of the Universe, Creator, Absolute, El, or Great Spirit are some of them.

Spirituality, of which prayer is a component, has been a part of nursing for centuries. The holistic perspective of nursing mandates that nurses assess the spiritual needs of a patient along with the physical, psychological, and social elements. Early hospitals and schools of nursing were often affiliated with specific religious organizations. Within this context, student nurses were taught to include prayer as part of care. With the increasing cultural diversity in American society it is necessary for nurses to be acquainted with prayer and religious practices found in multiple cultures.

DEFINITION

"Prayer" is from the Latin *precarius*, which means to obtain by begging, and from *precari*, which means to entreat. Dossey (1997) defined prayer as communication with the Absolute. A simple definition of prayer is the lifting up of the heart and soul to God or a Supreme Being.

Prayer and meditation (chapter 11) share many commonalities. Whereas the object of meditation is to focus attention on a word or an object so as to become more attentive and aware, the focus of prayer is on communication with a Higher Being. There are many forms of meditation and some of these, such as centering, incorporate prayer.

Many different types of prayer have been described in the literature. Table 12.1 provides a description of types of prayer that are commonly used. Prayer may be done on an individual basis, within a group, or as part of a faith or religious community. In the latter context, prayer often has prescribed words and rituals. However, this is not always true, as the Quaker prayer meeting does not use prescribed words. Prayer is unique to an individual in that each person establishes his or her relationship with the Absolute or Higher Being.

SCIENTIFIC BASIS

Some suggest that it is oxymoronic to explore the scientific basis of prayer because religion and science each have a different philosophical basis.

TABLE 12.1 Types of Prayer

Adoration or praise: acknowledging the greatness of a Higher Being
Colloquial: communicating informally with Higher Being
Directed: requesting a specific outcome
Intercessory: communicating with a Higher Being for another who has a need
Lamentation: communicating to a Higher Being during bereavement
Nondirected: requesting the best thing to occur in a given situation
Petition: asking a Higher Being for a personal request
Ritual: using set words and/or practices often within a specific religious faith
Thanksgiving: offering gratitude to a Higher Being for a request or gift received

However, studies have been conducted. Mueller, Plevak, and Rummans (2001) proposed a number of reasons persons experience positive results from religious involvement. Spiritual practices such as prayer engender positive emotions. These emotions in turn help to reduce a person's stress. Persons involved in religious experiences have been shown to have an enhanced immune function. Those with religious affiliations often have a support system that provides comfort and assistance. These suggestions are similar to those proposed by Dossey (1999). More studies are needed to validate these hypotheses.

Since the seminal research by Joyce and Welldon (1965), numerous studies on prayer have been conducted, and the findings from many of those studies support the benefits prayer has on health. Byrd (1997) randomized patients who were admitted to a critical care unit into a group that received intercessory prayer by Christians and a control group. All subjects agreed to be in the study and did not know to which group they were assigned. Findings showed that patients in the intercessory prayer group required less ventilatory assistance and fewer antibiotics and diuretics than did those in the control group. Harris and colleagues (1999) reported that patients in a coronary care unit who received inter- cessory prayer had an 11% reduction in critical care outcome scores, contrasted with a 4% reduction in the control group. In both of these studies, the length of hospital stay was not affected by prayer. In the MANTRA project conducted at Duke University (Mitchell & Krucoff, 1999), findings showed a 50% to 100% reduction in adverse outcomes in subjects undergoing cardiac catheterization who were prayed for com- pared with patients who had received the standard treatment without prayer.

Studies have also been conducted on the use of prayer for persons with chronic conditions. Sicher, Targ, Moore, and Smith (1998) found that the use of distant healing prayer with persons with AIDS resulted in the experimental group having a lower severity index after 6 months than subjects in the control group. Subjects in the prayer group showed improved mood; however, no differences in CD4+ counts were found between the two groups. O'Laire (1997) found positive differences on the measures of depression, self-esteem, or mood between persons in the control and the experimental group who received prayers.

Positive results from prayer have not been found in all of the reported studies. Walker, Tonigan, Miller, Comer, and Kahlich (1997) did not find any differences in alcohol consumption in chronic alcoholics between the group receiving intercessory prayer and the control group. In a review of studies on intercessory prayer, Roberts, Ahmed, and Hall (2000) con- cluded that the findings from their review provided no guidance to either uphold or refute the effects of intercessory prayer on health outcomes.

Likewise, Astin, Harkness, and Ernst (2000), in a review of distant healing interventions, found an average effect size of .25 in four studies that had used prayer as an intervention.

In the aforementioned studies, praying was done by persons other than the patients. A number of studies have documented the effectiveness of prayer as a coping strategy for patients themselves. Ai, Dunkle, Peterson, and Bolling (1998) found that patients who prayed following cardiac surgery had a significant decline in depression at one year compared to immediately after surgery and that they had less overall distress. The relationship between church attendance and health was examined by Strawbridge, Cohen, Shema, and Kaplan (1997). They found that people who frequently attended church had lower mortality rates than those who attended on an infrequent basis. Persons who went to church regularly also were more likely to engage in health-promoting behaviors such as exercising and not smoking.

How prayer works, whether intercessory on behalf of others or for oneself, is not known. Dossey (1999) has proposed that prayer is one of a number of nonlocal phenomena, that is, prayer is not constrained by space or time. The person praying does not have to be in proximity to the person being prayed for in order to be effective. A question also exists about whether the person being prayed for must believe in prayer or be receptive to it. In research studies, patients have given consent to be the recipients of prayers. However, in daily life, prayers are said for others without their knowledge. Roberts and colleagues (2000) noted that the understanding of prayer may be beyond our present scientific methods, and if the effects occur because of a Higher Being, determining the mechanism may be beyond our ability to prove or disprove the effects.

INTERVENTION

When prayer is discussed in terms of health, intercessory prayer (i.e., prayer for others or for self related to a particular problem) is often the type of prayer being used. Less attention has been given to exploring the impact of overall prayerfulness on the lives of individuals.

Assessment

Spiritual assessment should be part of a patient's health history obtained by nurses or other health professionals. Many spiritual assessments include information about the beliefs people hold, how they address the Higher Being, and settings and rituals that are important to them in order to pray. The spiritual assessment guide developed by O'Brien (1999, pp. 66–67) gathers information about belief in a Higher Being, religious practices, and spiritual contentment through agreement or disagreement with statements such as the following:

- I receive strength and comfort from my spiritual beliefs.

- My relationship with God is strengthened by personal prayer.

- I feel far away from God.

Findings from the spiritual assessment will guide the nurse in using prayer as an intervention. Times for discussing the use of prayer include when a diagnosis is given, when the person is fearful or anxious, before and after surgery, when giving birth, or at the end of life. Prayers of thanksgiving should not be forgotten in times of recovery or when the findings from a diagnostic test show no serious condition. Associated actions include providing an environment that will assist the person to pray; obtaining resources for the person; contacting a minister, rabbi, priest, or spiritual guide; or praying with the person if appropriate.

Increased attention is being paid to health professionals praying for their patients (Post, Puchalski, & Larson, 2000). Praying is closely linked to caring for a person. Praying for patients can be as simple as asking God (or the name you give to your Higher Being) to bless the patients and families you meet during the day, or it may be a short prayer as one enters a room. (We have little information about prayer dosage. Are long prayers better than short ones?) Remen (2000) commented that caring for the souls of our patients is as important as caring for their bodies.

Although prayer can be used outside of a religious context, knowledge about the beliefs and practices of the major religions is helpful. Such knowledge will help the nurse make patients feel comfortable in using practices that are part of their tradition and avoid proposing a prayer or ritual that may be offensive to the patient. Readers are referred to references such as *World Religions* (Bowker, 2003), which will provide them with information about religious traditions.

Technique

The form prayer takes should be the one the patient desires. If nurses feel comfortable doing so, they can ask if patients would like them to join them in praying. Reading scripture or from a holy book is one way to pray with a person. The nurse can also create an environment in which the person can pray. Many hospitals, nursing homes, and clinics have a chapel or room for prayer and meditation. Although the health status of many patients in acute care settings does not allow them to go to a chapel, family members may find peace and comfort in this space.

Patients with a religious affiliation may wish to use the formal prayers of their faith. For example, Christians may find the Lord's Prayer comforting. Patients of the Jewish faith may want to read the psalms or have them read to them, and Muslims may choose to read from the Qur'an (Koran). Giving praise to the four directions may be a prayer form people of Native American ancestry would like to use. Nurses need to respect whatever form or ritual the prayer takes. Table 12.2 provides short prayers from two faith traditions that were obtained from http://www.worldprayers.org. Numerous web sites provide prayers of many religions that can be used. For example, a web site containing Christian prayers and meditations for each day is http://www.sacredspace.ie.

Prayer circles or chains exist in many churches and groups. These provide a vehicle for intercessory prayer to be offered for a particular person or family. If nurses know about the existence of prayer circles,

TABLE 12.2   Examples of Prayers of Two Faith Groups

Muslim

O Allah, I supplicate you to grant me your Love
And the love of those who Love you
And the action that would lead me to win your Love
And make my love for you more dear to me
Than myself, my family, and cold refreshing water.

Hindu

From the point of Light within the Mind of God
Let light stream forth into the minds of men.
Let Light descend on Earth.
From the point of Love within the Heart of God
Let love stream forth into the hearts of men.
May Krishna return to Earth.
From the centre where the Will of God is known
Let purpose guide the little wills of men—
The purpose which the Masters know and serve.
From the centre which we call the race of men
Let the Plan of Love and Light work out
And may it seal the door where evil dwells.
Let Light and Love and Power restore the Plan on Earth.

From World prayers: http://www.worldprayers.org (Retrieved 11/15/04)

they could ask the patient or family members if they would like to have a group pray for them.

Measurement of Outcomes

The purpose for which prayer has been used will dictate what outcomes to measure. Because of the mind-body-spirit interaction, nurses may want to include more holistic elements than simply measurement of physiological or psychological status. For example, other indicators of effectiveness that could be pursued are the contentment of a person, overall well-being, and the person's relating that he or she is more at peace. The effect of prayer may be healing rather than curing an illness; this presents a challenge to Western measurement indices.

Precautions

Because of the highly personal nature of faith, spirituality, religious beliefs, and practices, it is important for nurses to assess both the prayer preferences of patients and their own personal beliefs and comfort with prayer. Knowledge about the beliefs and practices of other faith traditions is imperative in our pluralistic society. Used improperly, prayer may offend, awaken old antipathies, and make patients uncomfortable. Assessment and then offering possibilities are paramount.

Because prayer is to a Supreme Being and the "result" depends on what the Supreme Being determines is best for the person, the outcome is truly outside the realm of the person praying. When the outcome is not the one desired by the patient or family, the nurse must be careful not to use such platitudes as "God knows what is best," but rather provide comfort and support.

USES

Prayer has been used for persons with every type of illness, of all age groups, and from all cultures. Table 12.3 lists selected conditions for which studies on the use of prayer have been conducted. The literature also contains many anecdotal accounts about the efficacy of prayer. In a number of surveys, prayer has been found to be the most frequently used complementary therapy (Barnes, Powell-Griner, McFann, & Nahin, 2004; King & Pettigrew, 2004; Yeh, Eisenberg, Davis, & Phillips, 2002).

TABLE 12.3   Selected Studies Documenting the Effectiveness of Prayer

---

Addictive behaviors (Walker et al., 1997)

Cancer (Mcrviglia, 2002; VanderCreek, Rogers, & Lester, 1999)

Cardiac conditions (Ai et al., 1998; Harris et al., 1999)

Caregivers (Stolley, Buckwalter, & Koenig, 1999)

Depressive symptoms (Ellison, 1995)

Immunosufficiency syndrome (Sicher et al., 1998)

Post-stroke (Robinson-Smith, 2002)

Reduction of anxiety (Tloczynski & Fritzsch, 2002)

Renal transplantation (Martin & Sachse, 2002)

FUTURE RESEARCH

Prayer continues to be a frequently used complementary therapy. Conducting research on prayer, especially using randomized clinical trials, faces many challenges. The following are several areas in which research is needed:

1. Most of the reported studies have been from a Judeo-Christian perspective. Explorations on the impact of prayer on health outcomes need to reflect the many cultures and religions of the world.

2. Prayer has often been studied from the perspective of better health outcomes. Studies are needed that examine the impact of prayer on comfort, peace, and holistic healing. These latter studies are needed in persons with chronic illnesses or those approaching the end of life

3. What are methods that can be used to study prayer? How can scientific methods, if possible, be balanced with the philosophical basis of prayer?

REFERENCES

Ai, A. L., Dunkle, R. E., Peterson, C., & Bolling, S. F. (1998). The role of private prayer in psychological recovery among midlife and aged patients following heart surgery. *The Gerontologist, 38,* 591–601.

Astin, J. A., Harkness, E., & Ernst, E. (2000). The efficacy of "distant healing": A systematic review of randomized trials. *Annals of Internal Medicine, 132,* 903–910.

Barnes, P. M., Powell-Griner, E., McFann, K., & Nahin, R. L. (2004). Complementary and alternative medicine use among adults: United States, 2002. *Advance Data, 343*, 1–10.

Bowker, J. (2003). *World religions*. London: DK Publishing.

Byrd, R. C. (1997). Positive therapeutic effects of intercessory prayer in a coronary care unit population. *Southern Medical Journal, 81*, 826–829.

Dossey, L. (1997). The return of prayer. *Alternative Therapies in Health and Medicine, 3*, 10–17, 113–120.

Dossey, L. (1999). *Reinventing medicine*. New York: HarperSanFrancisco.

Dusek, J. A., Astin, J. A., Hibberd, P. L., & Krucoff, M.W. (2003). Healing prayer outcome studies. *Alternative Therapies in Health and Medicine, 9* (suppl), AA44–AA53.

Ellison, C. (1995). Race, religious involvement, and depressive symptomatology in a southeastern U.S. community. *Social Science and Medicine, 40*, 1561–1572.

Harris, W. S., Gowda, M., Kolb, J. W., Strychacz, C. P., Vacek, J. L., Jones, P. G., et al. (1999). A randomized, controlled trial of the effects of remote, intercessory prayer on outcomes in patients admitted to the coronary care unit. *Archives of Internal Medicine, 159*, 2273–2278.

Joyce, C. R., & Welldon, R. M. (1965). The objective efficacy of prayer. *Journal of Chronic Disease, 18*, 367–376.

King, M. O., & Pettigrew, A. C. (2004). Complementary and alternative therapy use by older adults in three ethnically diverse populations: A pilot study. *Geriatric Nursing 25*(1), 30–37.

Martin, J. C., & Sachse, D. S. (2002). Spirituality characteristics of women following renal transplantation. *Nephrology Nursing, 29*, 577–581.

McCaffrey, A. M., Eisenberg, D. M., Legedza, A. T., Davis, R. B., & Phillips, R. S. (2004). Prayer for health concerns: Results of a national survey on prevalence and patterns of use. *Archives of Internal Medicine, 16*, 858–862.

Merviglia, M. G. (2002). Prayer in people with cancer. *Cancer Nursing, 25*, 326–331.

Mitchell, W., & Krucoff, M. D. (1999). The MANTRA study project. *Alternative Therapies in Health and Medicine, 5*(3), 74–82.

Mueller, P. S., Plevak, D. J., & Rummans, T. A. (2001). Religious involvement, spirituality, and medicine: Implications for clinical practice. *Mayo Clinic Proceedings, 76*, 1225–1235.

National Center for Complementary/Alternative Medicine. Retrieved February 28, 2005, from http://www.nih.gov

O'Brien, M. E. (1999). *Spirituality in nursing: Standing on holy ground*. Sudbury, MA: Jones and Barlett.

O'Laire, S. (1997). An experimental study of the effects of distant, intercessory prayer on self-esteem, anxiety, and depression. *Alternative Therapies in Health and Medicine, 3*, 38–53.

Post, S. G., Puchalski, C. M., & Larson, D. B. (2000). Physicians and patient spirituality: Professional boundaries, competency, and ethics. *Annals of Internal Medicine, 132*, 578–583.

Remen, R. N. (2000). *My grandfather's blessings*. New York: Riverhead Books.

Roberts, L., Ahmed, I., & Hall, S. (2000). Intercessory prayer for the alleviation of ill health. *The Cochrane Library*, (3). (Update 2/23/00).

Robinson-Smith, G. (2002). Prayer after stroke: Its relationship to quality of life. *Journal of Holistic Nursing, 20*, 352–366.

Sacredspace. (2005). Retrieved from http://www.sacredspace.ie.

Sicher, F., Targ, E., Moore, D., & Smith, H. S. (1998). A randomized double-blind study of the effect of distant healing in a population with advanced AIDS: Report of a small scale study. *Western Journal of Medicine, 169*, 356–363.

Stolley, J. M., Buckwalter, K. C., & Koenig, H. G. (1999). Prayer and religious coping for caregivers of persons with Alzheimer's disease and related disorders. *American Journal of Alzheimer's Disease, 14*, 181–191.

Strawbridge, W. J., Cohen, R. D., Shema, S. J., & Kaplan, G. A. (1997). Frequent attendance at religious services and mortality over 28 years. *American Journal of Public Health, 87*, 957–961.

Tloczynski, J., & Fritzsch, S. (2002). Intercessory prayer in psychological well-being: using a multiple-baseline, across subjects design. *Psychological Reports, 91*, 731–741.

VanderCreek, L., Rogers, E., & Lester, J. (1999). Use of alternative therapies among breast cancer outpatients compared with the general population. *Alternative Therapies in Health and Medicine, 5*(1), 71–76.

Walker, S. R., Tonigan, J. S., Miller, W. R., Comer, S., & Kahlich, L. (1997). Intercessory prayer in the treatment of alcohol abuse and dependence: A pilot investigation. *Alternative Therapies in Health and Medicine, 3*, 79–85.

World prayers. Retrieved November 15, 2004, from http://www.worldprayers .org

Yeh, G. Y., Eisenberg, D. M., Davis, R. B., & Phillips, R. S. (2002). Use of complementary and alternative medicine among persons with diabetes mellitus: Results of a national survey. *American Journal of Public Health, 92*, 1648–1652.

CHAPTER 13

Storytelling

Roxanne Struthers*

All age groups engage in storytelling, a natural and common component of everyday conversation. It has been used for centuries as a powerful vehicle for communication (Koch, 1998). The ancient art of storytelling predated writing and was used by preliterate societies (Bowles, 1995). It is one of the oldest arts, having its roots in the beginning of articulate expression.

Stories are constructed to tell a tale, impart information to others, explain views, and share experiences. It is an intrinsic part of many cultures. African Americans make frequent use of storytelling (Banks-Wallace, 2002) and within our indigenous society storytelling takes precedence over written tradition (American Indian Research and Policy Institute, 1998). Representatives of many indigenous cultures argue that writing absolves individuals from remembering and therefore dilutes the complexity of knowledge that can be kept alive in any society (Thorne, 1993). The act of imparting oral knowledge and telling stories brings

---

*Dr. Roxanne Struthers, a leading nurse leader among Native Americans, died in December of 2005. We are privileged to have had Dr. Struthers as a contributor to the 4th and 5th editions. We extend our sympathy to her family and know that her memory will live on through her contributions to nursing among which is this chapter.

about a metaphysical presence and provides a natural, holistic, intuitive, and spiritual order to communication (Crazy Bull, 1997).

Storytelling serves multiple purposes across the life span and can be used by nurses. Nurses listen to stories whenever patients tell them what is going on in their lives and they tell and retell stories every time they pass on information about patients (Fairbairn & Carson, 2002). Whether we are the nursed or the nurse, we are the stories we tell (Sandelowski, 1994). It is in the unfolding, intertwining, and connecting that a story becomes my story, your story, our story. Stories are woven into the threads of life's fabric in our daily lives (Barton, 2004). We are all connected on a deeper, higher level and storytelling can take us to these levels.

DEFINITION

Storytelling depicts human memory and is an art and a science (Lawlis, 1995; Roberts, 1994). It involves an individual account of an event that creates a memorable picture in the mind of the listener (Kirkpatrick, Ford, & Castelloe, 1997). There are many forms of story, including the fairy tale, the legend, the personal incident, and the personal myth (Lawlis). Nevertheless, a factual or fictional story always has certain characteristics. William Labov, a sociolinguist, states that a complete story typically is composed of:

- an abstract—what the story is about
- an orientation—the "who, when, where, and what" of the story
- the complicating action—the "then-what-happened" part of the story
- the evaluation—the "so-what" of the story
- the resolution—the "what-finally-happened" portion of the story
- the coda—the signal a story is over
- the return to the present (Sandelowski, 1994, p. 25).

Margaret Newman (1994), a nurse theorist, defines stories or narratives as expressions of human consciousness and a means to expand this consciousness; thus, they help a person move toward the wholeness of health. Storytelling, as defined by Bowles (1995), is a descriptive medium by which personal experiences may be communicated to others with an immediacy and relevancy that can effect changes in the narrator as well as the audience. In other words, storytelling is an age-old healer.

Within the African American culture, storytelling is first and foremost about healing and nurturing through communion with the Great Spirit and one another; the collection and sharing of stories is considered sacred work (Banks-Wallace, 2002). According to an indigenous Canadian teacher, natural forms of indigenous healing include song, dance, ritual, and storytelling (C. Bird, personal communication, August 3, 2000). In indigenous healing workshops and retreats, storytelling is a major element used to assist with the healing process. Usually these storytelling sessions occur with the participants sitting in a talking circle, also known as a healing or sharing circle. According to Einhorn (2000), the circle is the most universally occurring shape; therefore, all healing ceremonies take place in a circle. The circle helps the person to gain insights about self and to tap into intuition. From this vantage point, process is crucial; the mind can exclaim with wonder and delight at what is revealed through the eyes of the heart, and intuitive knowledge discerns that things will occur when and how they are intended to happen.

SCIENTIFIC BASIS

Storytelling is regarded as an act or tool for prompting and influencing the health status of individuals and groups. Attributes of health that storytelling affects include (1) providing a connection to other people, (2) rendering a sense of connection between life events, (3) unlocking an opportunity for healing to occur, (4) helping to achieve the fullness of human potential, and (5) leading to an integrated sense of self (Sandelowski, 1994). Storytelling allows the person to gain perception about time; changes people's sense of place; articulates and stimulates strong emotions; helps resolve problems; facilitates change; and provides individuals with a forum for personal introspection in which to assess, understand, and change health-related behaviors (Banks-Wallace, 2002; Hodge, Pasqua, Marquez, & Geishirt-Cantrell, 2002; Sandelowski, 1991; Snyder, 1992). According to Lawlis (1995), anxiety is lowered in the listener, imagery is developed, relaxation ensues, pain may be relieved, and patients can become empowered. Nagai-Jacobson and Burkhardt (1996) state that storytelling can awaken spiritual forces and facilitate the release of energy, resulting in the healing of self and others. Students come alive when a teacher digresses and tells a story (Noddings, 1994). It is known that whenever an individual wants to provide an account of "what really happened," the natural impulse is to tell a story (Bowman, 1995) because stories depict what matters to people (Barton, 2004).

Although storytelling is utilized as a therapeutic and everyday tool across all ages, research on its effectiveness as a nursing intervention is in the beginning stages. In current qualitative and quantitative intervention research studies, various methods of storytelling have been used alone or in conjunction with other interventions, and there are multiple instruments to measure the effectiveness and outcomes that result.

Storytelling With Children

The therapeutic usefulness of storytelling with children has been explored in a number of studies. Walker (1988) used cartoon storytelling as one of several techniques to assess cognitive and behavioral coping strategies of siblings of pediatric cancer patients. Content analysis of the data revealed major stressor themes of loss, fear of death, and change among the siblings. In a descriptive correlation study, Collins (1991) used spontaneous storytelling to determine the stress levels in fourth graders. Differences were found in story themes among children with low, moderate, or high levels of stress. Werle (2004) used storytelling with middle-school students to explore the lived experience of violence. The students responded to the stories through a free writing style using open-ended questions as guides. School nurses may find storytelling helpful in violence prevention education programs.

Storytelling With Older Adults

Not only children benefit from storytelling. Lepp, Ringsberg, Holm, and Sellersjo (2003) conducted a pilot study among 12 elderly patients with moderate to severe dementia. Seven of their caregivers also participated in the research. Two groups received the intervention: one group focused on dance, rhythm, and songs familiar to this age group while the other group participated in storytelling. Quality of life improved in the drama and storytelling groups. Strickland (1996) used listening circles of 1¼ hours for four sessions in a nursing center. Each week, the residents shared personal stories, including much about "presence" and "caring" in the retirement community. Clark, Hanson, and Ross (2003) conducted focus groups among staff of a nursing home, community-dwelling older people, family caregivers, and practitioners to explore whether a biographical approach that incorporates storytelling can be used to enhance person-centered care. Findings revealed that life stories helped practitioners to see patients as people and to understand them more fully, and improved relationships with elders' families.

Storytelling Use in Hospice

Storytelling has been used with hospice patients and their families. Lehna (1999a) interviewed 4 mothers of sick children enrolled in hospice. Mothers used storytelling for two therapeutic purposes. This helped them to place the child in context of entire life. Telling stories helped them place the birth of their medically fragile children on a continuum connecting the time before their birth with the time after their birth and the life changes that occurred with diagnosis and/or birth. Telling the stories also helped the mothers understand and come to terms with their feelings. Storytelling provided this group of mothers with insight into their family's functioning and could be a powerful tool for health care providers.

Storytelling Use by African American and Native Indian Women

In a narrative analysis of 115 stories of women of African descent, Banks-Wallace (1998) found storytelling useful for learning more about the historical and contextual factors affecting the well-being of these women. The major functions storytelling served were: contextual grounding, bonding with others, validating and affirming experiences, venting and catharsis, resisting oppression, and educating others.

Rogers (2004) found storytelling at the heart of 11 Pacific Northwest African American widows, ages 55 and older, who described their experience of bereavement after their husbands' deaths. During the interviews, the widows took on various mannerisms and speech patterns of persons who were part of the story. These included changed tones, mimicking the voices of those involved, and use of hands, body language, and facial expressions. Nurses should be aware of storytelling as a means to gain in-depth understanding and cultural insight into African American experience.

Culturally appropriate communication methods, such as storytelling, have been found to be effective in health promotion activities. The talking circle is one format in which the art of storytelling occurs. Indigenous Ojibwa and Cree women healers use talking circles as instruments of healing and storytelling in their everyday traditional practice (Struthers, 1999). Studies have shown that the talking circle of American Indians can be used to promote health and convey health information. Using an experimental design, Hodge, Fredericks, and Rodriguez (1996) discovered that American Indian women responded favorably to the use of the talking circle, coupled with traditional stories, as a vehicle to disseminate cancer education and improve adherence to cancer screening. In another study, Hodge, Stubbs, Gurgin, and Fredericks (1998) also found that the talking circle was effective in teaching about cancer prevention. Storytelling was preferred as a natural pattern of communication for Yakima Indians to learn about health promotion related to cervical cancer prevention (Strickland, Squeoch, & Chrisman, 1999).

INTERVENTION

Inherent in each person's story is a key to healing (Roche, 1994), an opportunity for personal growth (Heiney, 1995), and the experience of interconnectedness while co-creating possibilities for change and growth (Milton, 2004). However, it is only within the past several decades in America and the Western world that telling one's personal story was recognized as a therapeutic healing modality (Sandelowski, 1994).

Techniques: How the Talking Circle Works

In a talking circle, participants sit in chairs placed in a circle in an environment that is conducive to healing; participants can number from 2 to 10, but groups of 5 to 10 are best. A facilitator opens the session by welcoming everyone and sharing a story. The information disclosed usually centers around a selected topic or reason for the talking circle. Then the circle is opened to all and each person is afforded the opportunity to talk. Typically, a feather, rock, or other item is passed from one participant to the next speaker, who holds the item while speaking. During this time, that particular person takes the lead and shares a story with the group. While the person is speaking, the facilitator and the other participants respect and support the person who is sharing the story by honoring that person, being present, and listening to the essence of the story. After each person has had a chance to contribute, the facilitator summarizes the events and the circle closes.

When one tells his or her story within a talking circle, several things happen simultaneously. A place is created where the following elements come together:

1. *A healing environment:* The first step necessary for healing to take place is to create an environment conducive to storytelling (Lindesmith & McWeeny, 1994). There can be no healing without an atmosphere conducive to it. Therefore, it is imperative that a comfortable physical environment be sought out, away from distractions. With chairs placed in a circle, participants can view each other and experience everyone's presence. The environment can be cleansed and kept clear with the assistance of purification rituals such as the use of candles, crystals, or feathers. In the Native American tradition sage, cedar, or sweet grass is commonly used for this purpose.

2. *Nonjudgment:* Individuals and groups must feel safe and supported in their surroundings (Bowman, 1995; Evans & Sev-

ertsen, 2001) in order to facilitate the healing process. We are often reluctant to reveal too much about ourselves because it makes us vulnerable. However, we cannot tell a story without self-disclosure (Kelly, 1995). Therefore, an atmosphere free from criticism, exploration, interpretation, or judgment must prevail and confidentiality must be assured.

3. *Listening:* It is of utmost importance that others listen to the story. Listening shows that one is valued as an individual (Clark et al., 2003; Koch, 1998). We need to cultivate the quality of listening carefully, patiently, attentively, and compassionately to other human beings while they tell their story. Simply put, this is caring enough about others to listen to what they have to say (Kelly, 1995) and to listen with one's heart (Heiney, 1995). While listening, we can let our imagination, our past experiences, and our various passions and problems help us form images to accompany the words we are hearing (Roberts, 1994).

4. *Spontaneity and creativity:* Storytelling requires no training or skill (Heiney, 1995). However, stories come alive when we let the story "lift and flow" and "laugh and cry" (Wilson, 1979, p. 3). Imagination, flexibility, and creativity flow forth naturally in storytelling (Kuhrik, 1995).

5. *Presence:* To be present is to consciously stay in the moment. Change takes place in the present, not in the past or in the future. When one is present in the moment, a state of non-interfering attention that allows natural healing to flow is generated (Dossey, Keegan, & Guzzetta, 2000). When a story is told, others can "settle into their bodies and become fully present" (Kimmel & Kazanis, 1995, p. 216).

6. *Empathy and caring:* Empathy is defined as "the action of understanding, being aware of, being sensitive to, and vicariously experiencing the feelings, thoughts, and experience of another . . . without having the feelings, thoughts, and experiences fully communicated in an objectively explicit manner" (Merriam-Webster, 1984, p. 407). Storytelling increases empathy (Heinrich, 1992). According to Diekelmann (1994/1995), as the story unfolds, participants in the narrative travel together to a place of intertwining where it is difficult to distinguish between the speaker and listeners. This sets up the possibility for one of us to dwell within the lived experience of another (Heinrich). To listen is to display caring, and caring is a factor Western society has a tendency to neglect.

7. *Community:* In the process of storytelling, a feeling of community is established. This feeling creates bonding or strengthening of intimate relationships with others like themselves and facilitates survival and well-being (Banks-Wallace, 1998). This sense of community decreases the invisibility and isolation of people (Heinrich, 1992). A feeling of belonging develops during the storytelling process that not only connects us to other people, but also connects us to higher truths (Heiney, 1995). This connection can be a liberating experience.

8. *Learning and sharing:* Learning occurs when stories are shared (Lindesmith & McWeeny, 1994) because storytelling provides a vehicle to share knowledge and wisdom (Banks-Wallace, 1998). According to Heiney (1995), part of this learning is becoming able to see things on many different levels through a prism. New perspectives may emerge as stories are told. In the process of storytelling, validation (Heinrich, 1992), recognition and self-knowledge (Kelly, 1995), and personal meaning develop. It is in these acknowledgments that the spirit evolves.

Measurement of Outcomes

A variety of tools can be used to measure outcomes of storytelling. Depending on the purpose for which storytelling is used, instruments that measure anxiety, depression, social isolation, spirituality, caring, and sense of well-being may be appropriate. Qualitative research methods may also be used to measure the effectiveness or changes brought about through storytelling.

Precautions

Those using storytelling need to be prepared to deal with the strong emotions stories may evoke. Health professionals should be ready to assist and support the participants, as diverse reactions can occur. A list of available resources to make referrals for follow-up may be helpful after the session ends. Only persons trained in psychotherapy should utilize storytelling with people who have psychological problems.

USES

Nurses can use storytelling in multiple situations across the life span for a variety of purposes. Stories can be used in family therapy and can assist members to tap into the flow of meaning of the past, present, and future, and help patients open up possibilities for making meaning and healing (Roberts, 1994). During storytelling, voices are found that become stronger and individualized and may be accompanied by visible signs of growth reflected in a straightening of the spine or release of tension (Kimmel & Kazanis, 1995). See Table 13.1 for storytelling uses in patient populations.

Stories can be used in self-help groups (Koch, 1998). Many 12-step self-help programs, such as Alcoholics Anonymous (AA), are based on storytelling (Davis & Jansen, 1998). Individuals tell about the development of their illness(es), identify how transformation occurs, and how subsequent recovery takes place. The stories people tell are powerful forms of communication both for themselves and others in AA (Davis & Jansen). Reach for Recovery for mastectomy patients is also based on a similar premise (Larkin & Zabourek, 1988).

FUTURE RESEARCH

Clearly, more research needs to be conducted to document storytelling as a proven therapeutic modality. Even though qualitative studies have

TABLE 13.1   Uses of Narrative Storytelling in Patient Populations

- To discover and uncover knowledge embedded in practice, recover the art of nursing, rediscover the "every-dayness" of nursing practice (Sandelowski, 1994; Walker, 1995), coordinate patient care, and prevent burnout (Lehna, 1999b).
- To enhance learning, professional development, and clinical practice among practicing nurses (Koch, 1998; Walker, 1995).
- To explain procedures, invoke hope, obtain information, resolve conflicts (Snyder, 1992), relieve tension (Kirkpatrick et al., 1997), and teach health behaviors (Lawlis, 1995) and morals and values (Kirkpatrick et al.).
- To frame healing encounters (Heiney, 1995; Struthers, 1999).
- To increase quality of care in long-term care settings (Heliker, 1999).
- To provide those in the storytelling relation with some distance from whatever threatens them when life is hard (Frank, 2000).
- To address diversity through understanding (Koch, 1998), assess cultural factors (Evans & Severtsen, 2001), and allow marginalized groups to have a voice (Koch, 1998).
- To help children master their feelings, act out unacceptable and/or fantasy feelings, support socialization (Lehna, 1999a).

been conducted that utilize storytelling to explore phenomena or to illuminate experiences in the discipline, storytelling must be viewed for its effect on patient outcomes. Examples of future research questions related to storytelling include the following:

1. Which are the characteristics of patients who benefit from storytelling?

2. How can nurses use storytelling to improve the quality of patient care?

3. How can stories assist in increasing identification of cultural factors, health behaviors, and health outcomes?

REFERENCES

American Indian Research and Policy Institute. (1998). *Reflections on traditional American Indian ways.* St. Paul, MN: Author.

Banks-Wallace, J. (1998). Emancipatory potential of storytelling in a group. *Image: Journal of Nursing Scholarship, 30*(1), 17–21.

Banks-Wallace, J. (2002). Talk that talk: Storytelling and analysis rooted in African American oral tradition. *Qualitative Health Research, 12*(3), 410–426.

Barton, S. S. (2004). Narrative inquiry: Locating Aboriginal epistemology in a relational methodology. *Journal of Advanced Nursing, 45*(5), 519–526.

Bowles, R. (1995). Storytelling: A search for meaning within nursing practice. *Nursing Education Today, 15*(5), 365–369.

Bowman, A. (1995). Teaching ethics: Telling stories. *Nursing Education Today, 15*(1), 33–38.

Clark, A., Hanson, E. J., & Ross, H. (2003). Seeing the person behind the patient: Enhancing the care of older people using a biographical approach. *Journal of Clinical Nursing, 12*(5), 697–706.

Collins, A. M. (1991). Perceived stress and stress projected into the spontaneous storytelling of two groups of fourth-grade children. *Journal of Child and Adolescent Psychiatric and Mental Health Nursing, 4*(3), 83–89.

Crazy Bull, C. (1997). A Native conversation about research and scholarship. *Tribal College: Journal of American Indian Higher Education, 9*(1), 17–23.

Davis, D. R., & Jansen, G. G. (1998). Making meaning of Alcoholics Anonymous for social workers: Myths, metaphors and realities. *Social Work, 43*(2), 169–182.

Diekelmann, N. (1994/1995, December/January). Sharing nursing work through stories. *Nursing New Zealand, 2*(11), 8.

Dossey, B. M., Keegan, L., & Guzzetta, C. E. (2000). *Holistic nursing: A handbook for practice* (3rd ed.). Gaithersburg, MD: Aspen.

Einhorn, L. J. (2000). *The Native American oral tradition: Voices of the spirit and soul.* Westport, CT: Praeger.

Evans, B. C., & Severtsen, B. M. (2001). Storytelling as a cultural assessment. *Nursing & Health Care Perspectives, 22*(4), 180–183.

Fairbairn, G. J., & Carson, A. M. (2002). Writing about nursing research: A storytelling approach. *Nurse Researcher, 10*(1), 7–14.

Frank, A. W. (2000). The standpoint of storyteller. *Qualitative Health Research, 19*(3), 354–365.

Heiney, S. P. (1995). The healing power of story. *Oncology Nursing Forum, 22*(6), 899–904.

Heinrich, K. L. (1992, March). Create a tradition: Teach nurses to share stories. *Journal of Nursing Education, 31*(3), 141–143.

Heliker, D. (1999). Transformation of story to practice: An innovative approach to long-term care. *Issues in Mental Health Nursing, 20*, 513–525.

Hodge, F. S., Fredericks, L., & Rodriguez, B. (1996). American Indian women's talking circle: A cervical cancer screening and prevention project. *Cancer (Suppl.), 78*(7), 1592–1597.

Hodge, F. S., Pasqua, A., Marquez, C. A., & Geishirt-Cantrell, B. (2002). Utilizing traditional storytelling to promote wellness in American Indian communities. *Journal of Transcultural Nursing, 13*(1), 6–11.

Hodge, F. S., Stubbs, H. A., Gurgin, V., & Fredericks, L. (1998). Cervical cancer screening: Knowledge, attitudes, and behavior of American Indian women. *Cancer (Suppl.), 83*(80), 1799–1802.

Kelly, B. (1995). Storytelling: A way of connecting. *Nursing Connections, 8*(4), 5–11.

Kimmel, E. B., & Kazanis, B. W. (1995). Explorations of the unrecognized spirituality of women's communion. *Women & Therapy, 16*(2–3), 215–227.

Kirkpatrick, M. K., Ford, S., & Castelloe, B. P. (1997). Storytelling: An approach to client-centered care. *Nurse Educator, 22*(2), 38–40.

Koch, T. (1998). Story telling: Is it really research? *Journal of Advanced Nursing, 28*(6), 1182–1190.

Kuhrik, M. (1995). Telling stories in the classroom. *Nurse Educator, 20*(5), 4–5.

Larkin, D. M., & Zabourek, R. P. (1988). Therapeutic storytelling and metaphors. *Holistic Nursing Practice, 2*(3), 45–53.

Lawlis, G. F. (1995). Storytelling as therapy: Implications for medicine. *Alternative Therapies in Health and Medicine, 1*(2), 40–45.

Lehna, C. (1999a). Storytelling in practice: Part one—mother's stories. *Journal of Hospice and Palliative Nursing, 1*(1), 21–25.

Lehna, C. (1999b). Storytelling in practice: Part two—professional storytelling. *Journal of Hospice and Palliative Nursing, 1*(1), 27–30.

Lepp, M., Ringsberg, K. C., Holm, A., & Sellersjo, G. (2003). Dementia—involving patients and their caregivers in a drama programme: The caregiver's experience. *Journal of Clinical Nursing, 12*(6), 873–881.

Lindesmith, K. A., & McWeeny, M. (1994, July/August). The power of storytelling. *The Journal of Continuing Education in Nursing, 25*(4), 186–187.

Merriam-Webster. (1984). *Merriam-Webster's New Collegiate Dictionary* (9th ed.). Springfield, MA: Author.

Milton, C. L. (2004). Stories: Implications for nursing ethics and respect for another. *Nursing Science Quarterly, 17*(3), 208–211.

Nagai-Jacobson, M., & Burkhardt, M. A. (1996, July). Viewing persons as stories: A perspective for holistic care. *Alternative Therapies in Health and Medicine, 2*(4), 54–58.

Newman, M. A. (1994). *Health as expanding consciousness.* New York: National League for Nursing.

Noddings, N. (1994). Learning to engage in moral dialogue. *Holistic Education Review, 7*(2), 5–11.

Roberts, J. (1994). *Tales and transformations: Stories in families and family therapy.* New York: Norton.

Roche, S. J. (1994). The story: A primary spiritual tool. *Health Progress, 75*(6), 60–63.

Rogers, L. S. (2004). Meaning of bereavement among older African American widows. *Geriatric Nursing, 25*(1), 10–16.

Sandelowski, M. (1991). Telling stories: Narrative approaches in qualitative research. *Image: Journal of Nursing Scholarship, 23*(3), 161–166.

Sandelowski, M. (1994). We are the stories we tell: Narrative knowing in nursing practice. *Journal of Holistic Nursing, 12*(1), 23–33.

Snyder, M. (1992). *Independent nursing interventions* (2nd ed.). Albany, NY: Delmar.

Strickland, C. J., Squeoch, M. D., & Chrisman, N. J. (1999). Health promotion in cervical cancer prevention among the Yakima Indian women of the Wa'Shat Longhouse. *Journal of Transcultural Nursing, 10*(3), 190–196.

Strickland, D. (1996). Applying Watson's theory for caring among elders. *Journal of Gerontological Nursing, 22*(7), 6–11.

Struthers, R. (1999). *The lived experience of Ojibwa and Cree women healers.* Unpublished dissertation, University of Minnesota, Minneapolis.

Thorne, S. (1993). Health belief systems in perspective. *Journal of Advanced Nursing, 18*, 1931–1941.

Walker, C. L. (1988). Stress and coping in siblings of childhood cancer patients. *Nursing Research, 37*(4), 208–212.

Walker, K. (1995). Nursing, narrativity and research: Toward a poetics and politics of orality. *Contemporary Nurse, 4*(4), 156–163.

Werle, G. D. (2004). The lived experience of violence: Using storytelling as a teaching tool with Middle School students. *The Journal of School Nursing, 20*(2), 81–87.

Wilson, J. B. (1979). *The story experience.* Metuchen, NJ: Scarecrow.

CHAPTER 14

Journaling

Mariah Snyder

Journal writing is one of a group of therapies that provide an opportunity for persons to reflect on and analyze their lives and the events and people surrounding them and to get in touch with their feelings. Reminiscence, life review, and storytelling are other interventions that utilize a similar scientific basis. Journal writing (journaling) requires the active involvement of the person in reflecting and analyzing his or her experiences.

Since the beginning of history, people have recorded the events of their lives, first in pictures and then in words. Libraries abound with volumes of personal journals, and countless others are stashed away in closets and attics. *Diary of a Young Girl* (Mooyaart, 1952), and *Markings* (Hammarskjold, 1964) are examples of journals that have had an impact on lives beyond that of the author. Journals provide a unique perspective on the thinking and struggles of individuals and on real life in a particular era. However, journaling as presented in this chapter will focus on writing for oneself and not for sharing with others via publication.

Although much anecdotal evidence exists about the beneficial effects of journaling, research on the use of journals is sparse. In nursing, studies have related primarily to journaling as an educational tool. Research by Pennebaker, a psychologist, and his colleagues provides evidence of the positive effects of journaling (Esterling, L'Abate, Murray, & Pennebaker, 1999; Pennebaker & Seagal, 1999; Petrie, Fontanilla, Thomas, Booth, &

Pennebaker, 2004). Although research on journaling is in the early stages of development, its pervasive use across the centuries and anecdotal accounts point to its value in promoting positive health outcomes.

DEFINITION

The terms *journal, diary,* and *writing* are often used interchangeably. Diaries focus on the recording of events and encounters whereas journals serve as a tool for recording the process of one's life (Baldwin, 1977). Events and experiences are noted in journals with emphasis placed on the person's reflections about these events and the personal meaning assigned to them. In journal writing, an interplay between the conscious and unconscious often occurs. Writing, another term, is used when the focus is on a theme or topic (Esterling et al., 1999). For example, people may be asked to write about their thoughts and feelings related to a specific stressful event in their lives. Poetry and stories are other forms that expressive writing may take. The term *journaling* will be used in this chapter to encompass writing for therapeutic purposes.

SCIENTIFIC BASIS

Journaling is a holistic therapy because it involves all aspects of a person: physical (muscular movements), mental (thought processes), emotional (getting in touch with feelings), and spiritual (finding meaning). Through journal recordings, people are able to connect with the continuity of their lives and thus enhance wholeness. Writing also assists persons in identifying unconscious ideas and emotions. Awareness of these is furthered when they reflect on specific events, thoughts, or feelings as they record them, link them with past feelings and meanings, and consider present and future implications.

Progoff (1975), a Jungian psychologist who developed a systematized method for journaling called the intensive journal, noted that this trans-psychological approach provided active strategies that enable persons to draw upon their inherent resources to become whole. Through journaling, Progoff maintained, people become more self-reliant as they develop their inner strengths and can use them when faced with problems and challenges such as stress or illness.

Journaling provides an opportunity for catharsis about highly emotional events (Pennebaker, 1997). Unlike merely venting feelings, journaling furnishes the avenue for a person to explore causes and solutions and to gain insights. A participant in a study by Pennebaker noted: "Although I have not talked with anyone about what I wrote, I was finally able to deal with it, work through the pain instead of trying to block it out. Now it doesn't hurt to think about it" (p. 38).

Inhibiting feelings about an event results in increased autonomic activity that often has long-lasting harmful effects on the body, such as hypertension. Therapies that assist in venting feelings may help to improve a person's health. Ulrich and Lutgendorf (2002) reported that students who journaled about cognitive and emotional aspects of a stressful event developed a greater awareness of the impact of the event as compared to students who wrote only about overall events. Further support for the efficacy of writing about traumatic events was documented in a second study in which persons with HIV infections journaled about emotional topics versus neutral topics; journaling about emotional topics resulted in a heightened immune function (Petrie et al., 2004). Spera, Buhrfeind, and Pennebaker (1994) found that 52% of persons in their study who had lost their jobs and engaged in journaling about the event had obtained employment after 8 months, compared to only 14% in the non-writing group and 24% in the group that wrote about superficial events.

Esterling and colleagues (1999) proposed three hypotheses for why journaling about a traumatic event may be helpful in bringing about positive physical and emotional outcomes:

1. Journaling allows the person to access multiple aspects of the event, including its significance and meaning.

2. Journaling makes the event more readily accessible. People can recall more of its dimensions, and as they deal with it over time, calling to mind the elements of the event becomes more automatic and thus less effort is needed to process information about the trauma.

3. Journaling transfers feelings into language. Applying a label to an emotion may help to reduce its intensity.

INTERVENTION

Techniques for journaling include free-flowing writing, topical or focused journaling, and creative writing. The period of time for which journaling is carried out (weeks, months, or years) will depend on its purpose. Sometimes people initially write during a specific stressful situation in their lives but become "hooked" and continue writing after the precipitating event has ended.

Some general guidelines for journaling or writing are found in Table 14.1. What is most important is for the person to be honest with him- or herself when writing. Knowing that the content is private and only to be shared if the writer so desires allows the person to write about very personal items. If one is required to share the entry, an internal monitor is activated that often censors what one will write.

Entries are made in a special notebook. This may be a fancy book purchased specifically for journaling or an inexpensive spiral notebook. Plain notebooks can be personalized by pasting pictures on the cover or using other artwork throughout the notebook. Because pencil recordings fade over time, a pen should be used as the person may want to re-read past entries. Some may prefer to use word processing for journaling. If this type of recording is done, strategies are needed to maintain privacy.

When and for how long to write are questions each person needs to answer. Establishing a specific time of day to make entries is helpful. Cameron (1992) suggested making entries in the early morning because it is easier to access the unconscious upon awakening. Many recommend making entries on a daily basis. The length of time devoted to journaling will vary. Pennebaker (1997) recommended 15 to 30 minutes. However, journaling needs to be the servant and not the master.

Techniques

Free-Flow Journaling

This is the most common type of journaling. Cameron (1992) describes it as "the act of moving the hand across the page and writing down

TABLE 14.1　Guidelines for Journaling

Date entries.

Write for 10–20 minutes each day.

Have a specific place to write that is private and where interruptions will not occur; you may wish to light a candle or play music.

Write with a pen.

Have a special notebook for writing.

Do not erase or black out words.

What you write is personal and you do not need to share what is written unless you wish to do so.

You may wish to personalize the journal with pictures, drawings, colored pens, and so forth.

---

whatever comes to mind. Nothing is too petty, too silly, too stupid, or too weird to be included" (p. 10). No attention is given to grammar, punctuation, or spelling. The main goal is to put one's thoughts and feelings on paper. Baldwin (1990) noted that flow writing is like the tip of the iceberg and allows us to begin to touch thoughts that are deep within us.

Dialogue Writing

Free-flow writing is like a monologue whereas dialogue journaling allows the person to view the situation or emotions from two perspectives. Dialogue writing may help individuals resolve conflicts and see the perspective of another person. This type of journaling can also be used for dialoguing with an event. Baldwin (1990) noted that in monologues we can avoid examining an issue whereas dialogue can get to the heart of the issue.

Using dialogue writing, one notes the question or issue and then proceeds to write from each perspective.

Me:	I am really upset that you did not show up for our walk.
Jane:	I just really forgot about it.
Me:	Forgot about it! I must not be that important in your life.
Jane:	You are, but there is so much going on now that I am having problems remembering.
Me:	Well, I was really teed off. Consider the time I have given to you when you needed to talk and last night was a time when I really needed to talk.
Jane:	What about?
Me:	Something that has been bugging me for a long time.

This written dialogue with Jane may open "Me" up to facing problems and exploring them and begin to see things from another's perspective.

Topical Journaling

This type of journaling focuses on a specific event or situation. The focus can be the person's illness or that of a family member. Journalers write about their feelings, how the illness will affect or has affected their lives, and fears they have about the treatment or outcome. Pennebaker has focused his research on using journaling to assist those dealing with trauma in their lives. They are instructed to consider multiple aspects of the event: who was involved, why they believe the event occurred, how it affected their lives, and the associated feelings. They just write, with no attention to the structure of what is written. No constraints are imposed.

Creative Writing

Some people may be more comfortable writing in story form or in poetry rather than focusing on specific events or emotions in their lives. This type of writing can assist persons to uncover deeper thoughts or emotions. Some may find that a picture or scene may help them focus on a topic. When they write about the picture or scene, inner feelings and thoughts come forth. Stories allow for feelings to emerge first in the people in the story and then in the self.

For those daunted by writing poetry, the Japanese forms of haiku or tanka may be used. Haiku consists of 17 syllables: lines of 5, 7, and 5 syllables (Haiku for People, 2004). Tanka poetry is an older form and consists of 31 syllables with lines of 5, 7, 5, 7, 7 syllables (American Tanka, 2004). One situation that comes up when using these poetry forms is that a person often needs to uncover new words of the appropriate syllabic length rather than using familiar words. These new words may reveal feelings the person has not previously considered.

Measurement of Outcomes

Many of the outcomes of journal writing may not be immediately discernable. Some of the possible areas to measure are improvement in self-esteem, reduction in anxiety, and acceptance of a chronic condition. Because journaling is very personal, it may be difficult for the nurse to evaluate specific outcomes, but patients doing journaling can report changes that have occurred.

Precautions

Fear that others will find and read journal entries is a common concern. This fear may prevent some persons from being completely open in expressing themselves. The heightened anxiety that the journal might be found may prevent unconscious thoughts from entering consciousness and thus decrease the efficacy of the intervention. Caution is needed in using journaling with those who are extremely introspective as the process may increase the turning inward.

USES

Journaling has been used to achieve a variety of outcomes. Table 14.2 lists some uses. One use is with people who are newly diagnosed with a chronic condition. Recording their perspectives may help them to uncover fears that could then be discussed with a health professional. Some fears may turn out to be unfounded. Journaling also provides an avenue for persons to increase knowledge about their own lives and to identify hidden resources or strengths that can be used in living with a chronic illness. Cameron (1992) urged people to provide positive affirmations to the self. Writing positive statements and then reading them may help them gain confidence in their ability to manage the chronic condition. Johnson and Kelly (1990) had patients with breast cancer use journaling to help them gain insights about their lives. Another group of researchers (Rancour & Brauer, 2003) used journaling to help patients with cancer adjust to changes in their body image.

Research and anecdotal evidence support the use of journaling to improve well-being. Runions (1984) instructed the mother of a seriously ill adolescent to keep a journal. She found that journaling helped her in coping with the stressful situation. Two authors (DiNapoli, 2004; Hall, 1990) used journaling with adolescents. DiNapoli found that journaling assisted adolescent girls with a smoking history to decrease their use of tobacco. Hall reported that journaling by high school students helped them identify their potential and develop techniques for managing conflict.

Although it is not specifically journaling, Storlie, Lind, and Viotti (2003) described the use of diaries in intensive care units. Nurses and families kept a record of the patients' stays. These were then used in a follow-up program to help patients gain an understanding of their time

TABLE 14.2   Uses of Journaling

Assisting with transitions (Spera et al., 1994)

Decreasing anxiety (L'Abate & Baggett, 1997; Ulrich & Lutgendorf, 2002)

Decreasing depression (L'Abate, Boyce, Frazier, & Russ, 1992)

Decreasing use of tobacco (DiNapoli, 2004)

Improving well-being (Booth, Petrie, & Pennebaker, 1997; Richards, Beal, Seagal, & Pennebaker, 2000)

Increasing creativity (Cameron, 1992)

Personal growth (Patton et al., 1997)

Spiritual growth (Chittister, 2004)

---

in the intensive care unit, including dreams and times when the patient was confused. The program has proved to be valuable for both patients and staff.

Journal writing has also been used extensively to help people develop spiritually (Baldwin, 1990; Writing the Journey, 2004). Growing spiritually requires reflection, and journaling is one intervention that will help people gain insight and discover new avenues to pursue. Chittister (2004) related how journaling on quotations or sayings of others helped her gain new perspectives.

FUTURE RESEARCH

Research on the efficacy of journaling is in its infancy. Few findings exist to guide clinicians in its use with patients. Several areas in which research is needed are as follows:

1. Identifying the characteristics of persons who will most benefit from journaling will assist health care workers to select persons for whom journaling may be helpful. Few of the studies on journaling have made reference to its use with minority groups, thus indicating that studies on use with these populations are needed.
2. Identification of outcome measures for journaling is needed. When and how should the measurements be made?
3. Studies using qualitative methodologies will help to identify the processes people use in journaling. Because a journal is private and to be shared only if the person so wishes, strategies are needed that will allow researchers to identify the topics or themes being recorded and how they relate to the outcomes.

REFERENCES

American Tanka. Retrieved October 11, 2004, from http://www.american tanka.com
Baldwin, C. (1977). *One to one*. New York: M. Evans.
Baldwin, C. (1990). *Life's companion*. New York: Bantam.
Booth, R. J., Petrie, K. J., & Pennebaker, J. W. (1997). Changes in circulating lymphocyte numbers following emotional disclosure: Evidence of buffering? *Stress Medicine, 13*, 23–29.
Cameron, J. (1992). *The artist's way*. New York: G. P. Putnam's Sons.
Chittister, J. (2004). *Called to question*. Oxford: Sheed & Ward.

DiNapoli, P. P. (2004). The lived experience of adolescent girls' relationship with tobacco. *Issues in Comprehensive Pediatric Nursing, 27*, 19–26.

Esterling, B. A., L'Abate, L., Murray, E. J., & Pennebaker, J. W. (1999). Empirical foundations for writing in prevention and psychotherapy: Mental and physical health outcomes. *Clinical Psychology Review, 19*, 79–96.

Haiku for People. Retrieved October 11, 2004, from http://www.toyomasu.com/haiku

Hall, E. G. (1990). Strategies for using journal writing in counseling gifted students. *The Gifted Child Today, 13*(4), 2–6.

Hammarskjold, D. (1964). *Markings.* London: Faber and Faber.

Johnson, J. B., & Kelly, A. W. (1990). A multifaceted rehabilitation program for women with cancer. *Oncology Nursing Forum, 17*, 691–695.

L'Abate, L., & Baggett, M. S. (1997). *Manual: Distance writing and computer assisted training in mental health.* Atlanta, GA: Institute for Life and Empowerment.

L'Abate, L., Boyce, J., Frazier, R., & Russ, D. (1992. Programmed writing: Research in progress. *Comprehensive Mental Health Care, 2*, 45–62.

Mooyaart, B. M. (trans.). (1952). *Diary of a young girl.* Garden City, NY: Doubleday.

Patton, J. G., Woods, S. J., Agarenzo, T., Brubaker, C. M., Metcalf, T., & Sherrer, L. (1997). Enhancing the clinical practicum through journal writing. *Journal of Nursing Education, 36*, 238–240.

Pennebaker, J. W. (1997). *Opening up: The healing power of expressing emotions.* New York: Guilford.

Pennebaker, J. W., & Seagal, J. D. (1999). Forming a story: The health benefits of a narrative. *Journal of Clinical Psychology, 55*, 1243–1254.

Petrie, K. J., Fontanilla, I., Thomas, M. G., Booth, R. J., & Pennebaker, J. W. (2004). Effect of written emotional expression on immune function in patients with human immunosufficiency virus infection: A randomized trial. *Psychosomatic Medicine, 66*, 272–275.

Progoff, I. (1975). *At a journal workshop.* New York: Dialogue House Library.

Rancour, P., & Brauer, K. (2003). Use of letter writing as a means of integrating body image: A case study. *Oncology Nursing Forum, 30*, 841–846.

Richards, J. M., Beal, W. E., Seagal, J. D., & Pennebaker, J. W. (2000). Effects of disclosure of traumatic events on illness behavior among psychiatric prison inmates. *Journal of Abnormal Psychology, 109*, 156–160.

Runions, J. (1984). The diary: A self-directed approach to coping with stress. *Canadian Nurse, 80*(5), 24–28.

Spera, S. P., Buhrfeind, E. D., & Pennebaker, J. W. (1994). Expressive writing and coping with job loss. *Academy of Management Journal, 37*, 722–733.

Storlie, S. L., Lind, R., & Viotti, I. (2003). Using diaries in intensive care: A method for following up patients. *Connect: The World of Critical Care Nursing, 2*(4), 103–108.

Ulrich, P. M., & Lutgendorf, S. K. (2002). Journaling about stressful events: Effects of cognitive processing and emotional expression. *Annals of Behavior Medicine, 24*, 244–250.

Writing the Journey. Retrieved October 11, 2004, from http://www.writingthejourney.com

CHAPTER 15

Animal-Assisted Therapy

Jennifer Jorgenson

Animal-assisted therapy (AAT) is grounded in research on the human–animal bond. Until recently this body of knowledge has been largely anecdotal, based on pet ownership and casual interactions between people and animals. Since the 1970s, research has begun to establish a link between animal companionship and improved health and well-being. The evolution of this research has promoted AAT as a therapeutic healing modality that can help promote physical, social, and psychological benefits. Today AAT has been implemented as an adjunctive therapy by nurses across the health care continuum in outpatient, acute care, and extended care facilities, as well as in all patient populations from pediatrics to geriatrics (Cole, 1999). It is important that nurses as advocates in the promotion of optimal holistic health care are aware of the role animals can play.

Throughout history animals have played a significant role in our customs, legends, and religions. Primitive people found that human–animal relationships were important to their very survival, and keeping pets was common in hunter-gatherer societies (National Institutes of Health [NIH], 1987). The process of domestication, which began more than 12,000 years ago, continues today as humans and domestic animals coexist, interact, and profoundly influence the shape of each other's social space (Young, 1985). National survey data on pet ownership indicate that approximately 58.9% of all U.S. households contain a companion animal (American Veterinary Medical Association, 1997).

The first recorded setting in which animals were used therapeutically was the York Retreat in England (Netting, Wilson, & New, 1987). Founded in 1792, the retreat kept small animals such as rabbits and poultry, which were cared for by psychiatric patients. The nursing establishment recognized the benefits of AAT early on. In 1860, Florence Nightingale observed that "a small pet is often an excellent companion for the sick, for long chronic cases especially" (Nightingale, 1860, p. 103). She suggested the use of a caged bird as the only pleasure an invalid confined for years to the same room might enjoy. The use of animals in a therapeutic setting began in the U.S. in 1944 at the Army Air Corps Convalescent Hospital at Pawling, New York. Patients recovering from war experiences were encouraged to work at the hospital's farm with hogs, cattle, horses, and poultry (NIH, 1987).

DEFINITION

AAT has had many names including pet-facilitated therapy, pet-assisted therapy, pet therapy, pet-oriented child psychotherapy, animal-facilitated therapy, animal-assisted activity, and animal visitation. These generic terms allude to programs that include visitation, attempts at milieu therapy, and animal-assisted psychotherapy (Berrisford, 1995). Today the terminology tends to differentiate between two distinct types of interventions: pet visitation and AAT.

The simplest use of animals in health care is pet visitation. This intervention is intended to foster rapport and initiate communication between therapists and patients. It is often effective in increasing patient responsiveness, giving patients a pleasurable experience, enhancing the treatment milieu, and helping to keep patients in touch with reality (Barba, 1995a). The animal initiates contact with patients, and the direction of the visit is determined by patients' needs at that particular time. Social interaction is often increased using the animal as a springboard for conversation. This therapeutic modality has demonstrated success in psychological counseling, as well as in long-term care facilities. Visitation may be provided by one or more animals and volunteer teams and may occur in individual or group settings. A variety of animals have been used favorably in this intervention including cats, rabbits, birds, and dogs.

By contrast, AAT is a goal-directed intervention in which an animal (usually a dog) that meets specific criteria is an integral part of the treatment process. This intervention, directed by a health or human-services provider, is designed to promote improvement in human physical, social, emotional, and cognitive functioning. AAT can be utilized in a variety of group or individual settings, often in acute care facilities, and is documented and evaluated (Delta Society, 1991). AAT exercises are purposeful, individually goal oriented, and can provide multiple benefits that include but are not limited to improvement in fine and gross motor skills; verbal, tactile, and auditory stimulation; verbalization skills; ambulating and equilibrium; following instructions and decision making; memory recall; and increased concentration and extended attention span. Often AAT interventions may occur during a visitation program, and the two terms are frequently used interchangeably.

SCIENTIFIC BASIS

Many theoretical frameworks support the use of AAT in health care. The most commonly cited is the social support theory (Barba, 1995b), which recognizes that buffers against stress are developed in relationships in which people gain a sense of security and a feeling of being needed. Using this framework, studies conducted with companion animals have demonstrated that animals promote well-being, health, and longevity and provide a source of relief, love, and companionship (Carmack, 1998). Willis (1997) applied Roy's Adaptation model to the extent that animals in the environment are factors that can influence adaptation and interdependence as a response. Studies by Calvert (1988) and Friedmann, Katcher, Lynch, and Thomas (1980) have supported the hypothesis that interaction between people and companion animals has a positive influence on loneliness. As early as 1965, family systems therapist Murray Bowen recognized the influence of animals in the dynamic family. Cain (1991) validated the notion that companion animals are often given "people-status," that pets can provide the emotional devotion that persons may be seeking from others, and that many family members believe that their pets are "tuned in" to their feelings.

The idea that human interactions with companion animals can result in physiological and psychological benefits is gradually gaining acceptance. Many research studies have indicated that people's health and well-being benefit from AAT. Table 15.1 lists research studies that support these conclusions in a variety of populations in a range of settings with many different types of interventions.

One of the first nursing studies to associate health benefits with animal contact was performed by Baun, Bergstrom, Langston, and Thoma (1983). Their study revealed a decrease in subjects' heart rate, respiratory

TABLE 15.1 Populations in Which Animals and Animal-Assisted Therapy Have Been Studied (Cole & Gawlinski, 1995)

Adolescents with special education needs (Cawley, Cawley, & Retter, 1994)

Adults in the community (Raina, Waltner-Toews, Bonnett, Woodward, & Abernathy, 1999; Sebkova, 1977)

Adult pet owners (Anderson, Reid, & Jennings, 1992; Serpell, 1991)

College students (Wilson, 1991)

Older persons in elder residences (Mugford & M'Comsky, 1975)

Older adult apartment residents (Riddick, 1985)

Heart patients (Friedmann et al., 1980; Friedmann, Katcher, Lynch, Thomas, & Messent, 1983; Friedmann & Thomas, 1995)

Hospice patients (Chinner & Dalziel, 1991)

Hospitalized psychiatric patients (Barker & Dawson, 1998)

Persons with Alzheimer's disease (Batson, McCabe, Baun, & Wilson, 1995; Kongable, Stolley, & Buckwalter, 1990)

Persons requiring wheelchair use (Allen & Blaskovich, 1966)

Pet-owning children (Triebenbacher, 1998)

Physically challenged school-aged children (Madder, Hart, & Bergin, 1989)

Women in prison

Older adults with dementia (Richeson, 2003)

Alzheimer patients with nutritional disparities (Edwards, 2002)

Elderly schizophrenic patients (Barak, Savorai, Majashev, & Beni, 2001)

---

rate, and blood pressure while petting a companion animal with which they had a bond. Allen (2002) conducted a trial of 30 men and 30 women and found a correlation between dog ownership and control of borderline hypertension. This study compared one group that adopted a dog from a shelter and those involved in a program of transcendental meditation. At the conclusion of the study it was demonstrated that the pet owners showed a significant reduction in resting and ambulatory blood pressure while at work. Those who practiced transcendental meditation showed no significant changes (Stanley-Hermanns & Miller, 2002).

Research conducted by Siegel (1990) suggested that pet ownership could influence physician utilization in older adults. Ownership of pets appeared to help these individuals in times of stress. The accumulation of stressful events was associated with increased physician contacts for respondents without pets; however, this association did not emerge for pet owners. Data revealed that owning a dog provided a stress buffer, whereas owning other types of pets did not. The advantages associated with dog ownership included the companionship functions of talking, spending more time outdoors, and having an increased sense of security.

An exciting study conducted by Heimlich (2001) attempted to provide a quantitative measure of the effects of animal-assisted therapy for severely disabled children. Although analysis of the data indicated a positive effect for all participants, no generalizations were made due to a number of confounding factors. Despite the lack of conclusive evidence, much was learned and tools for evaluation were developed.

More recently, Cole and Gawlinski (2000) explored the value of aquariums in promoting relaxation in patients awaiting heart transplants. Benefits included humanizing the hospital environment, and patients reported a sense of control in choosing feeding schedules and in performing the feeding ritual. Many patients described the fish as soothing and comforting at night. The aquariums also provided cognitive stimulation and became a bridge for communication among patients.

INTERVENTION

One of the newer and more exciting ways AAT has been utilized is in critical care settings. Several successful programs have been documented in the literature. Conner and Miller (2000) have implemented an extensive program at Trinity Mother Frances Health System in Tyler, Texas, as have Giuliano, Bloniasz, and Bell (1999) at Baystate Medical Center in Springfield, Massachusetts.

The author is involved in expanding an existing pet visitation program in pediatrics and rehabilitation at WakeMed Hospital to include the surgical intensive care unit (SICU). WakeMed is a 650-bed level-II trauma center with a nine-bed SICU located in Raleigh, North Carolina. The program was implemented in order to reduce patients' anxiety and stress, improve communication, aid in reality orientation, and provide a more humanistic environment.

The preparation for obtaining approval was fairly rigorous and involved many disciplines. Physicians were surveyed about their support for the program, staff in the SICU was educated, and the volunteer department was involved to refine the existing policies and protocols. An extensive literature search was performed, highlighting other successful programs around the country, and a final proposal was prepared and presented to the hospital's infection control committee. Approval was obtained for a 6-month pilot program. Next the actual volunteers and dog teams were oriented to the unit to ensure that the dogs and the volunteers would be comfortable in the ICU setting. Issues addressed were sights, smells, equipment, appearances of patients, and guidelines for prevention of disease transmission. The program was well received by patients and families as well as staff and physicians. During the first 6 months approximately 25 visits were provided, there were no untoward events, and the positive feedback was phenomenal. Because of the high degree of success initially generated, the program has evolved to include all of the adult intensive care units. There are approximately 21 canines in the program and there are 3 teams that visit the hospital each day (1 per shift) and weekend teams that come every other Saturday. Currently there are approximately 400 visits per month. Johnson (2005) states, "The visits are received very favorably by the patients, families and staff. It is as much a stress relief for the staff and families as it is for the patients. The patients will respond to the dogs, when they will not respond to the staff and other 'humans.' There has been no resistance to the expansion by physicians, families, staff or patients" (personal communication, February 8, 2005).

Guidelines

Policies and procedures were developed for pet visitation in the SICU at WakeMed. Visits in the unit were conducted twice a week, and each visit lasted approximately 20 minutes. These policies are unique to the facility, but may be viewed as general guidelines (Table 15.2).

Measurement of Outcomes

In the evaluation of AAT, there are frequent methodological limitations, often caused by the complexity of the subject area. Small sample sizes, failure to randomize subjects, and poor design are cited most often as the barriers to fully appreciating the results of many AAT studies (Brodie & Biley, 1999). Failure to correct and design appropriate studies will only slow the acceptance of AAT as a legitimate, research-based intervention.

Outcome measurements are assessed relative to the various types of interventions and their intended effects. To date, published material on AAT suggests that the human–animal bond could have positive effects on human physical, social, and psychological health. Brodie and Biley (1999) conducted a review of the literature on animal-induced health benefits and concluded that evidence exists to promote the use of AAT as a therapeutic intervention by nurses. Improvements in physical health included reduced risk of cardiac problems, lowered blood pressure, and

TABLE 15.2   Guidelines for Pet Visitation

Inclusion criteria for potential patients to receive pet visitation:

- Length of stay >72 hours
- Patient is awake and alert
- Patient is hemodynamically stable
- Patient meets the screening for exclusion criteria

Exclusion criteria: Any patients with the following diagnoses or conditions would be excluded from participating in a pet visitation:

- Fear of animals
- Any patient in the SICU with a documented allergy to dogs
- Pet visitation not supported by the attending physician
- Patient is diagnosed with any of the following:

  - Methicillin-resistant staphylococcus
  - Tuberculosis
  - Group A streptococcus
  - Hepatitis
  - Salmonella
  - Staphylococcus aureus
  - Ringworm
  - Shigella
  - Fever of unknown origin

- All patients in the SICU, who have been medically cleared and have guardian or patient permission, may participate in a pet visitation, unless otherwise ordered by the physician.
- Staff RNs in the SICU will be responsible to ask if patient/family members would like a pet visit. If they are agreeable, a note confirming verbal consent will be placed in the nursing notes.
- The charge RN will evaluate the unit acuity and level of activity to determine if a pet visitation is appropriate.
- The volunteer team will contact the charge RN for a list of appropriate patients prior to entering the unit.
- Prior to the visit, linen or bedding will be placed on the patient's bed as a barrier.
- The dog and the volunteer team will go directly to the appropriate room; once inside, the door will be closed with a sign posted outside to indicate that pet visitation is in progress.

better overall health. When AAT is employed, increased social interaction, happiness, and harmony appear elevated in the general population and in specific groups such as children, older adults, and those with disabilities. Decreased loneliness, improved morale, and increased levels of relaxation appear to be some of the psychological benefits.

Precautions

The strongest opposition to using AAT is found in acute care facilities. The major concern is the potential for transmitting disease. For this reason dogs are the most frequently used species as specific guidelines have been well established to ensure that the risk of disease transmission is minimized. The Delta Society (1991) and Therapet (Bernard, 1998) are two well-known programs that have developed standards for policy, protocol, and procedures that clearly outline the criteria for AAT visits. Protocols for the health and grooming of dogs are addressed, along with policies for patient selection and handler responsibilities. Dogs in the program are carefully screened by a veterinarian for any physical or behavioral problems. A primary concern is patient exposure to animal feces, saliva, blood, or parasites. Stool samples to screen for any enteric pathogens and parasites are taken from the dogs on entry to the program and on an ongoing basis thereafter. Patients and staff members must wash their hands after petting the dogs. In addition, the dogs never ride the elevators, thus avoiding encounters with people who may be allergic or phobic.

Dr. Sandra Wallace, an infectious disease specialist and chair of the infection control committee at Huntington Memorial Hospital, Pasadena, California, reports that thoroughly screened dogs in controlled programs can interact with hospital patients without transmitting zoonotic infections or serving as transient carriers of nosocomial pathogens. Huntington Memorial Hospital has been host to 3,281 dog visits to 1,690 patients over 5 years. In that time no zoonotic infections have been reported (Huntington Memorial Hospital, 1992). In addition, as of 2005, the WakeMed program reports no infection generated as a result of the pet visits.

Yamauchi and Olmsted (1996) have developed specific guidelines for AAT, which are presented in *APIC-Infection Control and Applied Epidemiology*. This comprehensive overview is an invaluable tool for creating policies for new or existing programs. It is noted that although the transmission of nosocomial infection associated with AAT programs is theoretically possible, there are no documented cases.

USES

In addition to the types of interventions already mentioned, the variety of ways and settings in which AAT can be used is almost limitless. One only has to be creative when designing this intervention. The following is a partial list of additional ways AAT can be utilized.

- "Hippotherapy," or horseback riding is used in a variety of ways to influence the physical and psychological well-being of a person with movement disorders. Specially trained physical and occupational therapists prescribe therapeutic riding to improve a patient's posture, balance, mobility, and function (NIH, 1987). Casady and Nichols-Larsen (2004) have performed a comprehensive study of the effect of hippotherapy on children with cerebral palsy. Positive improvement in functional motor performance was statistically significant.

- Porpoises and dolphins have helped autistic children become more responsive. A 1989 study demonstrated that dolphins, used as both stimulus and reinforcement, were 2 to 10 times more effective at increasing attention and language skills among children with mental disabilities than were other stimuli and reinforcements used in land-based classrooms (Nathanson & de Faria, 1993).

- Psychotherapy has utilized animals in an effort to decrease anxiety and open up the lines of communication. Often patients will more readily talk about painful experiences in their lives when they are petting a dog (Conner & Miller, 2000).

- Companion dogs have been used with great success for people who are blind and in recent years by those or are hearing impaired or using a wheelchair. Not only do service dogs provide for more independence and greater mobility, but the presence of a companion dog also creates a "magnet" effect that serves to increase the quantity and quality of attention directed toward those who are handicapped (Edney, 1992).

- Rehabilitation units in acute care facilities have begun to utilize AAT to increase motor skills through activities that challenge balance, fine and gross motor skills, and endurance; improve stress management and coping skills; improve cognitive function; and assist with adjusting to life changes (Jorgenson, 1997).

- Several prisons have recently begun limited trials in which inmates are given animals to raise for service programs or local shelters. These programs are carefully supervised. Pet visitation to inmates is also being used as a form of behavior modification (Connor & Miller, 2000).

FUTURE RESEARCH

Because the interventions available to AAT are virtually limitless, so too are the areas for further research. In critical care, the effect of therapy dogs on ventilatory weaning, pain medication requirements, length of stay, and body image are interesting areas for further research. Determining the most effective delivery aspects of AAT (i.e., timing and frequency of visits) and comparing AAT outcomes to other types of therapy should also be investigated. Finally, studies to determine cost effectiveness in improving recovery rates and long-term health benefits would substantially increase the acceptance of AAT.

Web Sites

Excellent information and resources can be found at:

- Delta Society, 580 Naches Avenue SW, Suite 101, Renton, WA 98055-2297 (425)226-7357, (800)869-6898 www.deltasociety .org.
- Therapet Animal Assisted Therapy Foundation, PO Box 1696, Whitehouse, TX 75791 (903)842-2150 www.therapet.com.

ACKNOWLEDGMENT

The author is grateful to Angie Bullock, RN, MSN, Nurse Manager, SICU, WakeMed, for her support in initiating the AAT program in the SICU. I am also grateful to Elizabeth VanHorn, RN, MSN, for her editorial help and encouragement throughout the project.

REFERENCES

Allen, K. (2002). Dog ownership and control of borderline hypertension: A controlled randomized trial. Delta Society: Retrieved from http://www.delta society.org

Allen, K. M., & Blaskovich, J. (1996). The value of service dogs for people with severe ambulatory disabilities. *Journal of the American Medical Association, 275,* 1001–1006.

American Veterinary Medical Association. (1997). *U.S. pet ownership & demographics sourcebook, 1997.* Schaumburg, IL: Center for Information Management.

Anderson, W. P., Reid, C. M., & Jennings, G. L. (1992). Pet ownership and risk factors for cardiovascular disease. *Medical Journal of Australia, 157,* 298–301.

Barak, Y., Savorai, O., Majashev, S., & Beni, A. (2001). Animal-assisted therapy for elderly schizophrenic patients: A one-year controlled trial. *American Journal of Geriatric Psychiatry, 9*(4), 439–442.

Barba, B. (1995a). The positive influence of animals: Animal-assisted therapy in acute care. *Clinical Nurse Specialist, 9*(4), 199–202.

Barba, B. (1995b). A critical review of research on the human-companion animal relationship 1988–1993. *Antrozoos, 8*(1), 9–15.

Barker, S. B., & Dawson, K. S. (1998). The effects of animal-assisted therapy on anxiety ratings of hospitalized psychiatric patients. *Psychiatric Service, 49,* 797–801.

Batson, K., McCabe, W., Baun, M. M., & Wilson, C. (1995). The effect of a therapy dog on socialization and physiologic indicators of stress in persons diagnosed with Alzheimer's disease. In C. C. Wilson & C. C. Turner (Eds.), *Companion animals in human health* (pp. 203–215). Thousand Oaks, CA: Sage.

Baun, M. M., Bergstrom, N., Langston, N. F., & Thoma, L. (1983). Physiological effects of human/companion animal bonding. *Nursing Research, 33*(3), 126–130.

Bernard, S. (1998). Animal assisted therapy: A guide for health care professionals and volunteers. Whitehouse, TX: Therapet. Retrieved from www.therapet.com

Berrisford, J. A. (1995). Implications of pet-facilitated therapy in palliative nursing. *International Journal of Palliative Nursing, 1,* 86–89.

Brodie, S. J., & Biley, F. C. (1999). An exploration of the potential benefits of pet-facilitated therapy. *Journal of Clinical Nursing, 8,* 329–337.

Cain, A. D. (1991). Pets and the family. *Holistic Nurse Practice, 5*(2), 58–63.

Calvert, M. (1988). Human-pet interaction and loneliness: A test of concepts from Roy's adaptation model. *Nursing Science Quarterly, 2*(4), 194–202.

Carmack, B. J. (1998). Companion animals: Social support for orthopedic clients. *Orthopedic Nursing, 33*(4), 701–711.

Casady, R. L., & Nichols-Larsen, D. S. (2004). The effect of hippotherapy on ten children with cerebral palsy. *Pediatric Physical Therapy, 16*(3), 165–172.

Cawley, R., Cawley, M. S., & Retter, M. (1994). Therapeutic horseback riding and self-concept in adolescents with special educational needs. *Anthrozoos, 7,* 129–134.

Chinner, T. L., & Dalziel, F. R. (1991). An exploratory study on the viability and efficacy of a pet-facilitated therapy project with a hospice. *Journal of Palliative Care, 7,* 13–20.

Cole, K. (1999). Animal-assisted therapy. In G. M. Bulechek & J. C. McCloskey (Eds.), *Nursing interventions: Effective nursing treatments* (3rd ed., pp. 508–519). Philadelphia: Saunders.

Cole, K. M., & Gawlinski, A. (1995). Animal-assisted therapy in the intensive care unit. *Nursing Clinics of North America, 30*(3), 529–537.

Cole, K. M., & Gawlinski, A. (2000). Animal-assisted therapy: The human-animal bond. *AACN Clinical Issues, 11*(1), 139–149.

Conner, K., & Miller, J. (2000). Animal-assisted therapy: An in-depth look. *Dimensions of Critical Care Nursing, 19*(3), 20–26.

Delta Society. (1991, February). Task force meeting of the standards committee. Renton, WA: Rowley Educational Consulting: Author.

Edney, A. T. B. (1992). Companion animals and human health. *Veterinary Record, 130*(4), 285–287.

Edwards, N. E. (2002). Animal-assisted therapy and nutrition in Alzheimer's disease. *Western Journal of Nursing Research, 24*(6), 697–712.

Friedmann, E., Katcher, A. H., Lynch, J. J., & Thomas, S. A. (1980). Animal companions and one-year survival of patients after discharge from a coronary care unit. *Public Health Reports, 95*(4), 307–312.

Friedmann, E., Katcher, A. H., Lynch, J. J., Thomas, S. A., & Messent, P. (1983). Social interaction and blood pressure: Influence of animal companions. *Journal of Mental Disorders, 171*, 461–465.

Friedmann, E., & Thomas, S. A. (1995). Pet ownership, social support, and one-year survival after acute myocardial infarction in the cardiac arrhythmia suppression trial (CAST). *American Journal of Cardiology, 76*, 1213–1217.

Giuliano, K. K., Bloniasz, E., & Bell, J. (1999). Implementation of a pet visitation program in critical care. *Critical Care Nurse, 19*(3), 43–50.

Heimlich, K. (2001). Animal-assisted therapy and the severely disabled child: A quantitative study. *Journal of Rehabilitation, 67*(4), 48–54.

Huntington Memorial Hospital. (1992, December). Patient's best friend? Hospital dogs raise spirits, not infection rates. *Hospital Infection Control.* Pasadena, CA: Interagency Communication: Author.

Jorgenson, J. (1997). Therapeutic use of companion animals in health care. *Image: Journal of Nursing Scholarship, 29*(3), 249–254.

Kongable, L. G., Stolley, J. M., & Buckwalter, K. C. (1990). Pet therapy for Alzheimer's patient: A survey. *Journal of Long-term Care Administration, 18*(3), 17–21.

Madder, B., Hart, L. A., & Bergin, B. (1989). Social acknowledgments for children with disabilities: Effects of service dogs. *Child Development, 60*(6), 1529–1534.

Mugford, R., & M'Comsky, J. (1975). Some recent work on the psychotherapeutic value of caged birds with old people. In R. Anderson (Ed.), *Pet animals and society* (pp. 54–65). London: Balliere Tindall.

Nathanson, D. E., & de Faria, S. (1993). Cognitive improvements to children in water with and without dolphins. *Anthrozoos 6*(1), 17–27.

National Institutes of Health. (1987). The health benefits of pets (1988-216-107). Washington, DC: U.S. Government Printing Office.

Netting, F. E., Wilson, C. C., & New, J. C. (1987). The human-animal bond: Implications for practice. *Social Work, 12*(1), 60–64.

Nightingale, F. (1860). *Notes on nursing.* New York: Dover, 1969.

Raina, P., Waltner-Toews, D., Bonnett, B., Woodward, C., & Abernathy, T. (1999). Influence of companion animals on the physical and psychological health of older people: An analysis of a one-year longitudinal study. *American Geriatric Society, 47*, 323–329.

Richeson, N. E. (2003). Effects of animal-assisted therapy on agitated behaviors and social interactions of older adults with dementia. *American Journal of Alzheimers Disorders and Other Dementias, 18*(6), 353–358.

Riddick, C. C. (1985). Health aquariums and the non-institutionalized elderly. In M. B. Sussman (Ed.), *Pets and the family* (pp. 163–172). New York: Haworth.

Sebkova, J. (1977). Anxiety levels as affected by the presence of a dog. Unpublished thesis, Lancaster, UK: University of Lancaster.

Serpell, J. (1991). Beneficial effects of pet ownership on some aspects of human health and behavior. *Journal of the Royal Society of Medicine, 84,* 717–720.

Siegel, J. M. (1990). Stressful life events and use of physician services among the elderly: The moderating role of pet ownership. *Journal of Personality and Social Psychology, 58*(6), 1081–1086.

Stanley-Hermanns, M., & Miller, J. (2002). Animal-assisted therapy: Domestic animals aren't merely pets. To some, they can be healers. *American Journal of Nursing, 102*(10), 69–76.

Triebenbacher, S. L. (1998). The relationship between attachment of companion animals and self-esteem: A developmental perspective. In C. C. Wilson & D. C. Turner (Eds.), *Companion animals in human health* (pp. 135–148). Thousand Oaks, CA: Sage.

Willis, D. A. (1997). Animal therapy. *Rehabilitation Nursing, 22*(2), 78–81.

Wilson, C. C. (1991). The pet as an anxiolytic intervention. *Journal of Nervous Disorders, 179,* 482–489.

Yamauchi, T., & Olmsted, R. N. (1996). Animal assisted therapy. In R. N. Olmsted (Ed.), *APIC infection control and applied epidemiology: Principles and practice* (pp. 1–5). St. Louis, MO: Mosby-Year Book.

Young, M. S. (1985). The evolution of domestic pets and companion animals. *The Veterinary Clinics of North America, 15*(2), 297–310.

PART III

Energy and Biofield Therapies

OVERVIEW

The classification of complementary/alternative therapies of the National Center for Complementary/Alternative Medicine combines biofield therapies and bioelectromagnetics into one category: energy therapies. These therapies focus on energy originating in or near the body and energy coming from other sources. The concept of energy and its use in healing is universal. Most cultures have a word to describe energy. Qi (pronounced chee) is a basic element of Traditional Chinese Medicine. The Japanese word is ki, whereas in India energy is prana, and in ancient Egypt it was called ankh. The Dakota Indians' word for energy is ton and the Lakota Indians call it waken.

Nurses have used energy therapies for many years. The most familiar is therapeutic touch, which Krieger described in the 1970s. Healing touch incorporates multiple therapies based on energy as a form of healing. The "touch" noted in these therapies may or may not involve actual physical touching of the body. Rather, the nurse or therapist seeks to bring energy into the patient or to balance the energy within the patient. Although persons other than nurses may administer these therapies, nurses continue to be the leaders in the use of and research on healing touch therapies.

Other energy therapies are less well known but are increasing in popularity. Some nurses have been educated in the administration of acupressure, the stimulation of pressure points of the body, from Traditional Chinese Medicine, in order to treat illness and promote health. Acupressure points can be used to decrease pain, nausea, and vomiting. Reflexology, the massage and stimulation of select parts of the body to promote the movement of energy to promote healing in targeted organs and tissues, is a therapy that has great potential for use by nurses. Reiki, originating in Japan, is another energy therapy that nurses are using to promote healing; energy is channeled through the practitioner to achieve healing of the total person.

A growing body of research is found on bioelectromagnetic therapies. A variety of therapies are based on the use of electromagnetic fields: pulsed fields, transcutaneous electrical nerve stimulation, low-energy emission therapy, and magnets. Magnets have been used to treat pain, especially back pain. Transcutaneous electrical nerve stimulation (TENS) likewise has been used to manage pain and to promote wound healing.

Establishing a scientific base to support the use of energy therapies has been challenging because many of the measurements and designs typically used in Western clinical trials can be difficult to apply when studying the effectiveness of energy therapies. It is difficult to observe energy, and some have questioned whether the effects are real or merely a placebo effect. However, strides have been made in developing techniques to measure energy. Nurse researchers can play a critical role in the ongoing research to document the efficacy of energy and biofield therapies.

CHAPTER 16

Magnet Therapy

Corjena K. Cheung

Magnets have been used for healing purposes for centuries in many countries such as China, Egypt, Greece, and India. It was mentioned in the oldest medical text ever found, the Yellow Emperor's *Classic of Internal Medicine* in 2000 BC as well as in the ancient Hindu scriptures, the *Vedas* (Whitaker & Adderly, 1998). Magnet therapy was popular in the United States in the 18th century. It was used for treating many ailments of the body, but with the introduction of antibiotics, cortisone, and other medications, magnet therapy lost its allure. Since the 1960s, there has been a resurgence of interest in magnet therapy by health professionals (Whitaker & Adderly). Currently, magnets have been marketed for a wide range of diseases and conditions such as soft tissue or muscle sprains, arthritis, respiratory problems, high blood pressure, circulatory problems, stress, and pain (National Center for Complementary and Alternative Medicine [NCCAM], 2000).

Today, energy healing remains a debatable subject in the scientific community. The scientific literature on magnet therapy, although it has conflicting findings in the limited studies, is slowing increasing. Scientists are trying to understand the healing power of magnets, and if, how, and why, magnets work on certain health problems.

DEFINITION

According to the classification of the National Center of Complementary and Alternative Medicine (NCCAM), magnet therapy is classified under the category of energy therapies. Energy therapies operate on the principle that health can be influenced by the subtle realignment of a person's "vital energy"—energy that is innate to all living beings and that, when disordered or blocked, theoretically creates disease (Kaptchuk, 1996).

Magnet therapy is the use of magnets that are applied to different parts of the body for specific therapeutic purposes. The term *magnet* comes from the legend of a Greek shepherd, Magnes, who about 2,500 years ago discovered mysterious iron deposits attracted to the nails of his sandals while walking in an area near Mount Ida in Turkey. These deposits, which were known to the ancients as lodestones or live-stones, are now known as magnetite (magnetic oxide, Fe_3O_4) (Macklis, 1993).

SCIENTIFIC BASIS

The existence of the earth's magnetic field as well as the body's own bioenergetic field is beyond all reasonable doubt. Magnet therapy is based on the premise that all living things exist in a magnetic field (the earth), and that the human body exists in and generates a magnetic field that has healing powers. For centuries, the effects of magnets and low-frequency electromagnetic fields on biological processes have been investigated and debated. The application of magnets is believed to restore the balance or flow of electromagnetic energy so as to restore health (Hinman, 2002). However, the mechanism of action is still not fully understood.

According to Oschman (1998), each of the great systems in the body—the musculoskeletal system, the digestive system, the circulatory system, the nervous system, the skin—is composed of connective tissues that have important roles in communication and regulation. The extracellular, cellular, and nuclear matrices throughout the body form an interconnected solid-state network of a "living matrix." Because the main structural components are helical piezo-electric semiconductors, the living matrix generates energetic vibrations, absorbs them from the environment, and conducts a variety of energetic signals from place to place. There are many energetic systems in the living body and many ways of influencing them. The western version of energy is similar to "Qi" in Traditional Chinese Medicine and "Prana" in Ayurveda.

Scientists suggest that magnetic fields can influence important biologic processes in the following ways: decrease the firing rate of certain neurons, particularly c-type chronic pain neurons; change the rate of enzyme-mediated reactions, which may play a role in inflammatory cascades and free radical generation; modulate intracellular signaling by affecting the functioning of calcium channels in cell membranes; and cause small changes in blood flow (Wolsko et al., 2004). The *Mayo Clinic Health Letter* reports that magnets may also work by blocking pain signals to the brain (Second Opinion, 1998). Yet another theory, the Hall effect, has been suggested. The Hall effect refers to positively and negatively charged ions in the bloodstream that become activated by a magnetic field and generate heat-causing vasoconstriction and an increased blood and oxygen supply to the affected area (Whitaker & Adderly, 1998).

INTERVENTION

Types of Therapeutic Magnets

A permanent magnet is either a natural or artificially made magnet that produces magnetic force by the movements of electrons in the atoms of the material that make up the magnet, such as iron or nickel. These materials can be ordered to all lie in one direction (referred to as "north" or "south"). Therefore one large magnetic field can be created where similar poles repel one another and opposing poles attract (Lawrence, Rosch, & Plowden, 1998). Permanent magnets can be unipolar (one pole of the magnet faces or touches the skin) or bipolar (both poles face or touch the skin, sometimes in repeating patterns).

There are a number of permanent magnets available commercially for therapeutic purposes in various shapes and forms. The three most common forms of permanent magnets are plastiform magnets, neodymium magnetic discs, and ceramic magnets. Plastiform magnets are flexible, rubberized magnetic rolls that can be wrapped around an affected extremity or lie along the full length of the spine. Neodymium magnetic discs are lightweight and can be used on the face and on various acupuncture points. Ceramic magnets can be made in any shape and size (Beattie, 2004). Typically, permanent magnets are placed directly on the skin or inside clothing or other materials that come into close contact with the body.

Electromagnets are magnets produced by electric current passing through a cylindrical coil of wire, also known as a time-varying magnetic field. The magnetic strength is directly proportional to the strength of the electric current. When the electric current is discontinued, the wire loses its magnetism. Pulsed electromagnetism is the process by which alternating electromagnetic fields are delivered in a time-varying manner. The electromagnetic field is primarily used in hospitals and clinics under the supervision of a health care provider. Medicare has recently announced the coverage of electromagnetic therapy for wound treatment (Medlearn Matters, 2004).

Two other electromagnets being used in clinical settings are Magnetic Molecular Energizer (MME) and Transcranial Magnetic Stimulation (TMS). They are considered experimental treatments, with ongoing studies being conducted to evaluate their efficacy. MME, which acts as a catalyst to improve chemical reactions occurring in the human body, is commonly used for neurological and neuromuscular ailments. TMS, a neurological technique for inducing motor movement by direct magnetic stimulation of the brain's motor cortex, is most often used as a diagnostic tool (NCCAM, 2000). TMS has been explored for treating depression in psychiatric settings (George et al., 1999).

Strength of Magnets

The strength of a magnet is measured in units referred to as gauss (G), which represents "the number of lines of magnetic force passing through an area of 1 square centimeter" (Whitaker & Adderly, 1998, p. 15). Currently, the earth's magnetic field is estimated to be about 0.5 G, whereas a refrigerator magnet ranges from 35–200 Gs. Magnets used for pain intervention usually measure from 300–5,000 Gs (Magnetic field therapy, 2003; Vallbona, Hazlewood, & Jurida, 1997). Manufacturers are not required to mark the strength of magnets on the magnets, so the G of a magnet can be checked against the weight a magnet can lift with a formula of 1 kg as equivalent to approximately 600 Gs. (Whitaker & Adderly). Although it is important to determine the correct strength of a magnet for a therapeutic effect, some practitioners believe that the right choice of polarity (north or south pole) is more crucial. However, the issue of the two poles remains controversial.

Methods and Duration of Application

Table 16.1 lists various ways in which magnets can be applied. Generally, it is safe to apply permanent magnets for a long period of time. The time of application largely depends on the type and nature of the disease, the age of the individual, and the strength of the magnet. It is thought that large magnets of more than 2,000 Gs should be used for short periods of time ranging from several seconds to about 60 minutes for one application (Beattie, 2004).

TABLE 16.1   Methods of Application of Magnets

Modes	Applications
Local	Magnets are placed directly on the skin over affected areas
Acu-Site	Local application with use of acupuncture points
General	Used for whole body or larger portion of the body ailments
Internal	Magnetic water (ionized water) is ingested
Remote	Wearing magnetic jewelry to treat an ailment remote from the point of application such as a magnetic necklace for stimulating the thymus to boost its own immune system

Measurement of Effectiveness

The type of measurement used to determine the effectiveness of a magnet therapy depends on the purpose for the intervention. A variety of outcome measures have been used. For instance, the progression of bone healing has been objectively measured by using X-rays, bone mineral density, and calcium content in bone. Pain relief or stress reduction has been measured by an individual's subjective report on a pain/stress rating scale. The improvement of a sleep disorder can be detected by using the Polysomnography, a diagnostic test that records a number of physiologic variables during sleep. Two objective measurements that have been used to indicate the change of magnetic field in the body are as follows:

1. The superconducting quantum interference device (SQUID), a sensitive magnetometer to map the magnetic fields around the human body, can be used to detect an increase or decrease of the biomagnetic field in the body (Oschman, 1997).

2. Kirlian photography is a tool that provides photographs, video, or computer images of energy flow. It introduces a high frequency, high voltage, ultra low current to the object being photographed. This influx of electrical energy amplifies as it travels through the object and makes visible the biological and energetic exchange (Cope, 1980).

USES

There are electromagnets that require professional administrations. Commercially available magnets exist in the form of wraps, belts, mattresses, and jewelry for the public for self-help treatments. Many people purchase magnets in stores or over the Internet to use on their own without consulting a health care provider. A 1999 survey indicated that the permanent magnet was the second most frequently used complementary and alternative medicine (CAM) therapy by arthritis patients (Rao et al., 1999). Table 16.2 lists conditions in which magnets have been used for treatment.

Health Conditions Treated With Magnetic Therapy

Pain

Although articles and books contain testimonials to support the efficacy of magnets on pain, there are only a few studies to support its use. Vallbona and colleagues (1997) reported that a single 45-minute treatment with 300 to 500 G bipolar magnets significantly reduced chronic pain in 50 postpoliomyelitis patients. Weintraub (1999) reported that magnetic foot insoles might be an effective way of relieving the pain of diabetic feet. However, a similar study (Caselli, Clark, Lazarus, Velez, & Venegas, 1997) showed that the placebo group reported better pain improvement in the heel (60%) than the subjects with magnetic insoles (58%). Brown, Parker, Ling, and Wan (2000) found that a majority of female patients with chronic refractory pelvic pain reported a 50% reduction in pain ratings after 4 weeks of treatment with pulsating magnets. Likewise, findings from a recent study on chronic knee pain indicated pain ratings, functional ratings, and gait speed improved significantly more in a magnet group than in a placebo group (Hinman, Ford, & Heyl, 2002). In a report of a pilot study, bipolar permanent magnets had no

TABLE 16.2   Conditions and Populations in Which Magnets Have Been Used

Bone and Wound Healing (Saltzman, Lightfoot, & Amendola, 2004; Szor & Topp, 1998)
Cancer (Raylman, Clavo, & Wahl, 1996)
Depression (George et al., 1999)
Improve Balance (Suomi & Koceja, 2001)
Inflammatory Disorders (Johnson, Waite, & Nindl, 2004; Wolsko et al., 2004)
Muscle Injury (Borsa & Liggett, 1998)
Neurological Disorder (Richards et al., 1997; Sandyk, 1999)
Pain (Hinman et al., 2002; Vallbona et al., 1997)
Growth in Pre-term Infants (Cody & Moran, 1999)

effect on subjects with chronic low back pain (Collacott, Zimmerman, White, & Rindone, 2000).

Inflammatory Disorder

Alfano and associates (2001) reported a significant decrease in pain and tender points and an increase in functional status in patients with fibromyalgia who had magnet therapy versus placebo and control groups. The study also found that unipolar mattress pads were more effective in reducing pain than bipolar pads. Colbert, Markov, Banerji, and Pilla (1999) also found significant improvement in pain and physical function in patients with fibromyalgia who slept for a 4-month period on a mattress pad containing 1100 G unidirectional magnets.

Wolsko and colleagues (2004) reported that magnets were significantly more effective in relieving knee pain in osteoarthritis patients in a treatment group than in those in a placebo group. In another study a significant decrease in pain, tenderness, and joint swelling was reported, along with improvements in the rheumatologist's global assessment of the disease activity in patients with osteoarthritis (Segal, Huston, Fuchs, Holcomb, & McLean, 1999). Although results of these studies are promising, their number is limited, and thus so are the generalizations that can be made about their use in improving inflammatory symptoms.

Wound/Bone Healing

Clinical tests have proven that pulsed electromagnetic field therapy will "jump-start" bone repair. Medical research has revealed that magnetic fields can activate a healing process even in patients who have suffered for as long as 40 years (Bassett, 1995). Because clinical trials have reported the absence of side effects, pulsating electromagnetic therapy for fracture "non-unions" was granted the "safe and effective" classification by the Food and Drug Administration (FDA) in 1979 (Horowitz, 2000). A case report of a chronic non-healing wound showed that the wound was healed 1 month after the application of magnet therapy over the wound dressing (Szor & Topp, 1998). A review article on PEMF in the treatment of bone fracture reported a success rate of 81% in bone healing among patients with ununited fractures (Bassett, 1995). However, a recent report indicated that PEMF, immobilization, and limited weightbearing did not promote healing in 19 post foot and ankle arthrodesis patients (Saltzman et al., 2004). More research is needed to support the use of magnet therapy in wound and bone healing.

Precautions

There are some precautions regarding the placement of magnets. Magnets should not be placed over (1) the heart as it may cause arrhythmia, (2) the carotid artery as it may cause lightheadedness and dizziness, (3) the stomach within 60 minutes after a meal as it may interfere with the normal contraction of the digestive tract, (4) any open wounds with active bleeding, or (5) any transdermal drug delivery system or patch as it may increase the amount of drug circulating in the body (Magnetic Field Therapy, 2003). Magnets should not be used with pregnant women or people with pacemakers or defibrillating regulators. Strong magnets are not recommended for small children.

RESEARCH QUESTIONS

Claims of magnet therapies vary greatly from promoting wound healing to growth of pre-term infants. However, findings from Western research are inconclusive. These findings could be attributed to the subjective nature of many of the outcome measures used, the inability to control the etiology and severity of the pathological condition, and variation in the types of magnets and treatment parameters. Furthermore, conducting controlled, scientific experiments on permanent magnet therapy is challenging because participants can notice if a metal device is magnetized or not. However, as there is little evidence that the application of magnets is harmful, it is reasonable to encourage the practice if a patient experiences symptom relief from their use, especially if they can reduce the patient's consumption of drugs. Continued efforts are needed to enhance our knowledge about the use of magnet therapy. Questions for further knowledge development include:

1. Why do magnets appear to be ineffective for some people?
2. What are the long-term effects of the use of magnets?
3. Which research methods are best for studying permanent magnet therapies?

WEB SITES

Advanced Magnetic Research Institute: www.amripa.com/
Biomagnetic Therapy; The science and history of using magnets to improve health: http://biomagnetictherapy.webwise-media.com/
Biomagnetic Therapy Association: www.biomagnetic.org/

REFERENCES

Alfano, A., Taylor, A., Foresman, P., Dunkl, P., McConnell, G., Conaway, M., et al. (2001). Static magnetic fields for treatment of fibromyalgia: A randomized controlled trial. *Journal of Alternative & Complementary Medicine, 7*(1), 53–64.

Bassett, C. (1995). Bioelectromagnetics in the service of medicine. In M. Blank (Ed.), *Electromagnetic fields: Biological interactions and mechanisms. Advances in chemistry series* (pp. 261–275). Washington, DC: American Chemical Society.

Beattie, A. (2004). *Magnet therapy.* New York: Barnes and Noble.

Borsa, P., & Liggett, C. (1998). Flexible magnets are not effective in decreasing pain perception and recovery time after muscle microinjury. *Journal of Athletic Training, 33*, 150–155.

Brown, C., Parker, N., Ling, F., & Wan, J. (2000). Effect of magnet on chronic pelvic pain. *Obstetric & Gynecology, 1*(95), S29.

Caselli, M., Clark, N., Lazarus, S., Velez, Z., & Venegas, L. (1997). Evaluation of magnetic foil and PPT insoles in the treatment of heel pain. *Journal of the American Podiatry Medical Association, 87*(1), 11–16.

Cody, D., & Moran, J. (1999). Use of biomagnetic therapy to encourage growth in preterm neonates. *Neonatal Network–Journal of Neonatal Nursing, 18*(6), 63–64.

Colbert, A., Markov, M., Banerji, M., & Pilla, A. (1999). Magnetic mattress pad use in patients with fibromyalgia: A randomized double-blind study. *Journal of Back and Musculoskeletal Rehabilitation, 13*, 19–31.

Collacott, E., Zimmerman, J., White, D., & Rindone, J. (2000). Bipolar permanent magnets for the treatment of chronic low back pain: A pilot study. *Journal of the American Medical Association, 283*(10), 1322–1325.

Cope, F. (1980). Magnetoelectric charge states of matter-energy. A second approximation. Part VII. *Physiological Chemistry & Physics, 12*(4), 349–355.

George, M., Nahas, Z., Kozel, F., Goldman, J., Molloy, M., & Oliver, N. (1999). Improvement of depression following transcranial magnetic stimulation. *Current Psychiatry Reports, 1*(2), 114–124.

Hinman, M. (2002). Therapeutic use of magnets: A review of recent research. *Physical Therapy Review, 7*(1), 33–43.

Hinman, M., Ford, J., & Heyl, H. (2002). Effects of static magnets on chronic knee pain and physical function: A double-blind study. *Alternative Therapies in Health & Medicine, 8*(4), 50–55.

Horowitz, S. (2000). Update on magnet therapy. *Alternative and Complementary Therapies, 12*, 325–330.

Johnson, M., Waite, L., & Nindl, G. (2004). Noninvasive treatment of inflammation using electromagnetic fields: Current and emerging therapeutic potential. *Biomedical Sciences Instrumentation, 40*, 469–474.

Kaptchuk, T. (1996). Historical context of the concept of vitalism in complementary and alternative medicine. In M. Micozzi (Ed.), *Fundamentals of complementary and alternative medicine* (p. 35). New York: Churchill Livingstone.

Lawrence, R., Rosch, P., & Plowden, J. (1998). *Magnet therapy: The pain cure alternative.* Roseville, CA: Prima.

Macklis, R. (1993). Magnetic healing, quackery, and the debate about the health effects of electromagnetic fields. *Annals of Internal Medicine, 18*(5), 376–382.

Magnetic field therapy. (2003). Retrieved January 20, 2005, from http://www.chclibrary.org/micromed/00055750.html

Medlearn Matters. (2004). Electrical stimulation and electromagnetic therapy for the treatment of wounds. Retrieved January 20, 1995, from http://www.cms.hhs.gov/medlearn/matters/mmarticles/2004/mm3149.pdf

National Center for Complementary and Alternative Medicine. (2000). Questions and answers about using magnets to treat pain. Retrieved January 20, 2005, from http://www.nccam.nih.gov/health/magnet/magnet.htm

Oschman, J. (1997). What is healing energy? Part 2: Measuring the field of life energy. *Journal of Bodywork & Movement Therapies, 1*(2), 117–121.

Oschman, J. (1998). What is healing energy? Part 6: Conclusions: Is energy medicine the medicine of the future? *Journal of Bodywork & Movement Therapies, 2*(1), 46–59.

Rao, J., Mihaliak, K., Kroenke, K., Bradley, J., Tierney, W., & Weinberger, M. (1999). Use of complementary therapies for arthritis among patients of rheumatologists. *Annals of Internal Medicine, 131*(6), 409–416.

Raylman, R., Clavo, A., & Wahl, R. (1996). Exposure to strong static magnetic field slows the growth of human CA cells in vitro. *Bioelectromagnetics, 17*(5), 358–363.

Richards, T., Lappin, M., Acosta-Urquidi, J., Kraft, G., Heide, A., Lawrie, F., et al. (1997). Double-blind study of pulsing magnetic field effects on multiple sclerosis. *Journal of Alternative & Complementary Medicine, 3*(1), 21–29.

Saltzman, C., Lightfoot, A., & Amendola, A. (2004). PEMF as treatment for delayed healing of foot and ankle arthrodesis. *Foot and Ankle International, 25*(11), 771–773.

Sandyk, R. (1999). Treatment with AC pulsed electromagnetic fields improves olfactory function in Parkinson's disease. *International Journal of Neuroscience, 97*(3–4), 225–233.

Second opinion. (1998, August). *Mayo Clinic Health Letter, 16*(8), 8.

Segal, N., Huston, J., Fuchs, H., Holcomb, R., & McLean, M. (1999). Efficacy of a static magnetic device against knee pain associated with inflammatory arthritis. *Journal of Clinical Rheumatology, 5*, 302–305.

Suomi, R., & Koceja, D. (2001). Effect of magnetic insoles on postural sway measures in men and women during a static balance test. *Perceptual & Motor Skills, 92*(2), 469–476.

Szor, J., & Topp, R. (1998). Use of magnet therapy to heal an abdominal wound: A case study. *Ostomy Wound Management, 44*(5), 24–29.

Vallbona, C., Hazlewood, C., & Jurida, G. (1997). Response of pain to static magnetic fields in postpolio patients: A double-blind pilot study. *Archives of Physical Medicine & Rehabilitation, 78*(11), 1200–1203.

Weintraub, M. (1999). Alternative medicine. Magnetic biostimulation in painful diabetic peripheral neuropathy: A novel intervention. *American Journal of Pain Management, 9*, 8–17.

Whitaker, J., & Adderly, B. (1998). *The pain breakthrough: The power of magnet.* Toronto, Canada: Little, Brown.

Wolsko, P., Eisenberg, D., Simon, L., Davis, R., Walleczek, J., Mayo-Smith, M., et al. (2004). Double-blind placebo-controlled trial of static magnets for the treatment of OA of the knee. *Alternative Therapies in Health & Medicine, 10*(2), 36–43.

CHAPTER 17

Healing Touch

Alexa W. Umbreit

All cultures, both ancient and modern, have developed some form of touch therapy as part of their desire to heal and care for one another. The oldest written evidence of the use of touch to enhance healing comes from China more than 5,000 years ago (Dossey, Keegan, Guzzetta, & Kolkmeier, 1995; Hover-Kramer, Mentgen, & Scandrett-Hibdon, 1996; Krieger, 1979). This therapeutic use of the hands has been passed on from generation to generation as a tool for healing. However, there have been philosophical and cultural differences that have influenced the way touch has been used throughout the world. The Eastern viewpoint has based its touch healing practices on energy channels (called meridians), energy fields (auras), and energy centers (chakras). Expert practitioners in energetic touch therapies use their hands to influence this flow of energy to promote balance and healing. The Western viewpoint focuses on physiological changes that occur at the cellular level from touch therapies that are believed to influence healing. A blending of both Eastern and Western techniques has led to an explosion of a wide variety of touch therapies (Dossey et al.). Nursing has used touch throughout its history and today's nurses are integrating many touch techniques into their practice. One of these therapies is Healing Touch, which now has more than 80,000 participants who have been trained during the past 15 years.

DEFINITION

Healing Touch (HT) is a type of complementary therapy that uses gentle energy-based techniques to influence and support the human energy system within the body (energy centers) and surrounding the body (energy fields) (Healing Touch International, 2005). Based on a holistic view of health and illness, HT focuses on creating an energetic balance of the whole body at the physical, emotional, mental, and spiritual levels rather than on a dysfunctional part. Through this process of balancing the energy system and therefore opening up energy blockages, an environment is created that is conducive to self-healing. Through the interaction of the energy fields between practitioner and client, the use of the HT practitioner's hands, an intention focusing on the client's highest good, and a centering process, non-invasive HT techniques specific for the client's needs are used to create this energetic balance (Umbreit, 2000). Krieger (1979) describes the centering process as a meditation in which one eliminates all distractions and concentrates on that place of quietude within which one can feel truly integrated, unified, and focused. Finding this "place of quietude within" is achieved by many through deep belly breathing, prayer, meditation, or any other technique that slows one down, calms the mind, and accesses a deeper spirit of compassion and strength. To be centered is to be fully present with another person or situation, with heart and mind, deeper feelings, and thoughts. The centered state of mind is maintained throughout the HT treatment.

Umbreit (2000) describes the role of the HT practitioner as observation, assessment, and repatterning of the client's energy field because it is disrupted when there is disease, illness, psychological stressors, and pain. Practitioners describe these disruptions in the energy field as blockages, leaks, imbalances, or congestion. The goal of the HT practitioner is to open up these blockages, seal the leaks, rebalance the energy field to symmetry, and release congestion.

The HT program, started in 1989 and endorsed by the American Holistic Nurses' Association, involves a formal educational program that teaches techniques including interventions described by Brugh Joy (1979), concepts presented by Rosalyn Bruyere (1989) and Barbara Brennan (1986), and original techniques developed by the founder of the healing touch program, Janet Mentgen, and her students (Scandrett-Hibdon, 1996). The six-level HT educational program in energy-based practice moves from beginning to advanced practice, certification, and instructor level. Advanced practice requires at least 105 hours of workshop instruction plus a 1-year course of study, as well as work in case studies, mentoring, ethics, client–practitioner relationships, establishment of a practice, and integration of activities within the health community (Healing Touch International, 2005). After this, students may apply for certification. Instructor status requires more education and mentoring. The HT course work is open to nurses, physicians, body therapists, counselors, psychotherapists, other health care professionals, and individuals desiring an in-depth understanding and practice of healing work using energy based concepts (Mentgen, 2003). Six thousand HT workshops have been taught over the past 15 years.

SCIENTIFIC BASIS

Nursing has long described the profession as dedicated to the art and science of human caring. Rogers (1990) and Watson (1985) have written extensively about caring as a central quality of the nursing profession, along with nursing's concern for the promotion of health and well-being, taking into account the individual's constant interaction with the environment. It was this concern that led nurse theorist Rogers to develop her concepts of the nature of individuals as energy fields in constant interplay with the surrounding environment (Hover-Kramer et al., 1996). The most concentrated part of the energy field is the physical body, but it also extends beyond the level of the skin, imperceptible to the untrained senses (Wright, 1987). Simply stated, Rogers' theoretical framework emphasizes that every living thing is composed of energy, and that living things are continually, simultaneously, and mutually exchanging energy with each other, striving toward the goal of balance and universal order (Sayre-Adams, 1994). Using the hands, intention, and centering, the HT practitioner assesses the client's energy field and helps direct it to a more open, symmetrical pattern that enhances the client's ability to self-heal. Results of scientific studies on energy-based healing, as initially researched in therapeutic touch, indicate that healers can interact with energy fields even without actually touching the client (Fedoruk, 1984; Keller & Bzdek, 1986; Quinn, 1984; Wirth, Richardson, Eidelman, & O'Malley, 1993). These findings support Rogers' concept that humans and environment are energy fields constantly interacting (Miller, 1979). However, it is still not clear how the energy of a practitioner balances the energy patterns of a recipient or how recipients utilize the energy to enhance their self-healing processes (Egan, 1998), but the effect of energy-based healing interactions are measurable and significant (Hover-Kramer, 2002). The fields of physics, engineering, biology, and physiology continue to research this area of energy exchange in an attempt to explain what occurs during an energetic interaction (Forbes, Rust, & Becker, 2004; Oschman,

2000; Stouffer, Kaiser, Pitman, & Rolf, 1998). Oschman reports that various energy therapies (including complementary therapies and those approved by current medical practice) actually stimulate tissue healing by the production of pulsating magnetic fields that induce currents to flow within the body's tissue. A superconducting quantum interference device (SQUID) has been used for more than 20 years to measure these biomagnetic fields emanating from the hands of energy field practitioners who use therapeutic touch, qi gong, yoga, and meditation. Motoyama (1997), a Japanese physicist, has developed electrode devices that measure the human bioelectrical field at different distances from the body (Hover-Kramer, 2002). Infrared energy (heat) and other forms of energy yet unnamed from the interaction of energy fields between practitioner and client may also affect the healing process.

This concept of energy systems as part of the human interactive environment and healing has been part of many cultures for centuries. Ancient East Indian traditions speak of a universal energy (prana) that flows and activates the life force (kundalini) (Hover-Kramer et al., 1996). In China, Japan, and Thailand, the basic life energy is called chi, qi, or ki. The Egyptians called it ankh and the Polynesians refer to it as mana. Multiple other cultures throughout the world have equivalent terms for describing human energies (Hover-Kramer, 2002). The belief is that an imbalance in this energy force can result in illness.

It is unknown precisely how symptoms are managed by HT interventions. What have been observed are changes in outcomes being measured in the nursing research. It may be postulated that because energy fields are in constant interaction within and outside the physical body, internal mechanisms are stimulated by this movement of energy (Umbreit, 2000). Studies specific to HT interventions and biological markers are limited by weak findings (Merritt, 1998; Stouffer, Duennes, & Pitman, 2000; Wilkinson, 2002; Wilkinson et al., 2002), due to the fact that HT research is in the early stages of development. However, over the past 30 years, most published studies of touch energy therapies have focused on the therapeutic touch technique in which changes in some internal mechanisms have been observed (Krieger, 1976; Krieger, Peper, & Ancoli, 1979; Olson, Sneed, Bonadonna, Ratliff, & Dias, 1992; Quinn & Strelkauskas, 1993; Wirth, Chang, Eidelman, & Paxton, 1996; Wirth et al., 1993), indicating that physiologic changes at the cellular level can be affected by working with the body's energy fields. Studies specific to other HT interventions and physiological changes are currently in process (Healing Touch International, Inc., 2004).

What has been reported in the HT literature is managing the symptoms of pain and anxiety; decreasing the side effects of cancer treatments;

promoting faster post-procedural recovery; improving mental health; using HT with the elderly to improve pain, appetite, sleep, behavior patterns, and functional abilities; increasing relaxation; and promoting a sense of well-being (Bulbrook, 2000; Cook, Guerrerio, & Slater, 2004; Geddes, 2002; Healing Touch International, Inc., 2004; Hutchison, 1999; Krucoff et al., 2001; Post-White et al., 2003; Scandrett-Hibdon, Hardy, & Mentgen, 1999; Silva, 1996; Umbreit, 1997, 2000; Wardell, 2000; Wardell & Weymouth, 2004; Wilkinson et al., 2002). In pediatrics, two small research studies have been completed (Speel, 2002; Verret, 2000) and four more are in progress (Healing Touch International, Inc., 2004) that examine various outcomes. As of May 2004, there were 63 completed HT studies and 25 in progress (Healing Touch International, Inc., 2004).

Umbreit (2000) proposed a model of how HT may promote positive changes in symptoms (Figure 17.1). A trained HT practitioner moves and repatterns a client's energy field, promoting a more open and symmetric pattern to enhance the client's perceived sense of well-being. This movement of energy may stimulate physiological, neurochemical, and psychological changes that promote positive impacts on pain, anxiety, wound healing, immune system function, depression, and sense of well-being.

INTERVENTION

Techniques

Nearly 30 HT techniques are taught in the HT program, from the simple to the complex. The HT practitioner determines which to use after an assessment of the client's expressed needs, symptoms presented, and results of an energy field hand scan. They range from localized to full-body techniques. Table 17.1 lists several basic techniques, including indications and brief descriptions of the procedures. These techniques, which treat a wide range of client symptoms, should be practiced in a supervised setting with an instructor before working with a client.

Most of the HT techniques involve two basic types of hand gestures (called magnetic passes) that are described in terms of hands in motion or hands still (Mentgen, 2003). In the hands in motion gestures, the hands make gentle brushing or combing motions, usually downward and outward, in order to remove congested energy from the field. The hands remain relaxed, palms facing downward toward the patient, between one to six inches above the skin or clothing. The hand strokes may be slow and sweeping or short and rapid. In the hands still position, the practitioner holds his or her hands over an area of the client's body for one

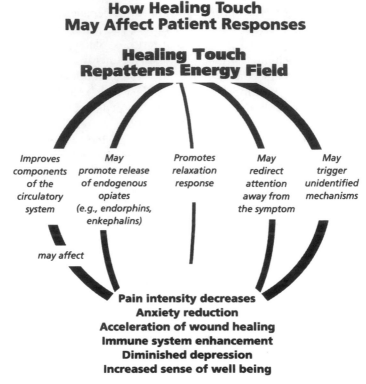

FIGURE 17.1 How healing touch may affect patient responses.

Note: From "Healing Touch: Applications in the Acute Care Setting," by A. Umbreit, 2000, *AACN Clinical Issues, 11*(1), 107. Copyright 2000 by A. Umbreit. Reprinted with permission.

to several minutes, either lightly touching or just above the skin. The practitioner uses intent to facilitate a transfer of energy to the specific body part of the client from a "universal source" of energy, with the practitioner as the conduit of this energy.

Although several of the HT techniques can be done in a seated position, most are done while the client is lying down in the most relaxed state possible, in order to promote a more profound effect. The practitioner briefly describes HT and what he or she plans to do, invites the client to ask any questions at any time, and receives permission to do the treatment and to touch the client.

Measurement of Outcomes

Measurement of HT outcomes have included patient satisfaction; anxiety and stress reduction; improved mood and less fatigue in cancer patients;

TABLE 17.1 Basic Healing Touch Techniques (Hover-Kramer, 2002; Mentgen, 2003)

Note: Each technique begins with determining the client's specific need for HT and obtaining client permission. This is followed by centering oneself, physically and psychologically, setting the intention for the client's highest good. Each technique ends with evaluating the client's experience and asking for feedback.

	Indications:	Brief Description of Procedure:
Full Body Techniques		
Basic Healing Touch (HT) Sequence	Promote relaxation Reduce pain Lower anxiety, tension, stress Facilitate wound healing Promote restoration of the body Promote a sense of well-being	1. Assess client's energy field with a hand scan over the body 2. Use magnetic passes in client's energy field (hands in motion and/or hands still) to move congestion and density from the field 3. Re-assess client's energy field with hand scan to determine effects of intervention 4. Ground the client to the present moment and to feel connection to the earth
Magnetic Clearing	Clear the body's energy field of congestion and emotional debris Used for: history of drug use, post-anesthesia, chronic pain, trauma, systemic disease, after breathing polluted air, history of smoking, environmental sensitivities, emotional clearing and release of unresolved feelings (e.g., anger, fear, worry, tension)	1. Assess client's energy field with a hand scan over the body 2. Place hands 12 inches above the top of client's head with fingers spread, relaxed and curled, thumbs touching or close together 3. Move hands very slowly in long continuous raking motions over the body from above the head to off the toes, one to six inches above the body, each sweep taking about 30 seconds (work the middle of the body first, followed by each side)

(continued)

TABLE 17.1 *(continued)*

	Indications:	Brief Description of Procedure:
		4. Procedure is repeated 30 times and takes about 15 minutes
		5. Re-assess client's energy field with hand scan to determine effects of intervention
		6. Ground the client to the present moment and to feel connection to the earth
Chakra Connection (Joy, 1979)	Connect, open, and balance the energy centers (chakras), enhancing the flow of energy throughout the body	1. Assess client's energy field with a hand scan over the body 2. Place hands on or over the minor energy centers (chakras) on the extremities and the major energy centers (chakras) on the trunk in a defined sequential manner, holding each area for at least 1 minute 3. Reassess client's energy field with hand scan to determine effects of intervention 4. Ground the client to the present moment and to feel connection to the earth
Chakra Spread	Open the energy centers (chakras) producing a deep clearing of energy blocks Used for: severe pain, pre- and post-medical procedures/surgery, severe stress reactions, the terminally ill, and assisting a client who has chosen to enter a profound spiritual state	1. Assess client's energy field with a hand scan over the body 2. Hold the client's feet, then hands, one by one in a gentle embrace for at least 1 minute 3. Place hands (palms up) above each energy center (chakra), moving the hands slowly downward toward the chakra, then spreading the hands out-

TABLE 17.1 *(continued)*

Indications:	Brief Description of Procedure:
	ward as far as possible; motion is repeated three times for each energy center, moving from the upper to the lower chakras
	4. Repeat entire sequence two more times
	5. Re-assess client's energy field with hand scan to determine effects of intervention
	6. End treatment with holding the client's hand and heart center (procedure is done in silence and takes 10–15 minutes; is used very carefully by experienced practitioners for special needs and sacred moments in healing)

Localized Techniques

	Indications:	Brief Description of Procedure:
Energetic Ultrasound	Break up congestion, energy patterns, and blockages Relieve pain Assist in stopping internal bleeding, sealing lacerations, healing fractures, and joint injuries	1. Hand scan client's localized area to assess energy field 2. Hold the thumb, first, and second fingers together, directing energy from the palm down the fingers 3. Imagine a beam of light coming from the fingers of one hand into the client's body 4. Place opposite hand behind the body part being worked on 5. Move the hand in any direction over the affected part continuously moving for 3–5 minutes 6. Repeat hand scan to determine effect of intervention

(continued)

TABLE 17.1 *(continued)*

	Indications:	Brief Description of Procedure:
Energetic Laser	Cuts, seals, and breaks up congestion in the energy field Relieves pain	1. Hand scan client's localized area to assess energy field 2. Hold one or more fingers still and pointed toward the problem area 3. Use for a few seconds to a minute 4. Repeat hand scan to determine effect of intervention
Mind Clearing	Promotes relaxation and focusing of the mind	1. Hold fingertips or palms on designated parts of the neck and head, holding each part 1–3 minutes 2. Gently massage mandibular joint 3. End with light sweeping touches across the forehead and cheeks three times, and a gentle hold around the jaw
Pain Drain	Eases pain or energy congestion	1. Place left hand on area of pain or energy congestion and right hand downward away from body 2. Siphon off congested energy from painful area through left hand and out right hand 3. Place right hand on painful or congested area and place left hand upward in the air to bring in healing energy from the universal energy field (each position is generally held for 3–5 minutes)

TABLE 17.1 *(continued)*

	Indications:	Brief Description of Procedure:
Wound Sealing	Repairs energy field leaks that occur from the physical body experiencing trauma, incisions, or childbirth	1. Hand scan body above a scar or injury to determine if any leaks of energy are felt coming from the site (may feel like a column of cool air) 2. Move hands over the area gathering energy 3. Bring gathered energy down to the client's skin over the injury and hold for a minute with hands 4. Re-scan the area to determine that the energy field feels evenly symmetrical over the entire body

pain reduction; improved sense of well-being; decrease in depression; positive changes in blood pressure, blood glucose, and salivary immunoglobulinA; decreased length of hospitalization and adverse periprocedural outcomes after cardiac procedures; diminished agitation levels in dementia patients; improved behaviors in Alzheimer's patients; and improved functional status for patients with mobility issues. Studies currently in progress are also examining cellular immune function and cancer treatment side effects comparing those who receive HT and those who do not; interpersonal connectedness, emotional well-being, functional quality of life, and sense of meaning between elders giving and receiving HT; cost effectiveness outcomes; and stress recovery in a neonatal intensive care unit. Until a reliable and easily available tool is developed to measure changes in the energy system, objective measuring of changes in the flow of an energy field is not possible. Practitioners do report a change in clients' energy field that they perceive through the use of their senses, most commonly through touch.

Outcomes measured must reflect the specific client need and presenting symptoms, and the particular HT technique used to treat. Tools that have been used to measure client outcomes have included measuring patient satisfaction and well-being using Likert-type scale responses; the Spielberger State/Trait Anxiety Inventory, Profile of Mood States, or an

Anxiety Visual Analog Scale; a Pain Visual Analog Scale, the McGill-Melzack Pain Questionnaire, or the Chronic Pain Experience Instrument; Beck's Depression Inventory; cardiovascular variables (heart rate, systolic/diastolic blood pressure, and mean arterial blood pressure); oxygenation variables (pH, CO_2, PO_2, and HCO_3); Recovery Index; goniometer readings; length of stay; Functional Behavioral Profile; the Cohen-Mansfield Agitation Inventory; Ashworth Scale for grading spasticity; the HELP Strands or Preschooler for assessing gross motor skills; SF-36 to measure health related quality of life; and immunoglobulin concentrations pre- and post-treatments.

It is difficult to determine whether the outcome of the HT intervention is solely due to the treatment or to other factors. The effect of the practitioner's presence has always been considered a confounding variable affecting client outcome, but this is also true in many nursing interventions.

Precautions

Precautions to be aware of when using HT techniques include the following:

- The energy field of infants, children, older people, the extremely ill, and the dying are sensitive to energy work, so treatments should be gentle and time limited.

- Gentle energy treatments are also required for pregnant women because the energy field also includes the fetus.

- Energy work with a cancer patient should be focused on balancing the whole field rather than concentrating on a particular area.

- The effect of medications and chemicals in the body may be enhanced with energy work so one must be alert to the possibility of side effects and sensitivity reactions to these substances.

It is recommended that experienced practitioners work with clients in the above situations. However, in order to help develop a knowledgeable practice, a student or an apprentice in HT can provide treatments in these situations if supervised by a mentor (Umbreit, 2000). Healing Touch is not considered a curative treatment and must always be used in conjunction with conventional medical care. However, practitioners and clients have reported that clients have experienced a sense of healing at a more holistic level of mind, body, and spirit, even if a cure is not possible.

Umbreit (2000) reports anecdotal comments from clients that include: "I feel wonderful," "relaxed," "peaceful," "in a meditative state," "warm," "soothed," "safe," "reassured," "more balanced," "mellow," "happier with life," "as if all my tension was melting," and a "sense of inner peace." Because HT is a noninvasive intervention, these clients' responses have enormous implications for improving quality of life in their striving toward wellness.

USES

Healing Touch interventions have been used on all age groups from the neonate to the elderly. Besides the general curriculum for learning HT, there are also classes available for specifically working with infants. Healing Touch has been taught in 21 countries in North, Central, and South America; Europe; Africa; Australia; and New Zealand, with more countries continuing to request HT education each year. In addition, HT is being utilized within diverse health care facilities: tertiary care, community hospitals, hospices, medical clinics, and long-term care. Models of delivering services range from volunteer to staff-provided programs. There are also well-established community service models that provide support for individuals with cancer while they are receiving conventional medical treatment (L. Anselme, personal communication, January 13, 2005). Healing Touch interventions have been supported by a limited number of rigorous research studies, with the majority of reports from anecdotal stories in a variety of clinical situations in all age groups and states of illness or wellness (Bulbrook, 2000; Hover-Kramer, 2002; Scandrett-Hibdon et al., 1999; Umbreit, 1997, 2000) and from studies that unfortunately were missing some vital information, which led to problems with both internal and external validity (Wardell & Weymouth, 2004). Healing Touch studies have shown positive results in the following clinical situations:

- Reduction of anxiety and stress
- Promotion of relaxation
- Reduction in acute and chronic pain
- Acceleration of postoperative recovery
- Aid in preparation for medical treatments and procedures
- Improvement of cancer treatment side effects
- Reduction in symptoms of depression

- Promotion of a sense of well-being

- Reduction in agitation levels

- Improvement in quality of life physically, emotionally, relationally, and spiritually

Table 17.2 lists several research studies that have supported the use of HT interventions in some of these clinical situations over the past 10 years. Many studies are not published in medical, nursing, or psychology

TABLE 17.2 Research Studies Using Healing Touch Interventions (1996–2004)

Uses	Selected sources
Anxiety/stress reduction	Dubrey (1997); Gehlhaart & Dail (2000); Guevara, Menidas, & Silva (2002); Taylor (2001); Wilkinson et al. (2002)
Promotion of relaxation/relief of spasticity in pediatric populations	Speel (2002); Verret (2000)
Acute and chronic pain reduction	Cordes, Proffitt, & Roth (1997); Darbonne & Fontenot (1997); Diener (2001); Merritt & Randall (1998); Peck (2001); Protzman (1999); Slater (1996); Wardell (2000); Welcher & Kish (2001); Weymouth & Sandberg-Lewis (2000)
Acceleration of postoperative recovery	Arom & MacIntyre (2002); Silva (1996)
Aid in medical procedures/treatments	Norris (2000)
Improvement of cancer treatment side effects	Cook et al. (2004); Post-White et al. (2003)
Diminished depression	Bradway (1998); Van Aken (2003)
Agitation level reduction/functional behavior improvement in elders	Ostuni & Pietro (1999); Wang & Hermann (1999)
Quality of life improvement: physically, emotionally, relationally, spiritually	Geddes (1999); Wardell (1999)

journals, but information can be accessed through Healing Touch International's research department (www.healingtouch.net/research/index. shtml). The research continues to be controversial because the exact mechanism of action cannot be seen or easily explained in our Western view of what constitutes sound scientific research, and few double-blind studies have been done in this area.

FUTURE RESEARCH

Research studies and anecdotal cases in HT offer promising, yet certainly not conclusive, data on the positive outcomes from this complementary therapy. Qualitative responses from clients have been especially important in helping guide the direction of the research and may provide insight into the phenomenon of energy exchange in the future. Some of the problems encountered in nursing research include insufficient funding to support the work, multiple variables that are hard to control in a clinical setting versus a laboratory setting, and the use of small sample sizes that can be easily affected by highly variable data and sampling error. There is the additional difficulty of testing the efficacy of an energy-based therapy in which the energy exchange between practitioner and client cannot be seen by most but is only observed as subjective responses from clients. The whole conceptual framework of energy fields and energy exchange does not fit the cause–effect model that Western science is focused on. Rogers' theory (1990) speaks about energy changing, exchanging, and patterning, one moment in time never replicating itself. The focus is on nature's restoring universal order and balance, and restoring energy balance is the goal of HT. This is a huge area of research that obviously will require a multidisciplinary effort by Western and Eastern medicine, quantum physics, biology, psychology, philosophy, spirituality, and nursing. Outcome studies, as well as studies of mechanism, will help support the development and understanding of the phenomenon of energy exchange. As shown in Figure 17.1, there are mediating factors that may contribute to decreases in pain intensity, anxiety reduction, acceleration of healing, immune system enhancement, diminished depression, and increased sense of well-being. More studies that measure some of these mediating mechanisms are recommended.

The choice of a valid instrument for measuring outcomes is critical in HT studies. Results can be skewed in either direction if the instrument is not reliable. However, in order to obtain subject cooperation when working with persons who are ill, the measuring instrument must be easy to use and not burdensome to patients who are already facing difficulties.

Other challenges to be controlled in conducting HT research studies include the experience of the HT practitioner, the presence phenomenon of the caregiver, the type of HT treatment modality chosen, the length and number of treatments, when the treatment is done, and when measurements are done. There is a wide range of skill levels of HT practitioners from novice to certified practitioner and comparable skill level is important in planning a research study. The phenomenon of presence of the HT practitioner may also affect the outcome of the research and needs to be controlled in the study design. Because there are many HT interventions that can be used, a research study would need to be consistent in the type of chosen therapy. The challenge with length and number of treatments is that under normal circumstances, a HT intervention is not used for a prescribed length of time or number of treatments. The practitioner does the work until he or she intuits that it is time to stop or that no more treatments are needed. Research could restrict this professional decision-making process. Choosing when to give a HT treatment and when to measure outcomes and ascertaining how long the outcome may last continue to be challenging. Experienced HT practitioners must have input into determining these time lines by observing patterns they may typically see in their own professional practice.

The next steps for research must build upon the small studies already completed. Replication of studies would help strengthen the validity of HT. The following are questions related to specific areas to build upon:

1. Is HT equally effective in acute versus chronic pain? How long and how often do treatments need to be for the client to report a decrease in pain? How long does this improvement last?

2. How is postoperative recovery affected by administering HT (pain relief, wound healing, restoring of bowel function, ease of physical activity, length of stay in the hospital)?

3. Does HT have a positive effect on degenerative diseases such as arthritis, multiple sclerosis, fibromyalgia, stroke, immune deficiency disorders, and chronic lung conditions?

4. Does HT assist in managing the side effects of treatments in cancer patients?

5. What are the psychological and spiritual benefits reported by HT recipients?

6. What tools are effective in measuring a change in energy in the recipient before and after HT or an exchange of energy between practitioner and recipient?

7. Does HT reduce medical costs for pharmaceuticals, hospital stays, and clinic time?

In the quest to examine the impact of HT scientifically, we must not be too quick to dismiss the overwhelming positive client feedback from its clinical application. Creativity is necessary in conducting research of this phenomenon that cannot be seen by the naked eye, but is so often felt by the human spirit.

WEB RESOURCES

For more information on healing touch:
Healing Touch International: www.healingtouch.net
Colorado Center for Healing Touch: www.healingtouch.net
American Holistic Nurses Association (AHNA): www.ahna.org

REFERENCES

Arom, D., & MacIntyre, B. (2002, January). *The effect of healing touch on coronary artery bypass surgery patients.* Paper presented at Healing Touch International 6th Annual Conference, Denver, CO.

Bradway, C. (1998). The effects of healing touch on depression. *Healing Touch Newsletter, 8*(3), 2.

Brennan, B. (1986). *Hands of light.* New York: Bantam.

Bruyere, R. L. (1989). *Wheels of light.* New York: Simon & Schuster.

Bulbrook, M. J. T. (2000). *Healing stories to inspire, teach and heal.* Carrboro, NC: North Carolina Center for Healing Touch.

Cook, C. A., Guerrerio, J. F., & Slater, V. E. (2004). Healing touch and quality of life in women receiving radiation treatment for cancer: A randomized controlled trial. *Alternative Therapies, 10* (3), 34–41.

Cordes, P., Proffitt, C., & Roth, J. (1997). The effect of healing touch therapy on the pain and joint mobility experienced by patients with total knee replacements. Compiled by Diane Wind Wardell in *Healing Touch Research Survey May 2004* (pp. 40–41). Lakewood, CO: Healing Touch International.

Darbonne, M., & Fontenot, T. (1997, January). *The effects of healing touch modalities on patients with chronic pain.* Paper presented at Healing Touch International Research Symposium, Denver, CO.

Diener, D. (2001). A pilot study of the effect of chakra connection and magnetic unruffle on perception of pain in people with fibromyalgia. *Healing Touch Newsletter, Research Edition, 01*(3), 7–8.

Dossey, B. M., Keegan, L., Guzzetta, C. E., & Kolkmeier, L. H. (1995). *Holistic nursing: A handbook for practice.* Gaithersburg, MD: Aspen.

Dubrey, R. (1997). Perceived effectiveness of healing touch treatments by healees. *Healing Touch Research Survey May 2004* (p. 52). Lakewood, CO: Healing Touch International.

Egan, E. C. (1998). Therapeutic touch. In M. Snyder & R. Lindquist (Eds.), *Complementary/alternative therapies in nursing* (3rd ed., pp. 49–62). New York: Springer Publishing.

Fedoruk, R. B. (1984). *Transfer of the relaxation response: Therapeutic touch as a method of reduction of stress in premature neonates.* Unpublished doctoral dissertation, University of Maryland, College Park.

Forbes, M. A., Rust, R., & Becker, G. J. (2004, May). *Surface electromyography (EMG) as a measurement for biofield research: Results of a preliminary investigation.* Paper presented at the 8th Annual Healing Touch International Conference, San Diego, CA.

Geddes, N. (1999). The experience of personal transformation in healing touch practitioners: A heuristic inquiry. *Healing Touch Newsletter, 9*(3), 5.

Geddes, N. (2002). Research related to healing touch. In D. Hover-Kramer (Ed.), *Healing touch: A guidebook for practitioners* (2nd ed., pp. 24–40). Albany, NY: Delmar.

Gehlhaart, C., & Dail, P. (2000). Effectiveness of healing touch and therapeutic touch on elderly residents of long term care facilities on reducing pain and anxiety level. *Healing Touch Newsletter, 0*(3), 8.

Guevara, E., Menidas, N., & Silva, C. (2002). The effect of healing touch therapy on post traumatic stress disorder (PTSD) symptoms on domestic violence abused Mexican women. *Healing Touch Research Survey May 2004* (pp. 62–63). Lakewood, CO: Healing Touch International.

Healing Touch International. (2004). *Healing Touch research survey.* Lakewood, CO: Author: Wardell, D.W.

Healing Touch International. (2005). What is Healing Touch? Retrieved from www.healingtouch.net/hti.shtml and www.healingtouch.net/ccht.shtml

Hover-Kramer, D. (2002). *Healing touch: A guidebook for practitioners* (2nd ed.). Albany, NY: Delmar.

Hover-Kramer, D., Mentgen, J., & Scandrett-Hibdon, S. (1996). *Healing touch: A resource for health care professionals.* Albany, NY: Delmar.

Hutchison, C. P. (1999). Healing touch: An energetic approach. *American Journal of Nursing, 99*(4), 43–48.

Joy, B. (1979). *Joy's way.* New York: G. P. Putnam's Sons.

Keller, E., & Bzdek, V. (1986). Effects of therapeutic touch on tension headache pain. *Nursing Research, 13*(2), 101–106.

Krieger, D. (1976). Healing by the laying on of hands as facilitator of bioenergetic change: The response of in-vivo hemoglobin. *Psychoenergetic Systems, 1,* 121–129.

Krieger, D. (1979). *The therapeutic touch: How to use your hands to help or to heal.* New York: Simon & Schuster.

Krieger, D., Peper, E., & Ancoli, A. (1979). Therapeutic touch: Searching for evidence of physiological change. *American Journal of Nursing, 79,* 660–662.

Krucoff, M. W., Crater, S. W., Green, C. L., Maas, A. C., Seskevich, J. E., Lane, J. D., et al. (2001). Integrative noetic therapies as adjuncts to percutaneous intervention during unstable coronary syndromes: Monitoring and actualization of noetic training (MANTRA) feasibility pilot. *American Heart Journal, 142*(5), 760–767.

Mentgen, J. (2003). *Healing touch level I syllabus.* Lakewood, CO: Colorado Center for Healing Touch.

Merritt, P. (1998). Effect of healing touch and other complementary therapies on diabetes. *Healing Touch International Research Survey May 2004* (pp. 32–33). Lakewood, CO: Healing Touch International.

Merritt, P., & Randall, D. (1998). The effect of healing touch and other forms of energy work on cancer pain. *Healing Touch Research Survey May 2004* (p. 16). Lakewood, CO: Healing Touch International.

Miller, L. A. (1979). An explanation of therapeutic touch using the science of unitary man. *Nursing Forum, 18*(3), 278–287.

Motoyama, H. (1997). *Treatment principles of Oriental medicine from an electrophysiological viewpoint.* Tokyo: Human Sciences Press.

Norris, R. (2000, January). *Evaluation of energy-based relaxation techniques as nursing interventions to improve outcomes in patients undergoing nurse-performed screening flexible sigmoidoscopy.* Paper presented at the Healing Touch International Conference, Kauai, HI.

Olson, M., Sneed, N., Bonadonna, R., Ratliff, J., & Dias, J. (1992). Therapeutic touch and post-Hurricane Hugo stress. *Journal of Holistic Nursing, 10,* 120–136.

Oschman, J. L. (2000). *Energy medicine: The scientific basis.* Dover, NH: Churchill Livingston.

Ostuni, E., & Pietro, M. J. (1999). Effects of healing touch on nursing home residents in later stages of Alzheimer's. *Healing Touch Research Survey May 2004* (pp. 25–26). Lakewood, CO: Healing Touch International.

Peck, S. (2001). A descriptive study of outcomes with the use of healing touch in elders and adults with chronic illness. *Healing Touch Research Survey May 2004* (pp. 26–27). Lakewood, CO: Healing Touch International.

Post-White, J., Kinney, E. E., Savik, K., Gau, J. B., Wilcox, C., & Lerner, I. (2003). Therapeutic massage and healing touch improve symptoms in cancer. *Integrative Cancer Therapies, 2*(4), 332–344.

Protzman, L. (1999). The effect of healing touch on pain and relaxation. *Healing Touch Research Survey May 2004* (p. 48). Lakewood, CO: Healing Touch International.

Quinn, J. (1984). Therapeutic touch as energy exchange: Testing the theory. *Advances in Nursing Science, 6*(2), 42–49.

Quinn, J., & Strelkauskas, A. (1993). Psychoimmunologic effect of therapeutic touch on practitioners and recently bereaved recipients: A pilot study. *Advances in Nursing Science, 15*(4), 13–26.

Rogers, M. (1990). Nursing: Science of unitary, irreducible, human beings: Update 1990. In E. A. M. Barrett (Ed.), *Vision of Rogers' science-based nursing* (pp. 5–11). New York: National League for Nursing.

Sayre-Adams, J. (1994). Therapeutic touch: A nursing function. *Nursing Standard, 8*(17), 25–28.

Scandrett-Hibdon, S. (1996). Research foundations. In D. Hover-Kramer, J. Mentgen, & S. Scandrett-Hibdon (Eds.), *Healing touch: A resource for health care professionals* (pp. 27–42). Albany, NY: Delmar.

Scandrett-Hibdon, S., Hardy, C., & Mentgen, J. (1999). *Energetic patterns: Healing touch case studies Vol. 1*. Lakewood, CO: Colorado Center for Healing Touch.

Silva, C. (1996). The effects of relaxation touch on the recovery level of postanesthesia abdominal hysterectomy patients. *Alternative Therapies, 2*(4), 94.

Slater, V. (1996). Safety, elements, and effects of healing touch on chronic nonmalignant abdominal pain. *Healing Touch Research Survey May 2004* (pp. 48–49). Lakewood, CO: Healing Touch International.

Speel, L. (2002). A pilot study on the effect of healing touch-mind cleaning and magnetic unruffling on high school students with mental and physical disabilities. *Healing Touch Research Survey May 2004* (pp. 54–56). Lakewood, CO: Healing Touch International.

Stouffer, D., Duennes, M., & Pitman, G. (2000, January). Paper presented at the 4th Annual Healing Touch International Conference, Kauai, HI.

Stouffer, D., Kaiser, D., Pitman, G., & Rolf, W. (1998, January). *Electrodermal testing to measure the effect of a healing touch treatment*. Paper presented at the Healing Touch Research Symposium, Denver, CO.

Taylor, B. (2001, February). The effect of healing touch on the coping ability, self esteem, and general health of undergraduate nursing students. *Complementary Therapies in Nursing and Midwifery*, 34–42.

Umbreit, A. (1997). Therapeutic touch: Energy-based healing. *Creative Nursing, 3*, 6–7.

Umbreit, A. (2000). Healing touch: Applications in the acute care setting. *AACN Clinical Issues, 11*(1), 105–119.

Van Aken, R. (2003, January). *Emerging from depression: The experiential process of healing touch*. Paper presented at the 7th Annual Healing Touch International Conference, Colorado Springs, CO.

Verret, P. (2000). Healing touch as a relaxation intervention in children with spasticity. *Healing Touch Newsletter Research Edition, 0*(3), 6–7.

Wang, K., & Hermann, C. (1999). Healing touch on agitation levels related to dementia. *Healing Touch Newsletter, 9*(3), 3.

Wardell, D. (1999). Spirituality in healing touch practice. *Healing Touch Newsletter, 9*(3), 4.

Wardell, D. W. (2000). The trauma release technique: How it is taught and experienced in healing touch. *Alternative and Complementary Therapies, 6*(1), 20–27.

Wardell, D. W., & Weymouth, K. F. (2004). Review of studies of healing touch. *Journal of Nursing Scholarship, 36*(2), 147–154.

Watson, J. (1985). *Nursing: The philosophy and science of caring*. Boulder: Colorado Associated University Press.

Welcher, B., & Kish, J. (2001). Reducing pain and anxiety through healing touch. *Healing Touch Newsletter, 1*(3), 19.

Weymouth, K., & Sandberg-Lewis, S. (2000). Comparing the efficacy of healing touch and chiropractic adjustment in treating chronic low back pain: A pilot study. *Healing Touch Newsletter, 0*(3), 7–8.

Wilkinson, D. (2002). The clinical effectiveness of healing touch on HIV-infected individuals. *Healing Touch Research Survey May 2004* (pp. 35–36). Lakewood, CO: Healing Touch International.

Wilkinson, D. S., Knox, P., Chatman, J., Johnson, T. L., Barbour, N., Myles, Y., et al. (2002). The clinical effectiveness of healing touch. *Journal of Alternative and Complementary Medicine, 8*(1), 33–47.

Wirth, D., Chang, R., Eidelman, W., & Paxton, J. (1996). Haematological indicators of complementary healing intervention. *Complementary Therapies in Medicine, 4*(1), 14–20.

Wirth, D., Richardson, W., Eidelman, W., & O'Malley, A. (1993). Full thickness dermal wounds treated with non-contact therapeutic touch: A replication and extension. *Complementary Therapies in Medicine, 1*(3), 127–132.

Wright, S. M. (1987). The use of therapeutic touch in the management of pain. *Nursing Clinics of North America, 22*, 705–714.

CHAPTER 18

Therapeutic Touch

Janet F. Quinn

Therapeutic Touch was developed from the laying-on of hands by Dora Kunz, a gifted healer, and Dolores Krieger, Ph.D., R.N. In 1979 Krieger outlined the steps of the practice in her first book (Krieger, 1979). She introduced the method to students in the graduate nursing program at New York University in the early 1970s in a course called "Frontiers of Nursing," which continues today. Krieger estimates that, as of 1990, "Therapeutic Touch has also been taught in more than eighty colleges and universities in the United States as well as in innumerable hospital and health facility in-service and continuing education programs. In addition, Therapeutic Touch has been taught in sixty-eight countries" (Krieger, 1993, p. 5).

DEFINITION

Therapeutic Touch (TT) is the use of the hands on or near the body with the intention to help or to heal. It is a contemporary intervention that is different from the laying-on of hands in several key ways. Perhaps most notable of these differences is that Therapeutic Touch need not take place within a religious or spiritual framework. It is seen as a natural human potential that can be actualized by anyone who has the intention to heal and makes the commitment to learning and practicing. Therapeutic Touch has as its focus the facilitation and acceleration of the natural healing potential within all living systems.

SCIENTIFIC BASIS

Therapeutic Touch is founded on three basic assumptions:

1. Human beings are energy fields and open systems.
2. Illness is an imbalance in energy flow and/or pattern.
3. Trained practitioners can perceive and intervene in the recipient's energy field to stimulate the recipient's own natural healing potential.

1. *Human beings are energy fields.* When Kunz and Krieger developed Therapeutic Touch, they called on understandings gained from knowledge of Eastern thought to explain both the method and its effects. Prana, the vital life force energy identified in Indian philosophy and healing systems, is posited to be the energy that surrounds and pervades every living system. According to Krieger, it is this prana that is directed and modulated by the healer for the healee (Krieger, 1973, 1979, 1993). Other theorists have further developed Krieger's original hypothesis by applying the theoretical framework postulated by Rogers. In her "Nursing: Science of Unitary Human Beings," Rogers (1990) defines people as irreducible, indivisible, multidimensional energy fields integral with the environmental energy field. In earlier conceptualizations of TT within this framework, the theory that there was an energy transfer or exchange between the practitioner and the recipient was a primary explanatory model (Heidt, 1981; Keller & Bzdek, 1986; Quinn, 1984) deriving from Rogers' conceptual system and consistent with theoretical explanations offered by earlier researchers (Grad, 1963, 1964, 1965; Grad, Cadoret, & Paul, 1961; Smith, 1972). More recently, it has been postulated that the Therapeutic Touch practitioner, knowingly participating in the mutual human/environment process by shifting consciousness into a state that may be thought of as a "healing meditation" (Krieger, Peper, & Ancoli, 1979), facilitates repatterning of the recipient's energy field through a process of resonance, rather than "energy exchange or transfer" (Cowling, 1990; Quinn, 1992).

Therapeutic Touch practitioners believe that human beings are energy fields; they also believe that people are open systems. Because neither practitioners nor recipients stop at their skin, the Therapeutic Touch exchange may occur with no physical contact at all, or with a mix of physical contact and no physical contact. This becomes most relevant when actual physical contact between practitioner and recipient is undesirable for either medical or sociocultural reasons.

2. *Illness is an imbalance in energy flow and/or pattern.* When there is illness or other dysfunction in the body-mind-spirit, there is a corresponding imbalance in the energy field. In the case of disease, the assumption is that a shift in the energy field probably preceded the onset of physical symptoms and clinical evidence of the disease. This assumption is consistent with current scientific theories concerning the relationship between the state of the resistance of the host when exposed to pathogens and the onset of disease. In an energetic framework, one assumes that there are patterns or flows of energy that are more, or less, consistent with health and that therefore provide greater, or lesser, resistance to disease.

3. *Trained practitioners can perceive and intervene in the recipient's energy field to stimulate the recipient's own natural healing potential.* Through the process of turning one's attention inward and becoming quiet, relaxed, and focused, one can begin to get a sense of the human energy field of another. The energy field is always there, but we are not always quiet enough and paying close enough attention to notice it. Through practice, TT practitioners can become extremely sensitive to even subtle changes in the field, and through gentle movements of the hands coupled with a very focused intention they can assist in repatterning the field in a direction more conducive to health.

A 1998 study conducted by Therapeutic Touch critics Rosa, Rosa, Sarner, and Barrett, and published in the *Journal of the American Medical Association*, attempted to test the assumption that TT nurses can perceive the human energy field. The authors concluded, using a one-tailed t-test to test their hypothesis, that there was no deviation from chance in nurses' ability to detect a human energy field when a hand was held over their hands out of their vision. Serious design and interpretation flaws are itemized by the skeptics' group to which the authors belong (Selby, 1998). Selby concludes that "the unequivocal conclusion drawn by *JAMA* in its Editor's Note: 'This simple, statistically valid study tests the theoretical basis for Therapeutic Touch: the human energy field. This study found that such a field does not exist . . . ' is simply not so. The work reported in the *JAMA* article does not support that conclusion."

Furthermore, the authors neglected to report that, in fact, there was a significant deviation from what chance would allow, but it was in the opposite direction from their predictions. The nurses performed significantly worse than chance would have predicted. Thus, something other than the nurses' ability to perceive the energy field influenced their performance or they would have gotten the correct answer at least as often as chance would allow. The study may represent an instance of negative intentionality, that is, the negative expectations of the investigators and others present that the nurses would fail actually influenced their performance. This would support, rather than refute, the theory that we are open systems interacting with all other energy fields and that intention directed at those interactions may produce effects. Of course, this is a hypothesis requiring further research, along with all three of the basic assumptions presented here.

A better test of human beings' ability to perceive the energy of other human beings is presented by Schwartz, Russek, and Beltran (1995). These authors report on several experiments in which blindfolded subjects were able to correctly guess when another person's hand was held 3 to 4 inches above, palm open and facing, the open palm of one of the (randomly assigned) hands of the subject at a rate statistically greater than chance would allow.

At this time there is no conclusive evidence that is acceptable in the Western scientific tradition that a human energy field exists. As long as Therapeutic Touch practitioners and practitioners of all so-called "energy medicines," including Acupuncture, Homeopathy, Qi Qong, and others, acknowledge this and continue to treat the theory of energy exchange as a working hypothesis, they are well within the bounds of responsible scientific practice. Theories, rather than confirmed facts, regarding the mechanisms by which interventions have effects are the rule, not the exception, across modern medical, pharmaceutical, and nursing practice. The scientific evidence for the efficacy of TT will be discussed in the section on uses.

INTERVENTION

Technique

The steps of Therapeutic Touch include centering, assessment of the energy field, clearing and mobilizing the energy field, directing energy for healing, and balancing the energy field. They are described in detail below.

Centering

The TT assessment of the human energy field is uncomplicated and simple, but developing a deep sensitivity to subtle cues and differences in the field will take practice. To facilitate this sensitivity, and to create the most healing environment for both practitioner and recipient, the Therapeutic Touch practitioner prepares for the assessment and treatment by centering.

Centering involves a shift from our ordinary state of being into a calm, relaxed, and focused healing presence. It is the turning inward of attention and the making of an intention to help or to heal. The mind is quieted, extraneous thoughts from the past or about the future are temporarily set aside, and the full awareness of the practitioner is brought into the present moment. For this reason, Therapeutic Touch has been called a "healing meditation" (Krieger et al., 1979).

The intention to heal is believed to be the key variable in the efficacy of the treatment. In a randomized, placebo-controlled study, cardiac patients were given a TT treatment by very experienced nurses, and a control group received a mimic sham treatment, provided by nurses with no training in TT. The nurses who were doing the real treatments centered themselves in the moment and made the intention to heal before beginning and during the movement of their hands. The nurses in the sham condition were taught how to mimic the hand movements of the nurses doing real Therapeutic Touch but were doing mental arithmetic while they simply went through the motions, rather than holding the intent to heal. Both groups of nurses were videotaped and the tapes were reviewed by naïve observers. No one could tell the difference in the treatments by the way they looked. In the experimental group, receiving Therapeutic Touch, there was a highly significant decrease in anxiety on posttest. In the mimic group, anxiety didn't change (Quinn, 1984). This type of control has been used in other Therapeutic Touch research and demonstrates the same phenomenon, namely, that the intention of the practitioner seems to be the critical variable, not the hand movements. This is why centering is the most important step of the process. All of the movements of TT are done within this context of the intention for healing, wholeness, and balance.

Assessing

The goal of the assessment is to gain information about the pattern and flow of energy in the field. During the entire TT session the patient can be seated sideways in an armless chair, so that his or her back is unobstructed. To complete an assessment the practitioner, standing behind the clothed patient, extends the hands over the top of the patient's head, with palms turned toward the patient, and holds them about 2 to 4 inches above the skin. Maintaining this distance, the hands, held somewhat parallel to each other and palms parallel to the patient's body, are moved gently from the top of the head to the level of the hips, while the practitioner mentally notes any areas in which the energy field feels different from the rest of the field. Next, the practitioner moves to the front of the patient and repeats the assessment process from head to toe, again noting areas where the field feels different. Alternatively, the practitioner can assess front and back at the same time, and compare them, by using one hand behind the patient and one hand in front and moving both hands from head to foot simultaneously. Patients can also be assessed while lying in bed or on an exam table.

In the healthy person, the energy field should feel essentially symmetrical from left to right and from top to bottom. There should be a sense of smoothness or evenness and there should not be areas where there is a sharp difference in temperature or rhythm or flow. In illness, there are often areas of the field in which the smoothness is broken, or where there is a sharp change in perceived temperature over the area. In the person with serious systemic illness or depression the assessment may reveal a generalized disturbance over the entire field, such as a weakness, a thickness, a dullness, or a sense of decreased flow or increased temperature. For an excellent discussion of the various perceptions and their meanings as developed by one expert Therapeutic Touch practitioner see Macrae's primer (1988).

Clearing and Mobilizing the Energy Field

Krieger refers to this step as *unruffling* whereas Macrae uses the language employed here. The unruffling or clearing process prepares the field for further treatment and is also an extremely effective method of inducing a profound relaxation response. The practitioner again begins by holding the hands 2 to 4 inches above the body at the top of the head and moves the hands above the body, palms toward the patient, from head to foot in a gently sweeping motion. The intention of the practitioner remains focused on wholeness and balance, imagining that the patient is becoming more and more relaxed and that his or her energy is flowing easily and freely, from head to toe, in a balanced and harmonious way. This process is repeated over the front of the patient's body, ending with the feet. When the practitioner is at the feet, it is useful to gently massage the bottoms of the feet to assist in the outward flow of energy.

Directing Energy for Healing

Using the assessment data as a guide, the practitioner now begins to direct energy with the intention of restoring the imbalances in the field to order and harmony. The direction of energy is accomplished by placing the hands on or over the area of imbalance and allowing a sense of the healing energy to flow out through the practitioner and toward the patient. If it is useful, the practitioner may hold an image of the desired outcome in mind while directing this energy.

Balancing

The practitioner systematically treats each area of imbalance detected during assessment, as well as new areas uncovered through the clearing process. When the practitioner perceives that the imbalances have been eliminated or that the patient's system has taken as much energy as it can, the treatment ends with a general balancing and grounding process. The balancing consists of an additional head to toe clearing as before, but with the intention of smoothing and balancing the whole field. This process ends with the practitioner touching the feet and imagining the patient as being whole, balanced, and grounded or rooted—steady and strong like a tree with roots deep into the earth.

Measurement of Outcomes

Because the focus of Therapeutic Touch is broader than the cure of physical disease, outcomes of the process are not uniformly predictable. In general, most patients experience Therapeutic Touch as calming, integrating, and balancing. A strong relaxation response, characterized by the usual indicators of this response, is usually seen within minutes of the start of the treatment and deepening over its full course.

The Therapeutic Touch practitioner will be assessing the patient's energy field throughout the treatment. The practitioner is looking for changes in the pattern of the energy field compared to the initial assessment. These changes may be large or small, and may or may not be perceived by the patient. There are also times when the practitioner may assess that, although the pattern of imbalance has not shifted, the treatment is, nevertheless, over; the patient has gotten all that he or she can in this session. The intuitive capacity of the Therapeutic Touch practitioner helps to guide this process.

In addition to the energetic assessment, the Therapeutic Touch practitioner carefully monitors the patient's response throughout, and at the end of the treatment asks for feedback. Patients describe felt changes in their energetic, physical, emotional, and spiritual being. Some patients cannot report their perceptions, but the practitioner can observe them, like the neonate in the NICU who promptly falls asleep during the treatment after crying for an extended period of time, or the combative patient with Alzheimer's disease who becomes quiet and relaxed. Sometimes there is no immediate response, but the patient will experience a decrease in physical symptoms in the 15 to 20 minutes following treatment. Sometimes the change will manifest as a good night's sleep.

When Therapeutic Touch is used over time as a course of therapy, these kinds of changes can be monitored by having the patient keep a treatment journal and reviewing it with the practitioner before each session. Cumulative physical, emotional, and/or spiritual effects may become more obvious as a result. Again, because the focus in Therapeutic Touch is beyond, but including, the physical, changes in attitude, philosophy, and general well-being are all part of the process. These changes can be assessed best in dialogue with the patient over time.

Precautions

The safety of Therapeutic Touch is borne out in clinical practice. Since its introduction by nurses into mainstream health care institutions there have been no reported incidents of harm to a patient related to Therapeutic Touch. However, because we do not know the effects of energetic forms of healing on unborn children, Therapeutic Touch practitioners recommend that it not be used by inexperienced practitioners on pregnant women. Caution when treating the very old or the very young is also appropriate, and treatments with people in these age groups should be shorter and carefully modulated. Some people find direct treatment of the head to be uncomfortable and so the hands should be kept moving when working around the head.

USES

There is no way to know at the outset how any given person will respond to TT. What we do know is that Therapeutic Touch is a treatment for the whole person, not just an illness or a disease, and so is appropriate for use on anyone. Therapeutic Touch is almost always best used as a complement to standard medical and nursing care. As such, it has been found to be very useful clinically in musculoskeletal conditions such as sprains, strains, muscle spasms, and fractures. Practitioners report that the sooner treatment is given in these cases the more effective TT seems to be. Research data supporting efficacy remains preliminary. Peters (1999) reports in a meta-analytic review of TT studies that "it is impossible to make any substantive claims [about the efficacy of Therapeutic Touch] at this time because there is limited published research and because many of the studies had significant methodological issues that could seriously bias the reported results" (p. 52).

Nevertheless, there have been observed effects demonstrated through well-designed, placebo-controlled research and also reported from clinical practice that suggest uses for TT (Table 18.1). Therapeutic Touch may be useful in the treatment of tension headache pain (Keller & Bzdek, 1986), migraine headache pain (Hoffmeyer, 2000), pain in burn patients (Turner, Clark, Gauthier, & Williams, 1998), in extending the time between pain medicine requests of postoperative patients (Meehan, 1993; Meehan, Mersmann, Wiseman, Wolff, & Malgady, 1990), in managing chronic pain in the elderly (Lin & Taylor, 1998), and in treating both pain and functional ability in patients with osteoarthritis (Gordon, Merenstein, D'Amico, & Hudgens, 1998; Peck, 1997, 1998). A pilot study by Dennison (2004) suggests that TT may be helpful in decreasing pain and improving quality of life in women with fibromyalgia syndrome. Engle and Graney (2000) found that TT produced a significant decrease in total pulse amplitude (indicating vasoconstriction) and a shift in time perception, with effect sizes of large and medium respectively.

Therapeutic Touch may also be useful in any situation where anxiety or stress contributes to physical and/or psychological symptoms and where relaxation could be curative or at least palliative (Gagne & Toye, 1994; Heidt, 1981; Lafreniere et al., 1999; Larden, Palmer, & Janssen, 2004; Lin & Taylor, 1998; Olson et al., 1997; Quinn, 1984; Quinn & Strelkauskas, 1993; Simington & Laing, 1993; Turner et al., 1998). This includes all of those conditions generally thought of as psychosomatic. A pilot study by Woods and Dimond (2002) demonstrated that there was a significant decrease in overall agitation, vocalization, and pacing during treatment and posttreatment with TT in persons with Alzheimer's disease.

A pilot study where the immune systems of both practitioners and recipients were examined before and after a course of Therapeutic Touch treatments suggests that TT may have an immuno-enhancing effect in bereaved adults (Quinn & Strelkauskas, 1993). Turner and colleagues (1998) found a similar effect in burn patients. Smith, Reeder, Daniel, Baramee, and Hagman (2003) found that TT increased scores on a comfort scale in patients undergoing bone marrow transplant. However, no effects were noted on other variables in the study.

FUTURE RESEARCH

In 1989, three critical directions for future research efforts in TT were proposed and are still relevant and appropriate as guidelines (Quinn,

TABLE 18.1 Selected Therapeutic Touch Research (1980–2005)

Author/Yr.	Design	N	Variables/Population	Intervention	Control	Result
Heidt (1981)	Experimental Pre-Posttest	90	Anxiety (STAI)/cardiac patients	TT	Casual touch; presence	Significant ↓ in TT group
Keller & Bzdek (1986)	Experimental Pre-Posttest	60	Tension headache pain (McGill-Melzack)/ college students	Non-Contact TT (NCTT)	Mimic TT	Significant ↓ in TT group immediately after treatment
Quinn (1984)	Experimental Pre-Posttest	60	Anxiety (STAI)/cardiac patients	NCTT	Mimic NCTT	Significant ↓ in TT group
Quinn & Strel-kauskas (1993)	Descriptive Pre-Posttest; Pilot	6	Immune status; anxiety (STAI); positive and negative affect (ABS)/recently bereaved patients and TT nurses	TT	None	20% mean ↓ Suppressor T-cells; 29% ↓ anxiety; increased positive affect, decreased negative affect in bereaved. (not statistically analyzed)
Meehan (1993)	Experimental Pre-Posttest	159	post-op pain (VAS); analgesia consumption	NCTT with narcotic	Mimic NCTT; standard care	TT group waited significantly longer time before requesting re-medication

234

TABLE 18.1 (continued)

Author/Yr.	Design	N	Variables/Population	Intervention	Control	Result
Meehan et al. (1990)	Experimental Pre-Posttest	108	Post-op pain (VAS)	NCTT with narcotic	Mimic NCTT; standard care	Non-significant in pain (p < .06); TT group waited significantly longer time before re-questing re-medication
Simington & Laing (1993)	Experimental Posttest only	105	Anxiety (STAI)/institu-tioralized elderly	TT with backrub	Back rub with-out TT; Mimic TT with backrub	Significant ↓ in TT with backrub group com-pared to backrub with-out TT group
Gagne & Toye (1994)	Experimental Pre-Posttest	31	Anxiety (STAI)/inpa-tient psychiatric patients	TT; Relax-ation therapy	Mimic TT	Significant ↓ in anxiety in both TT and relax-ation therapy
Peck (1997)	Experimental repeated mea-sures	82	Pain and distress (VAS)/ elderly arthritis pa-tients)	TT; Progres-sive Muscle Re-laxation (PMR)	Subjects served as own con-trols: routine care for baseline	Significant ↓ in both pain and distress with both TT and PMR
Olson et al. (1997)	Experimental Pre-Posttest	20	T-lymphocyte function (CD25); immunoglobu-lin level/stressed college students	TT	No treatment	Significant differences between groups in IgA and IgM (immunoglobu-lins); differences in CD25 non-significant

(continued)

235

TABLE 18.1 *(continued)*

Author/Yr.	Design	N	Variables/Population	Intervention	Control	Result
Gordon et al. (1998)	Experimental	25	Pain (West Haven-Yale Multidimensional Pain Inventory; VAS); level of functioning (Stanford Health Assessment Questionnaire) general well-being (VAS)/patients with osteoarthritis of knee	T	Mimic TT; standard care	Significant ↓ in pain and ↑ functional ability in TT group compared to controls
Lin & Taylor (1998)	Experimental Pre-Posttest	95	Chronic muskuloskeletal pain (numeric rating scale) anxiety (STAI), salivary cortisol/elderly	TT	Mimic TT; standard care	Significant ↓ in pain and anxiety in TT group compared to controls; no differences in cortisol
Peck (1998)	Experimental repeated measures	82	Functional ability (VAS)/elderly arthritis patients	TT; Progressive Muscle Relaxation (PMR)	Subjects served as own controls: routine care for baseline	Significantly ↑ functional ability after TT and PMR; significantly better functional ability in TT group

TABLE 18.1 *(continued)*

Author/Yr.	Design	N	Variables/Population	Intervention	Control	Result
Turner et al. (1998)	Experimental Pre-Posttest	99	Pain (McGill Pain Questionnaire; Anxiety (VAS); lymphocytes subsets for 11 patients/ burn patients	TT	Mimic TT	Significant ↓ in pain and anxiety in TT group; ↓ in CD8 (suppressor T-cells)and lymphocyte concentration in TT group
Lafreniere et al. (1999)	Experimental Pre-Posttest	41	Biochemical and mood indicators (multiple measures)/healthy women	TT	No treatment	Significant ↓ in mood disturbance, levels of nitric oxide in TT group
Engle (2000)	Quasi-experimental, repeated measures Pre-Post-test	11	Pulse amplitude; BP; pulse, temperature; stress; self-assessment of health, time perception	TT	Mimic TT	Significant ↓ in total pulse amplitude and time perception in TT group
Hoffmeyer (2000)	Multiple single-case study, experimental repeated measures	9	Frequency, duration and intensity of migraine headaches, medications use; relaxation levels; perception of quality of life; hope	TT	Subjects served as own controls	Significant ↓ in frequency; Significant ↑ in relaxation level post-treatment

(continued)

237

TABLE 18.1 *(continued)*

Author/Yr.	Design	N	Variables/Population	Intervention	Control	Result
Woods & Diamond (2002)	Within-subject, interrupted time-series	10	Physical activity, salivary and urine cortisol	TT	Patients served as own controls	Significant ↓ in overall agitated behavior during treatment and post-treatment
Smith et al. (2003)	Randomized clinical trial	88	Time for engraftment, complications, patient perception of benefit	TT; massage (MT)	Friendly visit	Higher scores on comfort subscale in TT and MT groups
Denison (2004)	Quasi-experimental, Pre-Posttest	15	Pain (McGill Pain Questionnaire); Quality of life (Fibromyalgia Health Assessment Questionnaire; EIT)	TT	Sat quietly, listened to informational tape	Significant ↓ in pain and significant ↑ in QOL in TT group
Larden et al. (2004)	Experimental repeated measures	54	Anxiety (STAI); withdrawal symptoms checklist	TT	Shared activity with a nurse; standard care	Significant ↓ in anxiety in the TT group

1989). These are: new outcome/efficacy studies, replication of existing studies, and theory development studies. Whereas it is clear that the rigorous work of explicating outcomes of and an explanatory framework for TT has begun with serious and careful explorations by a small cadre of researchers, much remains to be done. TT researchers must continue to explore the effects of TT in controlled outcome studies, testing competing theoretical explanations for the outcomes observed, in addition to participating in interdisciplinary efforts related to basic research about the postulated human energy field. Of particular urgency are studies of the use of TT with children, as there has been so little work in this area. Because there are so few clinical situations in which TT has actually been researched related to outcomes, we should also expect that a significant amount of work will be done using simple descriptive designs, the most appropriate starting point when attempting to study a new area.

WEB RESOURCES

The Nurse Healers—Professional Associates International (NH-PAI): www.therapeutic-touch.org
Therapeutic Touch Network Ontario: www.therapeutictouchnetwk.com

REFERENCES

Cowling, R. W. (1990). A template for unitary pattern-based nursing practice. In E. A. M. Barrett (Ed.), Visions of Rogers' science-based nursing (pp. 45–66). New York: National League for Nursing.

Dennison, B. (2004). Touch the pain away: New research on therapeutic touch and persons with fibromyalgia syndrome. Holistic Nursing Practice, 18(3), 142–151.

Engle, V. F., & Graney, M. J. (2000). Biobehavioral effects of therapeutic touch. Journal of Nursing Scholarship, 32(3), 287–293.

Gagne, D., & Toye, R. C. (1994). The effects of Therapeutic Touch and Relaxation Therapy in reducing anxiety. Archives of Psychiatric Nursing, 8(3), 184–189.

Gordon, A., Merenstein, J. H., D'Amico, F., & Hudgens, D. (1998). The effects of therapeutic touch on patients with osteoarthritis of the knee. Journal of Family Practice, 47(4), 271–277.

Grad, B. (1963). A telekinetic effect on plant growth. International Journal of Parapsychology, 5, 117–133.

Grad, B. (1964). A telekinetic effect of plant growth II. International Journal of Parapsychology, 6, 473–485.

Grad, B. (1965). Some biological effects of the laying-on of hands: Review of experiments with animals and plants. Journal of the American Society for Psychical Research, 59, 95–127.

Grad, B., Cadoret, R. J., & Paul, G. I. (1961). An unorthodox method of wound healing in mice. *International Journal of Parapsychology, 3,* 5–24.

Heidt, P. (1981). Effect of therapeutic touch on anxiety level of hospitalized patients. *Nursing Research, 30,* 32–37.

Hoffmeyer, C. A. (2000). *A multiple single-case study experimental design exploring the effect of therapeutic touch on women with migraine headaches.* Doctoral dissertation, University of Colorado Health Sciences Center, Denver, CO.

Keller, E., & Bzdek, V. M. (1986). Effects of therapeutic touch on tension headache pain. *Nursing Research, 35*(2), 101–106.

Krieger, D. (1973). *The relationship of touch, with intent to help or heal, to subjects' in-vivo hemoglobin values: A study in personalized interaction.* Proceedings, Ninth American Nurses Association Nursing Research Conference, 39–58. San Antonio, TX.

Krieger, D. (1979). *The therapeutic touch: How to use your hands to help or to heal.* Englewood Cliffs, NJ: Prentice-Hall.

Krieger, D. (1993). *Accepting your power to heal: The personal practice of therapeutic touch.* Santa Fe, NM: Bear & Company.

Krieger, D., Peper, E., & Ancoli, S. (1979). Physiologic indices of therapeutic touch. *American Journal of Nursing, 4,* 660–662.

Lafreniere, K. D., Mutus, B., Cameron, S., Tannous, M., Giannotti, M., Abu-Zahra, H., et al. (1999). Effects of therapeutic touch on biochemical and mood indicators in women. *Journal of Alternative & Complementary Medicine, 5*(4), 367–370.

Larden, C. N., Palmer, M. L., & Janssen, P. (2004). Efficacy of therapeutic touch in treating pregnant inpatients who have a chemical dependency. *Journal of Holistic Nursing, 22*(4), 320–332.

Lin, Y., & Taylor, A. G. (1998). Effects of therapeutic touch in reducing pain and anxiety in an elderly population. *Integrative Medicine, 1*(4), 155–162.

Macrae, J. (1988). *Therapeutic Touch: A practical guide.* New York: Knopf.

Meehan, T. C. (1993). Therapeutic Touch and postoperative pain: A Rogerian research study. *Nursing Science Quarterly, 6*(2), 69–78.

Meehan, T. C., Mersmann, C. A., Wiseman, M., Wolff, B. B., & Malgady, R. (1990). The effect of Therapeutic Touch on postoperative pain [Abstract]. *Pain* (Suppl. 5), 149.

Olson, M., Sneed, N., LaVia, M., Virella, G., Bonadonna, R., & Michel, Y. (1997). Stress-induced immunosuppression and therapeutic touch. *Alternative Therapies in Health & Medicine, 3*(2), 68–74.

Peck, S. D. (1997). The effectiveness of Therapeutic Touch for decreasing pain in elders with degenerative arthritis. *Journal of Holistic Nursing, 15*(2), 176–198.

Peck, S. D. (1998). The efficacy of therapeutic touch for improving functional ability in elders with degenerative arthritis. *Nursing Science Quarterly, 11*(3), 123–132.

Peters, R. M. (1999). The effectiveness of therapeutic touch: A meta-analytic review. *Nursing Science Quarterly, 12*(1), 52–61.

Quinn, J. F. (1984). Therapeutic Touch as energy exchange: Testing the theory. *Advances in Nursing Science, 6,* 42–49.

Quinn, J. (1989). Future directions for Therapeutic Touch research. *Journal of Holistic Nursing, 7*(1), 19–25.

Quinn, J. F. (1992). Holding sacred space: The nurse as healing environment. *Holistic Nursing Practice, 6*(4), 26–35.

Quinn, J. F. (1996). *Therapeutic Touch: Healing through human energy fields: A 3 tape video course for health care professionals.* New York: National League for Nursing, distributed by HaelanWorks, Boulder, CO.

Quinn, J. F., & Strelkauskas, A. J. (1993). Psychoneuroimmunological effects of Therapeutic Touch on practitioners and recently bereaved recipients: A pilot study. *Advances in Nursing Science, 15*(4), 13–26.

Rogers, M. E. (1990). Nursing: Science of unitary, irreducible, human beings: Update 1990. In E. A. Barrett (Ed.), *Visions of Rogers' science-based nursing.* New York: National League for Nursing.

Rosa, L., Rosa, E., Sarner, L., & Barrett, S. (1998). A closer look at Therapeutic Touch. *Journal of the American Medical Association, 279*(13), 1005–1010.

Schwartz, G. E., Russek, L. G., & Beltran, J. (1995). Interpersonal hand-energy registration: Evidence for implicit performance and perception. *Subtle Energies, 6*(3), 183–200.

Selby, C. (1998). The *JAMA* article critiqued by Carla Selby. *Rocky Mountain Skeptic,* March/April. Retrieved from http://bcn.boulder.co.us/community/rms/rms-jamacrit.html

Simington, J. A., & Laing, G. P. (1993). Effects of Therapeutic Touch in the institutionalized elderly. *Clinical Nursing Research, 2*(4), 438–450.

Smith, M. J. (1972). Paranormal effects on enzyme activity. *Human Dimensions, 1,* 12–15.

Smith, M. C., Reeder, F, Daniel, L., Baramee, J., & Hagman, J. (2003). Outcomes of touch therapies during bone marrow transplant. *Alternative Therapies in Health and Medicine, 9*(1), 40–49.

Turner, J. G., Clark, A. J., Gauthier, D. K., & Williams, M. (1998). The effect of Therapeutic Touch on pain and anxiety in burn patients. *Journal of Advanced Nursing, 28*(1), 10–20.

Woods, D. Y., & Dimond, M. (2002). The effect of therapeutic touch on agitated behavior and cortisol in persons with Alzheimer's disease. *Biological Research for Nursing, 4*(2), 104–114.

CHAPTER 19

Reiki

Debbie Ringdahl and Linda L. Halcón

Reiki is an energy healing method that can be used as an alternative or complementary therapy for a broad range of acute and chronic health problems. Increasingly, it is gaining acceptance as an adjunct to management of chronic conditions: pain management, hospice and palliative care, and stress reduction. Miles and True (2003) identified hospitals and community-based programs in the United States that utilize Reiki in the areas of general medicine, surgery, treatment of HIV/AIDS and cancer, elder and hospice care, and for staff and family members.

According to the National Center for Complementary and Alternative Medicine (NCCAM) of the National Institutes of Health, Reiki is a biofield therapy. Therapies in this category affect energy fields that both surround and interpenetrate the human body. Bioenergy therapies involve touch or placement of the hands into a biofield, the existence of which has not been scientifically proven (Miles & True, 2003). The NIH is currently investigating the effectiveness of Reiki in the treatment of fibromyalgia, diabetic neuropathy, AIDS, and prostate cancer (Miles, 2004). A Reiki practitioner does not need to be prepared as a health care practitioner, but nurses and doctors who practice Reiki may have greater access to patients and acceptability within the health care system in performing hands-on treatments.

The origins of Reiki are unclear, but Reiki historians generally agree that this therapy may have its roots in hands-on healing techniques that were used in Tibet or India more than 2,000 years ago. Reiki emerged in modern times around 1900 through the work of a Japanese business-man and practitioner of Tendai Buddhism, Mikao Usui (Miles & True, 2003). According to William Rand, founder of the International Center for Reiki Training (2000), Usui searched for many years for knowledge of healing methods until he had a profound, transformative experience and received direct revelation of what became known as Reiki. Following this experience, Usui worked with the poor in Kyoto and Tokyo, teaching classes and giving treatments in what he called "The Usui System of Reiki Healing." One of Dr. Usui's students, Chujiro Hayashi, wrote down the hand positions and suggested ways of using them for various ailments.

Mrs. Hawayo Takata is credited with the spread of Reiki in the Americas and Europe. In 1973, Mrs. Takata began to train Reiki teachers (Miles & True, 2003). The Reiki Alliance, a professional organization of Reiki masters, grew from 20 to nearly 1,000 members from 1981 to 1999 (Horrigan, 2003). Currently, the International Center for Reiki Training estimates that there are more than 50,000 Reiki masters and 1 million Reiki practitioners worldwide (Federally funded, 2004).

DEFINITION

The word *Reiki* is composed of two Japanese words—Rei and Ki. Rei is usually translated as "universal," although some authors suggest that it also has a deeper connotation of all-knowing spiritual consciousness. Ki refers to life force energy that flows throughout all living things, known in certain other parts of the world as Ch'i, prana, or mana. When Ki energy is unrestricted, there is thought to be less susceptibility to illness or imbalances of mind, body, or spirit (Rand, 2000). In its combined form, the word *Reiki* is taken to mean spiritually guided life force energy or universal life force energy.

A mind–body component to Reiki healing is evidenced in the underly-ing belief that the deepest level of healing occurs through the spirit. The emphasis is on healing, not cure, which is believed to occur by Reiki energy connecting individuals to their own innate spiritual wisdom. Reiki flows through, but is not directed by, the practitioner, leaving the healing component to the individual receiving the treatment (Miles & True, 2003).

Reiki is not only a healing technique, but also a philosophy of living that acknowledges mind-body-spirit unity and human connectedness to all things. This philosophy is reflected in the Reiki principles for living: Just for today do not worry. Just for today do not anger. Honor your teachers, parents, and elders. Earn your living honestly. Show gratitude to all living things (Mills, 2001).

The ability to practice Reiki is transmitted in stages directly from teacher to student via initiations called attunements. This attunement process differentiates Reiki from other hands-on healing methods. During attunements, teachers open up the students' energy channels by using specific visual symbols that were revealed to Dr. Usui. There are three degrees of attunement necessary in order to achieve the status of Master Teacher, at which stage the practitioner is considered fully open to the flow of universal life force energy. By tradition, the Usui Reiki symbols and their Japanese names are confidential. This arises from the sacred nature of the technique rather than from proprietary motives; the symbols are not believed to carry power if used by non-initiates.

Level I Reiki is taught as a hands-on technique that includes basic information about Reiki principles and hand positions. In Level II, students are taught symbols that allow transfer of energy through space and time, also known as absentee or distance healing. The higher vibration of energy available at Level II is considered to work at a deeper level of healing. Level III, or the mastery level, is typically achieved through an apprenticeship with a Reiki Master, and includes more in-depth study of Reiki practice and teaching. At all levels, Reiki skill develops through committed practice.

In recent years additional branches of Reiki with further degrees of attunement have developed; two of these are Karuna Reiki and Reiki Seichim. There are currently no uniform standards in Reiki education. Because of the non-invasive nature of the treatments, this does not present problems in personal practice. However, the lack of standardization does pose problems when working to integrate Reiki into the conventional health care system (Horrigan, 2003).

SCIENTIFIC BASIS

An emerging body of evidence confirms the existence of energy fields and suggests new ways of measuring energy; these are not specific to Reiki. Traditional electrical measurements such as electrocardiograms and electroencephalograms can now be supplemented by biomagnetic field mapping to obtain more accurate information about the human condition. Superconducting quantum interference devices have been used to show the effect of disease on the magnetic field of the body, and pulsating magnetic fields have been used to improve healing (Oschman, 2002). In a small experimental study concerning the effects of one type of energy therapy, researchers found consistent, marked decreases in gamma rays measured at several sites within the subjects' electromagnetic fields during treatment (Benford, Talnagi, Doss, Boosey, & Arnold, 1999). To a lesser extent, the findings indicated a decrease during sham treatment but not among control subjects. The authors hypothesized that the effect among sham treatment recipients resulted from human touch. Brewitt, Vittetoe, and Hartwell (1997) studied electrical skin resistance at selected body points to measure effects of Reiki treatments. Charman's research (2000) suggests that intention to heal transmits measurable wave patterns to recipients. These studies indicate that in the future it may be possible to directly measure subtle elements of the human energy field in order to elucidate mechanisms by which Reiki and other energy healing techniques lead to changes in health outcomes.

Methodological problems have been identified in studies of Reiki. It is difficult to demonstrate validity in studies of energy therapies. Although case studies and anecdotal examples have been relatively consistent in reporting positive responses to Reiki treatments, this does not represent the scientific rigor that is demanded within an evidenced-based health care system. Mansour, Beuche, Laing, Leis, and Nurse (1999), in an effort to standardize treatments, demonstrated that it is possible to blind subjects to real vs. placebo Rieki, opening the door to placebo-controlled studies in Reiki research.

It has also been speculated that energy healing has an impact on outcomes in a way that is difficult to measure. Engebretson and Wardell (2002) concluded that many research models are not complex enough to capture the experience of a Reiki session. In their qualitative study they found that participants had a diverse and descriptive language that accompanied their experience. They also measured the effects of Reiki on objective measures for stress and anxiety. These measures demonstrated a decrease in perceived anxiety, an increase in signs of relaxation, and an increase in humoral immunological functioning (Wardell & Engebretson, 2001). These two studies demonstrate the potential for increasing the understanding of Reiki energy by utilizing more qualitative research designs.

INTERVENTIONS

Technique

The Reiki practitioner acts as a conduit for healing-intended energy to self or others. During treatments, a level I Reiki practitioner employs a series of 12 to 15 hand positions. A level II Reiki practitioner also uses hand positions but may use various Reiki symbols to focus the Ki energy or to perform distance healings. If touch is contraindicated for any reason, the hands can be held 1 to 4 inches above the body. A full Reiki session usually lasts 45 to 90 minutes. Reiki practitioners, especially if they are nurses working in a clinical setting, often do not have the luxury of providing a full session. At such times, shorter and more targeted treatments may be offered for specific purposes. In the original Reiki handbook of Usui the use of particular hand positions is recommended for addressing specific health problems (Petter, 1999).

Unlike other energy healing modalities, Reiki energy flows through the hands without employing cognitive, emotional, or spiritual skills. The attunement process provides access to the energy without requiring ongoing practice or conscious intention. In this respect, it has the advantage of simplicity (Nield-Anderson & Ameling, 2001). Potter (2003) compared her experience with therapeutic touch after receiving a level I attunement. She found that her work became less directive and the effort to stay centered was no longer a concern.

Guidelines for Full Hands-On Reiki Sessions

The recipient may sit or lie down, but because Reiki tends to be very relaxing, it is often preferable to lie down. Patients may remain clothed during a Reiki treatment. A massage table or hospital bed is frequently used, as this provides for both client and practitioner comfort. After practitioners center themselves and establish an intent to heal with Reiki, the energy flows automatically from their hands without cognitive effort. The hands rest gently on the person's body with the fingers straight and touching so that each hand functions as a unit. The sequence of hand positions may vary, but will generally include all seven major chakras and the endocrine glands.

Measurement of Outcomes

Recipients' subjective feelings during a Reiki session are not considered indications of effectiveness. Patients may feel sensations similar to those of the practitioner, but they may also feel nothing. Sensations may include heat, cold, numbness, involuntary muscle twitching, heaviness, buoyancy, trembling, throbbing, static electricity, tingling, color, and heightened or decreased awareness of sound (Engebretson & Wardell, 2002). This author found that it is not uncommon for clients to fall asleep during a treatment, and that they frequently reported feelings of increased relaxation, peacefulness, and reconnecting to their center.

Physiologic outcome measures examined in other healing touch studies are also appropriate for Reiki, such as hematology tests, blood pressure and heart rate, bioelectric measures, wound healing rate, inhibition of harmful microorganisms, and body temperature changes. Psychological measures are equally important, including perceived pain; cognitive function; memory; and levels of anxiety, depression, anxiety, or hostility.

Precautions

No serious adverse effects of Reiki treatments have been published. Some patients, however, may experience emotional release that may be uncomfortable or disturbing. Therefore, practitioners must be prepared to provide assistance and appropriate referrals if emotional distress persists. Moreover, some individuals may dislike being touched. Practitioners can avoid this discomfort by assessing the person's comfort level with touch and taking into account gender and cultural considerations. Few patients who are fully informed object, and even among vulnerable populations such as victims of torture, responses to hands-on energy healing methods have been found to be very favorable (Kennedy, 2001). The success of a Reiki treatment does not depend on the use of certain hand positions, for the Ki energy goes where it is needed.

USES

The range of potential practical applications with patients is broad and depends on the setting (Lipinski, 1999). Reiki has been used in hospice and palliative care (Bullock, 1997; Lewis, de Vedia, Reuer, Schwan, & Tourin, 2003; Mramor, 2004), among cancer patients (Mills, 2003; Olson & Hanson, 2003), introduced into HIV/AIDS programs (Horrigan, 2003; Schmehr, 2003), for pre- and post-operative patients (Alandydy & Alandydy, 1999; Sawyer, 1998), and in stroke rehabilitation (Hall, 2004; Shiftlett, Nayak, Bid, Miles, & Agostinelli, 2002). The common theme described in many of these programs is the benefit of Reiki for pain relief, stress and anxiety reduction, and relaxation. Miles, founding director of the Institute for the Advancement of the Studies of Complementary Studies, has been involved in research looking specifically at pain and anxiety reduction in HIV/AIDs clients (Vanderbilt, 2004). Shore (2004) recently provided evidence that Reiki may reduce symptoms of depression, with favorable outcomes that last as long as 1 year following treatment.

Table 19.1 provides a list of populations/settings in which Reiki has been used. In a biomedical treatment setting Reiki is best regarded as a complementary healing modality, whereas in other circumstances it can either be used alone or with other approaches.

Self-Treatment and Practitioner Benefits

One of the unique features of Reiki therapy is the capacity to self-treat. The concepts of empowerment and self-treatment have particular value when considering chronic health problems. For some Reiki practitioners, teaching their clients level I Reiki provides the clients with a greater sense of control over some of their health problems, including pain management and stress reduction (Miles & True, 2003; Mills, 2001). This author has taught level II Reiki to a client with advanced amyotrophic lateral sclerosis, which increased the practitioner's ability to self-treat and also to perform distant healing.

TABLE 19.1 Suggested Applications for Reiki in Clinical Settings

Application	Reference
Promoting relaxation in labor and delivery	(Mills, 2001)
HIV/AIDs	(Schmehr, 2003; Vanderbilt, 2004)
Supporting pre- and post-operative surgical patients	(Alandydy & Alandydy, 1999; Sawyer, 1998)
Hospice and palliative care	(Bullock, 1997; Lewis et al., 2003; Mramor, 2004)
Pain management	(Olson & Hanson, 2003; O'Mathuna, 2003)
Decreasing anxiety and stress levels	(Dressen & Singg, 2000; Shore, 2004; Witt & Dundes, 2001)
Enhancing immune function	(Wardell & Engebretson, 2001)
Promoting wound healing	(Papantonio, 1998)
Stroke rehabilitation	(Hall, 2004; Shiftlett et al., 2002)
Addiction and chemical dependency treatment	(Burkert, 1999)
Improving hematology measures	(Wirth, Chang, Eidelman, & Paxton, 1996)

Reiki energy, by moving through the practitioner's crown and out through the hands, also has positive effects on the practitioner. Reiki practitioners report feeling energized, relaxed, and more centered after performing a treatment. Whelan (2003) found in her research that performing Reiki on clients increased nurses' satisfaction with their nursing role. With Reiki use, nurses have reported an increase in touch sensitivity, perception, and assessment skills. Fortune and Price (2003) have identified Reiki as an energy therapy that can be used to prevent and treat burnout among nurses.

FUTURE RESEARCH

Most published research on Reiki has been conducted with small, non-controlled, convenience samples, raising questions about the validity and generalizability of findings. Clinical evaluation of Reiki represents a challenge, using our current standards of assessment. New models of research that enlarge our definition of outcomes need to be explored (Schiller, 2003). Combining subjective and physiological measures in such research studies will allow broader assessment of the effects of Reiki (Liverani, Minelli, & Ricciuti, 2000). Because the goals of Reiki may be broader than symptom relief and include concepts of physiologic and psychological balance, qualitative studies that can address values and meaning are also important (Wardell & Engebretson, 2001).

Although both hands-on and distant healing are forms of energy healing, the presence of touch has the capacity to confound the results, as all touch may have some healing properties. A review of studies of the efficacy of distant healing (Astin, Harkness, & Ernst, 2000) identified both methodological limitations and positive outcomes meriting further study. Shore (2004) compared outcomes between hands-on and distant Reiki healing and found a greater reduction in depression symptoms with distance healing.

There is a need to develop research designs that consider more subtle and lasting outcomes than those that have typically been used. If energy treatment works on a different level than the conventional medical model, the results may not be as dramatic and may require larger groups and a longer treatment period to show a positive outcome (Nield-Anderson & Ameling, 2000).

Suggested questions for future research include:

1. What are the physiologic and/or psychological effects of Reiki treatments for specific conditions when used alone or in conjunction with other therapies?

2. What is the relative effectiveness of non-contact Reiki (distant healing) as compared to hands-on Reiki?

3. What role does Reiki have in providing stress reduction for health care providers?

4. Are there differences in selected outcome measures between Reiki and other energy therapies?

REIKI WEB SITES

IARP-International Association of Reiki Professionals: www.iarp.org
The International Center for Reiki Training: www.reiki.org
The Reiki Page: www.reiki7gen.com
Usui Reiki: www.usuireiki.com

REFERENCES

Alandydy, P., & Alandydy, K. (1999). Performance brief: Using Reiki to support surgical patients. *Journal of Nursing Care Quality, 13*(4), 89–91.

Astin, J., Harkness, E., & Ernst, E. (2000). The efficacy of "distant healing": A systematic review of randomized trials. *Annals of Internal Medicine, 132*(11), 903–910.

Benford, M. S., Talnagi, J., Doss, D. B., Boosey, S., & Arnold, L. E. (1999). Gamma radiation fluctuations during alternative healing therapy. *Alternative Therapies in Health and Medicine, 5*(4), 51–56.

Brewitt, B., Vittetoe, T., & Hartwell, B. (1997). The efficacy of Reiki hands-on healing: Improvements in spleen and nervous system function as quantified by electrodermal screening. *Alternative Therapies in Health and Medicine, 5*(4), 51–56.

Bullock, M. (1997). Reiki: A complementary therapy for life. *American Journal of Hospice and Palliative Care, 14*(1), 31–33.

Burkert, L. (1999). *Reiki for the recovering alcoholic and addict.* International Center for Reiki Training. Retrieved August 22, 2000, from http://www.reiki.org/reikinews/reikin20.html

Charman, R. A. (2000). Placing healers, healees, and healing into a wider research context. *Journal of Alternative and Complementary Medicine, 6*(2), 177–180.

Dressen, L. J., & Singg, S. (2000). Effects of Reiki on pain and selected affective and personality variables of chronically ill patients. *Subtle Energies and Energy Medicine, 9*(1), 51–82.

Engebretson, J., & Wardell, D. W. (2002). Experience of a Reiki session. *Alternative Therapies in Health and Medicine, 8*(2), 48–53.

Federally funded Reiki study underway in Washington. (2004). *Acupuncture Today, 5*(3), 1, 8.

Fortune, M., & Price, M. (2003). The spirit of healing: How to develop a spirituality based personal and professional practice. *Journal of the New York State Nurses Association, 34*(1), 32–38.

Hall, M. (2004). Treating stroke and other neurological disorders. *Reiki News Magazine, 3*(2), 38–42.

Horrigan, B. (2003). Pamela Miles: Reiki vibrational healing. *Alternative Therapies in Health and Medicine, 9*(4), 75–83.

Kennedy, P. (2001). Working with survivors of torture in Sarajevo with Reiki. *Complementary Therapies in Nursing and Midwifery, 7*(1), 4–7.

Lewis, C., de Vedia, A., Reuer, B., Schwan, R., & Tourin, C. (2003). Integrating complementary and alternative medicine (CAM) into standard hospice and palliative care. *American Journal of Hospice and Palliative Care, 20*(3), 221–228.

Lipinski, K. (1999). *Enhancing nursing practice with Reiki.* International Center for Reiki Training. Retrieved February 5, 2005, from http://www.reiki.org/reiknews/NursingandReiki.htm

Liverani, A., Minelli, E., & Ricciuti, A. (2000). Subjective scales for the evaluation of therapeutic effects and their use in complementary medicine. *Journal of Alternative and Complementary Medicine, 6*(3), 257–264.

Mansour, A. A., Beuche, M., Laing, G., Leis, A., & Nurse, J. (1999). A study to test the effectiveness of placebo Reiki standardization procedures developed for a planned Reiki efficacy study. *Journal of Alternative and Complementary Medicine, 5*(2), 153–164.

Miles, P. (2004). Palliative care service at the NIH includes Reiki and other mind body modalities. *Advances, 20*(2), 30–31.

Miles, P. (in press). *Reiki: The definitive guide.* New York: Jeremy Tarcher.

Miles, P., & True, G. (2003). Reiki—review of a biofield therapy: History, theory, practice, and research. *Alternative Therapies in Health and Medicine, 9*(2), 62–72.

Mills, J. (2001). *Tapestry of healing: Where Reiki and medicine intertwine.* Green Valley, AZ: White Sage. Retrieved from www.TapestryofHealing.com

Mills, J. (2003). How I introduced Reiki treatments into my obstetrics and gynecologic practice. *Reiki News, 2*(2), 16–21.

Mramor, J. (2004). Reiki in hospice care: Miranda's story. *Massage and Bodywork, 19*(1), 51–59.

Nield-Anderson, L., & Ameling, A. (2000). The empowering nature of Reiki as a complementary therapy. *Holistic Nursing Practice, 14*(3), 21–29.

Nield-Anderson, L., & Ameling, A. (2001). Reiki: A complementary therapy for nursing practice. *Journal of Psychosocial Nursing, 39*(4), 42–49.

Olson, K., & Hanson, J. (2003). A Phase II trial of Reiki for the management of pain in advanced cancer patients. *Journal of Pain and Symptom Management, 26*(5), 990–997.

O'Mathuna, D. (2003). Reiki for relaxation and pain relief. *Alternative Therapies in Women's Health, 5*(4), 29–32.

Oschman, J. (2002). Clinical aspects of biological fields: An introduction for health care professionals. *Journal of Bodywork and Movement Therapies, 6*(2), 117–125.

Papantonio, C. (1998). Alternative medicine and wound healing. *Ostomy/Wound Management, 44*(4), 44–55.

Petter, F. (1999). *The original Reiki handbook of Dr. Mikao Usui.* Twin Lakes, WI: Lotus Press.

Potter, P. (2003). What are the distinctions between Reiki and therapeutic touch? *Clinical Journal of Oncology Nursing, 7*(1), 89–91.

Rand, W. (2000). *Reiki, the healing touch: First and second degree manual.* Southfield, MI: Vision Publications.

Sawyer, J. (1998). The first Reiki practitioner in our OR. *AORN Journal, 67*(3), 674–676.

Schiller, R. (2003). Reiki: A starting point for integrative medicine. *Alternative Therapies in Health and Medicine, 9*(2), 20–21.

Schmehr, R. (2003). Enhancing the treatment of HIV/AIDS with Reiki training and treatment. *Alternative Therapies in Health and Medicine, 9*(2), 120–121.

Shiftlett, S., Nayak, S., Bid, S., Miles, P., & Agostinelli, M. (2002). Effect of Reiki treatment as functional recovery in patients in poststroke rehabilitation: A pilot study. *The Journal of Alternative and Complementary Medicine, 8*(2), 755–763.

Shore, A. G. (2004). Long-term effects of energetic healing on symptoms of psychological depression and self-perceived stress. *Alternative Therapies in Health and Medicine, 10*(3), 42–48.

Vanderbilt, S. (2004). Somatic research: Moving energy forward in the scientific realm. *Massage and Bodywork, 19*(1), 136–139.

Wardell, D., & Engebretson, J. (2001). Biological correlates of Reiki touch healing. *Journal of Advanced Nursing, 33*(4), 439–445.

Whelan, K. M. (2003). Reiki therapy: The benefits to a nurse-Reiki practitioner. *Nursing Practice, 17*(4), 209–217.

Wirth, D. P., Chang, R. J., Eidelman, W. S., & Paxton, J. B. (1996). Hematological indicators of complementary healing intervention. *Complementary Therapies in Health and Medicine, 4*, 4–20.

Witt, D., & Dundes, L. (2001). Harnessing life energy or wishful thinking: Reiki, placebo, placebo reiki, meditation, and music. *Alternative and Complementary Therapies, 7*(5), 304–309.

CHAPTER 20

Acupressure

Pamela Weiss

Touch has been central to the practice of nursing since its inception. This chapter will discuss a Traditional Chinese Medicine form of touch known as acupressure and its application in nursing care. This method of treatment is common in many cultures. As Dossey, Keegan, and Guzzetta (2000) note, "All cultures have demonstrated that some form of rubbing, pressing, massaging or holding are [sic] natural manifestations of the desire to heal and care for one another" (p. 615). Acupressure is also integral to the practice of shiatsu, tui na, tsubo, and jin si ju jitsyu.

DEFINITIONS

Acupressure is defined by Gach (1990) as "an ancient healing art that uses the fingers to press certain points on the body to stimulate the body's self-curative abilities" (p. 3). To assist the reader, the following other definitions are provided.

> *Acupuncture:* "A procedure used in or adapted from Chinese Medical Practice in which specific body areas are pierced with fine needles for therapeutic purposes or to relieve pain or produce regional anesthesia" (Freedictionary, 2005).

Auriculotherapy: "also called ear acupuncture, applies the principles of acupuncture to specific points on the ear" (Firsthealth, 2005).

Jin Shin Jyutsu: "a non-massage form of shiatsu . . . using pressure points to 'harmonize' the flow of 'energy' through the body" (Heall, 2005).

Meridians: "specific interconnected channels through which Qi circulates" (Answers.com, 2005).

Moxibustion: "The burning of moxa or other substances on the skin, to treat diseases or to produce analgesia" (Freedictionary, 2005).

Qi: Pronounced "chee," "The vital force believed in Taoism and other Chinese thought to be inherent in all things. The unimpeded circulation of chi and a balance of its negative and positive forms in the body are held to be essential to good health in traditional Chinese medicine" (Freedictionary, 2005).

Shiatsu: "A form of therapeutic massage in which pressure is applied with the thumb and palms to those areas of the body used in acupuncture. Also called acupressure 9" (Freedictionary, 2005).

TRADITIONAL CHINESE MEDICINE

Traditional Chinese Medicine (TCM) is an ancient system of health developed more than 3,000 years ago in Asia. This system is based on the concept that qi that flows throughout the body and that balance of yin and yang forces represents health and well-being. As Kaptchuk (1983) describes it:

> This system of care is based on ancient texts and is the result of a continuous process of critical thinking, as well as extensive clinical observation and testing. It represents a thorough formulation and reformulation of material by respected clinicians and theoreticians. It is also, however, rooted in the philosophy, logic and sensibility, and habits of a civilization entirely foreign to our own. It has therefore developed its own perception of the body and health and disease. [p. 2]

The focus of care within this system is to restore balance in the body. To do so, yin and yang must be balanced. Yin aspects are associated with cold, passivity, interiority, and decreases. Yang aspects are associated with warmth, activity, external forces, and increases. Yin and yang are always in relation to each other (Kaptchuk, 1983). According to this conceptualization, they are in continuous flux and there is always yin within yang and yang within yin.

Unschuld (1999) reflects that TCM theory is a mixture of beliefs that pathogenic influences from the outside combine with the lack of balance or harmony within the person and result in illness. TCM is also concerned with the concept of qi. Qi flows in the body through specific pathways identified as meridians or channels. If the qi is blocked or diminished, a person experiences pain or illness.

There are 12 bilateral meridians and 8 extra meridians. All meridians have an exterior and an interior pathway and are named according to the organ system. Located on the meridians are specific points. In the 12 major meridians, the points are bilateral and in the West are called acupuncture points. This nomenclature implies that the points are designated for needle insertion and does not fully reflect the TCM concept of the point.

Acupuncture points are used for acupressure. The points do not have a corresponding anatomic structure but are described by their location relative to other anatomical landmarks. This contributes to the skepticism of many Western-trained scientists about their existence. In Chinese, the name of the point usually is descriptive of its function or location. Mistranslation over the years has often limited the substantial amount of anatomical basis for the nomenclature of points and the apparent knowledge of anatomy of Chinese scholars (Schnorrenberger, 1996).

There are 365 (Kaptchuk, 1983) to 700 (Jwing-Ming, 1992) major points on the meridians. Jwing-Ming stated that 108 could be stimulated using the fingers. In a traditionally formulated TCM treatment plan, whether the modality is needles or pressure, the points are combined to achieve maximum benefit for the patient. Rarely is only one point used. There are points that should not be stimulated, especially during pregnancy, which are referred to as "forbidden points."

SCIENTIFIC BASIS

Western medicine is the dominant system of health care in the United States. It is characterized by hospitals, clinics, pharmaceutical resources, and by a workforce of physicians, nurses, specialized therapists, and various support service personnel. There are many differences between Western medicine and TCM, which become more evident as nurses seek to add TCM modalities to their practice. Western medicine emphasizes disease, causal agents, and treatments that are designed to control or destroy the cause of disease (Kaptchuk, 1983). Once a causal agent or mechanism is identified, treatment plans are developed that focus on the agent or mechanism as a consistent factor in all human manifestations of the disease. In Western journals, almost all studies using the modality of acupuncture and acupressure emphasize the specific effects of needling one point known to address a specific symptom. Medical researchers are eager to find the mechanism by which acupuncture alleviates the symptoms. Some of the mechanisms have been suggested in Western medical research (National Center for Complementary/Alternative Medicines [NCCAM], 2000; National Institutes of Health [NIH], 1997). Stimulation of the points with needles or with pressure may produce a therapeutic effect due to the following:

1.   Conduction of electromagnetic signals that may start the flow of pain-killing biochemicals, such as endorphins, and of immune system cells to specific sites in the body that are injured or vulnerable to disease (Dale, 1997; Takeshige, 1989)

2.   Activation of opioid systems, thereby reducing pain (Han, 1997)

3.   Changes in brain chemistry, sensation, and involuntary responses by changing the release of neurotransmitters and neurohormones in a health-promoting way (Wu, 1995; Wu, Zhou, & Zhou, 1994).

The scientific research into an underlying mechanism demonstrates one of the differences between Western medicine and the TCM system. The focus in TCM is the imbalance in the patient, and the causality is always multifactorial. The function of the points is described in terms of TCM diagnosis. For example, Western medicine research has focused on pericardium 6, or nei guan, for the treatment of nausea. In English its name means inner border gate. Lade (1986) describes the point:

> The name refers to the point's role as the gateway or connecting point of the triple burner channel and the yin-linking vessel. Inner refers to the palmar aspect of the forearm and to the point's location on the yin channel. The actions of this point are: to regulate and tonify the heart, transform heart phlegm, facilitate qi flow, regulate the yin-linking vessel and clear heart fire, redirect rebellious qi downward, expand and relax the chest and benefit the diaphragm. [p. 196]

> The indications for use of the point are: asthma, bronchitis, pertussis, hiccups, vomiting, diaphragmatic spasms, intercostal neuralgia, chest fullness, and pain and dyspnea. [p. 197]

Whereas Western medicine focuses on the treatment of nausea for this point, the TCM paradigm suggests multiple uses. In TCM theory, nausea is considered rebellious qi (qi that flows in the wrong direction). Nausea and vomiting are examples of this. Nei guan (pericardium 6) is used as one of the points in the treatment of a patient who presents with nausea. In TCM theory, nausea is considered one of the external manifestations of the imbalance, but in an authentic TCM treatment, a practitioner would evaluate the imbalances that set up the manifestation and treat the underlying condition. Therefore, a combination of points to treat nausea would be used, possibly including other primary points for antiemesis (Hoo, 1997): Stomach 36 on the stomach meridian located on the knee, Ren 12 on the ren/conception meridian located on the upper abdomen, or the Spleen 4 on the spleen meridian located on the foot. Application of multiple acupoints may be more effective for the treatment of nausea; however, in Western medicine, the focus on finding the single active point or the mechanism creates an almost insurmountable challenge to the fullest application of the therapy.

In 1997, the National Institutes of Health held the first consensus conference on acupuncture. The conference concluded that

> Acupuncture is effective in the treatment of adult nausea and vomiting in chemotherapy and probably pregnancy and in postoperative dental pain. The conference members stated there is an indication that acupuncture may be helpful in the treatment of addiction, stroke rehabilitation, headache, menstrual cramps, tennis elbow, fibromyalgia, myofascial pain, osteoarthritis, low back pain, carpal tunnel syndrome, and asthma, in which acupuncture may be useful as an adjunct treatment or an acceptable alternative or be included in a comprehensive management program. [NIH, 1997]

Research evidence underlying the use of the point called nei guan (pericardium 6) for nausea is reviewed below. This NIH statement was the springboard for increasing the number of studies completed for the treatment of nausea and vomiting that include the use of devices to apply pressure or stimulation to pericardium 6. These devices included an elastic bracelet with a pressure button called SeaBands® or an electrical stimulation device called a Reliefband®. Table 20.1 demonstrates that studies continue to find conflicting results about the effectiveness of using pericardium 6 for the treatment of nausea and vomiting from any condition.

There are many limitations to the research done in acupuncture, and therefore acupressure. Harris (1997) frames the ongoing debate about the studies and results.

> The scientific quality of most of the published studies examining the effectiveness of multipoint acupressure, predominantly auriculotherapy, has been poor, without adequate control groups, randomization,

TABLE 20.1 Sample of Studies Using P6 for Treating Nausea

Condition Causing the Nausea	Modality	Author/Date	Conclusion
Nausea of chemo-therapy	Acupressure on P6 and Stomach 36	Dibble, Chapman, Mack, & Shih (2000)	During the first 10 days of the chemotherapy cycle, women with breast cancer who were taught and prac-ticed acupressure of P6 experi-enced a decreased intensity and frequency of nausea.
All nausea studies	Acupressure	Cochrane Collab-orative (2000)	The studies on nausea are lim-ited and the results are equivo-cal.
Nausea of chemo-therapy	Acupressure	Klein & Griffiths (2004)	Acupressure may decrease nau-sea among patients undergo-ing chemotherapy but further study is required.
Nausea of chemo-therapy	Acupressure	Shin, Kim, Shin, & Juan (2004)	Acupressure on P6 point ap-pears to be an effective ad-junct treatment.
Nausea of pregnancy	Acupressure and acu-stimulation bands	Roscoe et al. (2003)	This review article concludes that stimulation of the point is positive, but many of the studies have limitations that leave questions about effective-ness.
Nausea of chemo-therapy	Acupressure	Collins & Thomas (2004)	Acupressure in addition to antiemetics provides better control of the nausea of chemotherapy.
Nausea of HIV/AIDS	Acupressure	Capili (2002)	Symptoms of nausea were de-creased; however reports of the quality of life did not im-prove.
Postopera-tive nausea and vom-iting	Acupressure	Ming, Kuo, Lin, & Lin (2002)	In view of the absence of side effects, acupressure is a safe alternative to treatment of nausea and vomiting.

placebos, blinding, and statistical analyses. There seems to be a cultural divide between theory and methodological rigor. The scientifically rigorous studies have tended to be atheoretical in selecting the acupoint for treatment and in explaining how the points may work. [p. 157]

Table 20.2 presents a brief overview of recent studies examining the use of acupressure in a variety of patients. The conditions treated include wandering in Alzheimer's disease, dyspnea, sleep in elderly patients, pain of labor, dysmenorrhea, and stress of patients transported by emergency vehicles. The number of studies continues to increase, and yet scarce funding has yielded studies with small sample sizes, thus limiting their generalizability. However, these limited studies do provide the incentive for nurses to consider incorporating acupressure techniques into their practices as it is a non-invasive treatment that may have an impact on patient outcomes.

INTERVENTION

A diagnostic process is used to choose the correct points to stimulate. In TCM, the process includes an extensive history, observing the patient's appearance and demeanor, noticing the patient's odor, checking the tongue, palpating the abdomen and points on the body, and palpating the pulses at the radial location on the wrists. A diagnosis is formulated and a treatment plan, which may use a variety of techniques, is implemented. Nurses will not follow this process and will therefore be using a Western symptom-based system of determining the correct treatment plan.

Guidelines for Use

Nurses can incorporate acupressure into the care of patients by using some common points that have specific actions to relieve common symptoms. The nurse can treat the patient with acupressure or teach the patient or family members how to use acupressure as part of a care plan.

Prior to touching any patient, the nurse must assess the readiness of the client. Shames and Keegan recommend the following assessment of clients:

- perception of mind–body situation

- pathophysiological problems that may require referral

- history of psychological disorders

TABLE 20.2 Sample of Studies of Effective Uses of Acupuncture/
Acupressure

Condition	Modality	Author/Date	Conclusion
Wandering behaviors in Alzheimer's disease	Foot acupressure	Sutherland, Reakes, & Bridges (1999)	Foot acupressure may produce a decrease in wandering and an increase in quiet time.
Dyspnea of COPD	Acupressure	Wu, Wu, Lin, & Lin (2004)	Pulmonary function, dyspnea scores, and other physiological measures were improved with the use of acupressure of appropriate points
Sleep of elderly	Magnetic auricular beads	Suen, Wong, & Leung (2002)	Three-week treatment of placing magnetic beads in the ear significantly increased sleep time in the elderly.
Dysmenorrhea	Relief Brief® (a brief that puts pressure on acupuncture points)	Taylor, Miaskowski, & Kohn (2002)	Wearing of the acupressure brief relieved pain symptoms and reduced the need for medication in subjects.
Low back pain	Acupressure	Hsieh, Kuo, Yen, & Chen (2004)	Acupressure is another effective alternative medicine for reducing low back pain. However, careful assessment should be made in future studies.
Pain of labor	Ice massage at the Large Intestine 4 (LI 4) point	Waters & Raisler (2003)	Ice massage assisted women in reducing their pain perception on a scale from distressing to uncomfortable.
Pain of labor	Acupressure using Large Intestine 4 (LI 4) and Bladder 67 (BL 67) points	Chung, Hung, Kuo, & Huang (2003)	Acupressure reduced the pain of labor while not diminishing the quality of contractions in first stage labor.
Stress experienced during transport in EMS vehicle	Auricular acupressure	Kober et al. (2003)	Auricular acupressure reduced anxiety, decreased pain, and resulted in more positive attitudes about potential outcomes.

- cultural beliefs about touch

- previous experience with body therapies (2000, p. 264)

Each point is located using an anatomical marker. There are many books describing point location. The standard measure is the cun, which is different for each individual. One cun for a particular patient is defined as the "width of the interphalangeal joint of the patient's thumb or as the distance between the two radial ends of the flexor creases of a flexed middle finger of the patient. Two cun is the width of the index finger, the middle finger and the ring finger" (Hoo, 1997).

Stimulating the Point

There are several different types of techniques to stimulate the points, according to Gach:

- *Firm stationary pressure* using the thumbs, fingers, palms, the sides of hands, or knuckles

- *Slow motion kneading* using the thumbs and fingers along with the heels of the hands to squeeze large muscle groups

- *Brisk rubbing* using friction to stimulate the blood and lymph

- *Quick tapping* with the fingertips to stimulate muscles on unprotected areas of the body such as the face (1990, p. 9)

Evaluating Acupressure's Effect

Gach has developed guidelines for assessing results. The elements of the assessment include:

- Identifying the problems being addressed with acupressure

- Identifying the points being used for the treatment

- The length of time for the acupressure

- Identifying what makes the condition worse (e.g., standing, cold weather, menstruation, constipation, lack of exercise, stress, traveling, and others) (Gach, 1990, p. 13)

- Describing the changes experienced by the patient after 3 days and after 1 week of treatment

- Describing the changes in the condition and overall feeling of well-being

USES

There are many uses for acupressure. Some conditions for which it has been used are shown in Table 20.2. The use of acupuncture for nausea, pain, and gastrointestinal disorders is described below.

Nausea

Point: Pericardium 6 (nei guan, "inner gate")

Location: Pericardium 6 is located on the inner aspect of the wrist 2 cun (units) proximal to the transverse crease of the wrist between the tendons of the palmaris longus and flexor carpi radialis muscles (Lade, 1986). Have the patient place the middle three fingers (index, middle, and ring fingers) on the opposite hand that is palm upward. The point under the ring finger between the two tendons is pericardium 6 (see Figure 20.1).

Functions: Its functions were outlined previously in the discussion on the research on this point.

Method of stimulation: The point can be stimulated using firm pressure either with a rotating pattern with the thumb or the static pressure of a SeaBand.

Indications in nursing: This point can be used for the treatment of nausea in many situations, but research, as cited previously, has focused on postoperative nausea, the nausea of pregnancy, and the nausea accompanying chemotherapy.

Pain and Gastrointestinal Disorders

Point: Large intestine 4 (LI 4) (hoku, "joining the valley")

Location: This point is on the back of the hand halfway between the junction between the first and second metacarpal bones, which form a depression or valley when the thumb is abducted (Lade, 1986). There are two ways to locate this point easily. Have the patient hold the hand with the thumb touching the index finger; hold the hand at eye level and the highest mound at the base of the thumb and index finger is the location of LI 4. Or instruct the patient to place the thumb of one hand in the web between the thumb and index finger of the opposite hand. The patient should match the first crease on the thumb of one hand to the web of the other and then rotate the thumb to touch the fleshy area between the index finger and thumb. The point is where the tip of the thumb touches the area between the thumb and the index finger.

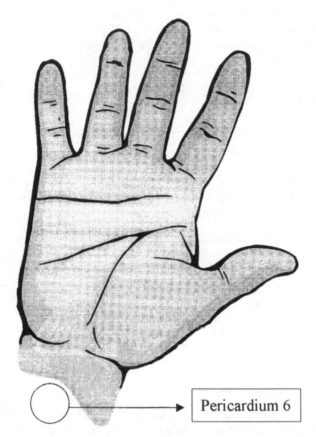

Pericardium 6

FIGURE 20.1 Pressure point pericardium 6.

Functions: This point has multiple functions and is one of the most important points of the body. It alleviates pain, tones qi, and protective qi (in Western medicine this would be considered an immune system building function); moistens the large intestine and in so doing relieves diarrhea or constipation; clears the nose; regulates the lungs in asthma, bronchitis, or the common cold; and expedites labor. This point is contra-indicated in pregnancy because of this function (Lade, 1986, pp. 40–41).

Indications in nursing: This point will relieve any pain in the body. In addition, persons with diarrhea or constipation may feel relief because stimulating the point balances the gastrointestinal functions. This point can be used to induce labor and, coupled with its pain-relieving effect, may be helpful.

Method of stimulation: Firm pressure can be applied on this point with a rotating thumb massage technique. This point is often sensitive and the patient will report a feeling of discomfort. This is normal and not indicative of a problem.

Precautions

There are overall guidelines and precautions carefully outlined by Michael Reed Gach (1990) in his book, *Acupressure Potent Points.*

- Never press any area in an abrupt, forceful, or jarring way. Apply finger pressure in a slow, rhythmic manner to enable layers of tissues and the internal organs to respond (p. 11).

- Use abdominal points cautiously, especially if the patient is ill. Avoid the abdominal area altogether if the patient has a life-threatening disease, especially intestinal cancer, tuberculosis, or leukemia. Avoid the abdominal area during pregnancy (pp. 11–12).

- During pregnancy, strong stimulation of certain points should be avoided: LI 4 (four point on the large intestine meridian), K 3 (third point on the kidney meridian), and SP 6 (sixth point on the spleen meridian). Each of these points may have an effect on the pregnancy (p. 192).

- Lymph areas such as the groin, the area of the throat just below the ears, and the outer breast near the armpits are very sensitive. Touch these areas lightly (p. 12).

- Do not work directly on a serious burn, ulcer, or area of infection.

- Do not work directly on a newly formed scar. New surgical or other wounds should not be touched directly. Continuous holding on the periphery of the injury will stimulate the injury to heal (p. 12).

- After an acupressure treatment, tolerance to cold is lowered and the energy of the body is focused on healing, so advise the patient to wear warm clothes and keep out of drafts (p. 12).

- Use acupressure cautiously in persons with a new acute or serious illness (Gach, 1990).

- Acupressure is not a sole treatment for cancer, contagious skin disease, or sexually transmitted disease (Gach, 1990, pp. 11–12).

- Brisk rubbing, deep pressure, or kneading should not be used for persons with heart disease, cancer, or high blood pressure (Gach, 1990, p. 9).

FUTURE RESEARCH

There are many areas of research in which the methods of traditional Chinese medicine and the underlying theory can be tested using Western medical research techniques. Research questions about the usefulness of acupressure techniques can be posed in many areas of nursing including their use for palliative care, rehabilitation nursing, support of women in labor, and health promotion and disease prevention.

Acupressure is used by millions of persons around the world. Incorporating this technique into nursing care plans will unite us in the commonality we share—the desire to relieve human suffering (Serizawa, 1976).

REFERENCES

Answers.com (n.d.). Retrieved October 26, 2005, from http://www.answers.com

Capili B. (2002). Testing acupressure for the relief of nausea and vomiting in persons with HIV/AIDS. Columbia University, D.N.Sc. 2002.

Cardini, F., & Weixin, H. (1998). Moxibustion for correction of breech presentation: A randomized controlled trial. *Journal of the American Medical Association, 280*(18), 1580–1584.

Cho, Z. H., Chung, S. C., Jones, J. P., Park, J. B., Park, H. J., Lee, H. J., et al. (1998). New findings of the correlation between acupoints and corresponding brain cortices using functional MRI. *Proceedings of the National Academy of Science, U.S.A. 95*, 2670–2673.

Chung U., Hung L., Kuo, S., & Huang, C. (2003). Effects of LI4 and BL 67 acupressure on labor pain and uterine contractions in the first stage of labor. *Journal of Nursing Research, 11*(4), 251–260.

Cochrane Collaborative. (2000). *Overview of Cochrane Collaborative.* Retrieved from http://www.cochrane.de/cochrane/cc-broch.htm

Collins, K. B., & Thomas, D. J. (2004). Evidenced-based practice: Acupuncture and acupressure for the management of chemotherapy-induced nausea and vomiting. *Journal of the American Academy of Nurse Practitioners, 16*(2), 76–80.

Dale, R. A. (1997). Demythologizing acupuncture, Part 1: The scientific mechanisms and the clinical uses. *Alternative and Complementary Therapies Journal, 3*(2), 125–131.

Dibble, S. L., Chapman, J., Mack, K. A., & Shih, A. S. (2000). Acupressure for nausea: Results of a pilot study. *Oncology Nursing Forum, 27*(1), 41–47.

Dossey, B. M., Keegan, L., & Guzzetta, C. E. (2000). *Holistic nursing: A handbook for practice.* Gaithersburg, MD: Aspen.

Education Yahoo. (n.d.). Retrieved October 26, 2005, from http://education.yahoo.com

Firsthealth. (n.d.). Retrieved October 26, 2005, from http://www.firsthealth ofandover.com

Freedictionary. (n.d.). Retrieved October 26, 2005, from http://www.thefree dictionary.com

Gach, M. (1990). *Acupressure potent points.* New York: Bantam Books.

Han, J. S. (1997). *Acupuncture activates endogenous systems of analgesia.* National Institutes of Health Consensus Conference on Acupuncture: Program and Abstracts. Bethesda, MD: National Institutes of Health.

Harris, P. E. (1997). Acupressure: A review of the literature. *Complementary Therapies in Medicine, 5*(3), 156–161.

Heall. (n.d.). Retrieved October 26, 2005, from http://www.heall.com

Hochberg, M. (1999). A randomized trial of acupuncture as an adjunctive therapy in osteoarthritis of the knee. *Rheumatology, 3*(4), 346–354.

Hoo, J. J. (1997). Acupressure for hyperemesis gravidarum. *American Journal of Obstetrics and Gynecology, 176*(6), 1395–1396.

Hsieh, L. L., Kuo, C., Yen, M., & Chen, T. H. (2004). A randomized controlled clinical trial for low back pain treated by acupressure and physical therapy. *Preventive Medicine, 39*(1), 168–176.

Jewell, D., & Young G. (2001). *Interventions for nausea and vomiting in early pregnancy.* Cochrane Database Systematic Review, Oxford, England.

Jwing-Ming, Y. (1992). *Chinese qigong massage.* Jamaica Plain, MA: Yangs' Martial Arts Association.

Kaptchuk, T. J. (1983). *The web that has no weaver.* New York: Congdon & Weed.

Klein, J., & Griffiths, P. (2004). Acupressure for nausea and vomiting in cancer patients receiving chemotherapy. *British Journal of Community Nursing, 9*(9), 383–386, 388.

Kober, A., Scheck, T., Schubert, B., Strasser, H., Gustorff, B., Bertalanffy, P., et al. (2003). Auricular acupressure as a treatment for anxiety in prehospital transport settings. *Anesthesiology, 98*(6), 1328–1332.

Lade, A. (1986). *Images and functions.* Seattle, WA: Eastland.

Ming, J., Kuo, B. I., Lin, J., & Lin, L. (2002). The efficacy of acupressure to prevent nausea and vomiting in post-operative patients. *Journal of Advanced Nursing, 39*(4), 343–351.

National Center for Complementary/Alternative Medicines. (2000). Acupuncture information and resources. Retrieved from http://nccam.nih.gov/fcp/factsheets/acupuncture/acupuncture.htm

National Institutes of Health. (1997). NIH Consensus Development Conference Statement. Acupuncture. Retrieved from http://odp.od.nih.gov/consensus/cons/107/107_statement.htm

Roscoe, J. A., Morrow, G. R., Hickok, J. T., Bushunow, P., Pierce, H. I., Flynn, P. J., et al. (2003). The efficacy of acupressure and acustimulation wrist bands for the relief of chemotherapy-induced nausea and vomiting: A University of Rochester Cancer Center Community Clinical Oncology Program Multicenter Study. *Journal of Pain and Symptom Management, 26*(2), 731–742.

Schnorrenberger, C. C. (1996). Morphological foundations of acupuncture: An anatomical nomenclature of acupuncture structures. *Acupuncture in Medicine, 14*(2), 89–103.

Serizawa, K. (1976). *Tsubo*. Tokyo: Japan Publications.

Shames, K. H., & Keegan, L. (2000). Touch: Connecting with the healing power in 2000. In B. Dossey, L. Keegan, & C. E. Guzzetta (Eds.), *Holistic nursing* (3rd ed., pp. 613–635). Gaithersberg, MD: Aspen.

Shin, Y. H., Kim, T. I., Shin, M. S., & Juan, H. (2004). Effect of acupressure on nausea and vomiting during chemotherapy cycle for Korean postoperative stomach cancer patients. *Cancer Nursing, 27*(4), 267–274.

Suen, L. K., Wong, T. K., & Leung, A. W. (2002). Effectiveness of auricular therapy on sleep promotion in the elderly. *American Journal of Chinese Medicine, 30*(4), 429–449.

Sutherland, J. A., Reakes, J., & Bridges, C. (1999). Foot acupressure and massage for patients with Alzheimer's disease and related dementias. *Image: The Journal of Nursing Scholarship, 31*(4), 347–348.

Takeshige, C. (1989). *Mechanism of acupuncture analgesia based on animal experiments: Scientific bases of acupuncture*. Berlin: Springer-Verlag.

Taylor, D., Miaskowski, C., & Kohn, J. (2002). A randomized clinical trial of the effectiveness of an acupressure device (Relief Brief) for managing symptoms of dysmenorrhea. *Journal of Alternative and Complementary Medicine, 8*(3), 357–370.

Tsay, S. (2004). Acupressure and fatigue in patients with end-stage renal disease—a randomized controlled trial. *International Journal of Nursing Studies, 41*(1), 99–106.

Unschuld, P. (1999). The past 1,000 years of Chinese medicine. *Lancet, 354*(Suppl.), SIV9.

Waters, B. L., & Raisler, J. (2003). Ice massage for the reduction of labor pain. *Journal of Midwifery & Women's Health, 48*(5), 317–321.

Wu, B. (1995). Effect of acupuncture on the regulation of cell-mediated immunity in patients with malignant tumors. *Chen Tzu Yen Chiu Acupuncture Research, 20*(3), 67–71.

Wu, H., Wu, S., Lin, J., & Lin, L. (2004). Effectiveness of acupressure in improving dyspnoea in chronic obstructive pulmonary disease. *Journal of Advanced Nursing, 45*(3), 252–259.

Wu, B., Zhou, R. X., & Zhou, M. S. (1994). Effect of acupuncture on interleukin-2 level and NK cell immunoactivity of peripheral blood of malignant tumor patients. *Chung Kuo Chung Hsi I Chieh Ho Tsa Chich, 14*(9), 537–539.

CHAPTER 21

Reflexology

Thora Jenny Gunnarsdottir

Although reflexology is ancient, it is one of a number of complementary therapies that has gained popularity in recent years. In reflexology the entire body has been mapped out in the hands and in the feet and can be manipulated directly from there with specific massage technique. The corresponding areas on the feet are easier to locate because they cover a larger area and are more specific, rendering them easier to work on than the hands. Therefore reflexology for the feet will be the main subject in this chapter. Reflexology shares the philosophical base of holism congruent with nursing. As such, it provides the nurse an opportunity to show caring and presence with the idea of helping the patient to become more whole within a fragmented health care system. This gentle intervention has been shown to affect symptoms, but the scientific basis behind reflexology needs to be further established.

DEFINITION

Reflexology is a holistic healing technique that aims to treat the individual as an entity, incorporating the body, mind, and spirit. It is a specific pressure technique that targets precise reflex points on the feet, based on the premise that reflex areas on the feet correspond with all other body parts. Figure 21.1 shows the areas on the foot and their corresponding body parts. Because the feet represent a microcosm of the body, all organs, glands, and other body parts are laid out in an arrangement similar to that on the feet (Dougans, 1999).

The International Institute of Reflexology defines it as a manual technique based on the theory that there are reflex areas in the feet and hands that correspond to all glands, organs, and parts of the body (Byers, 1983). Kunz and Kunz (2003) stipulate that the pressure techniques stimulate specific reflex areas on the feet and hands with the intention

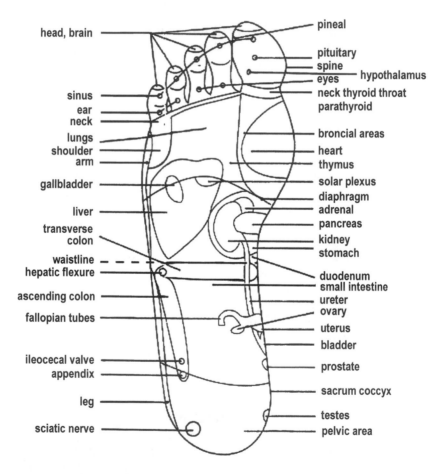

FIGURE 21.1 Relationship of body parts with reflexology points on the foot. (Retrieved from http://www.ivy-rose.co.uk, May 25, 2005)

of invoking a beneficial response in other parts of the body. Vennells (2001) articulates the word *reflex* as stimulus or reaction in the form of an increase, decrease, or rebalance of a particular physical, mental, or emotional function in the body.

Other definitions of reflexology have been presented, but they all carry the basic principle that the sole of the foot and the hand are connected to all parts of the human body and internal organs, and that there is a relationship among organs, systems, and processes. By using specific pressure techniques on the foot or hand, healing the whole body is possible. The left foot/hand represents the left site of the body and the right foot/hand represents the right site of the body.

SCIENTIFIC BASIS

The foundations of reflexology can be traced from two different theories or schools of thought that have been documented in the reflexology literature. The first theory originates from Traditional Chinese Medicine and the second one from Zone Therapy.

Traditional Chinese Medicine

The Chinese first began using reflexology roughly 5,000 years ago; however, its reputation has since declined in China. Its decline is believed to have been due to a rise in the popularity of acupuncture, which emerged from similar roots (Kunz & Kunz, 2003). Reflexology is thought to be of Eastern origin (Dougans, 1999), and it is congruent with the principle of organ representation from Traditional Chinese Medicine (TCM): the whole represents itself in the parts (Kaptchuk, 2000). This statement means that the feet are a microcosm, or holographic image of the body, where all organs, glands, and other body parts are laid out in a similar arrangement on the feet as they are in the body. The idea that the whole body can be represented in the parts is not new. For example, tongue diagnosis has been documented in China for at least 2,000 years. It is also evident in the iris of the eye, the face, and the ear (Omura, 1994).

TCM stipulates that there are a number of invisible energy pathways, or meridians within the body, that carry energy called Qi, which is the vital energy behind all processes. All organs are interconnected with each other by a meridian network system, and to maintain health, energy needs to be flowing in balance. Factors impeding the free circulation of Qi are divided into categories of "excess" and "deficiency." Excess refers to the presence of something that is "too much" for the individual to handle–too much food to digest, too much waste to eliminate, and so forth. Deficiency refers to the absence or relative insufficiency of one or more aspects of the life energies necessary for sustaining health and well-being. A deficiency or excess of life energy can allow outside factors to overwhelm the individual, thus inducing pathology and leading to pain and illness (Ehling, 2001; Kaptchuk, 2000).

In a healthy person with energy in balance, the feet feel soft when palpated and should have the same texture in every area. When an area is felt to be "empty" or is lacking in texture when palpated, it is an indication of deficiency in the energy of the corresponding organ or area in the body. If an area feels stiff and hard in texture when palpated, it indicates an excess of energy. If a lack of energy is found in one area, that means that some other area has too much energy. On empty areas, more aggressive pressure is needed to increase the energy flow, and more outgoing pressure is applied on the area that has too much energy in order to direct the flow out and away from this area. In that way, reflexology redirects excess energy in one area to another where there is an apparent deficiency in order to supplement a deficiency or to sedate an excess pattern. This process guides the client back to balancing the whole.

Zone Therapy

The second theory originates from the West, and is often referred to as *zone therapy*. At the beginning of the 20th century Dr. William H. Fitzgerald found that pressure applied to some parts of the feet of his clients induced anesthesia in a specific part of the body. Hence he found that the body and organs were laid out in a similar arrangement to that in the soles of the feet. He divided the body into 10 longitudinal zones, running from the top of the head to the toes, and proposed that parts of the body within a certain zone were linked with one another; thus this idea became known as zone therapy. An American therapist, Eunice Ingham, is credited for establishing reflexology in its present form. She used the zones as a guiding map, but began to chart the feet according to where pressure would produce distinct effects in the body. She evolved a map of the entire body on the feet and called the areas reflexes. Her proposition was that when the bloodstream becomes blocked with waste materials or excess acid, calcium deposits start to form in the nerve endings, thus impeding the normal circulation of the blood and creating an imbalance in the various parts of the body, depending on where the blockage is. She believed that by using the specific pressure of reflexology, the calcium deposits on the feet can be detected as "gritty areas," and the client may feel pain in those areas when touched. Ingham describes these as resembling particles of frost when examined under a microscope. The pressure and massage techniques taught in reflexology are designed to dissipate these crystal blocks and to break down their crystalline structures. By doing so, the corresponding area connected with this particular nerve ending will receive an added supply of blood. In this way, the circulatory and lymphatic systems are stimulated, thus encouraging the release and removal of toxins, and the body starts to heal itself (Ingham, 1984).

Neither of these theories has been directly proven, which may explain why there is little agreement on how to classify reflexology. The NCCAM (National Center for Complementary and Alternative Medicine) classifies reflexology as a manipulative and body-based method (NCCAM, 2003), but many reflexologists see their practice as an energy therapy (Dougans, 1999; Vennells, 2001).

INTERVENTION

The client will be lying comfortably, covered with a blanket, on a table somewhat higher than the chair in which the reflexologist sits, and will have pillows under the knees and the head to induce relaxation. In addition the client will be barefoot, with any tight clothes loosened so as not to hinder circulation. Then the client will be assessed continuously for tolerance of the amount of pressure applied. The pressure needs to be firm enough to activate the body's healing potentials, but must also be suitable for the client. Sensitivity varies in each individual, and the feet usually become more sensitive with subsequent treatments. Each area is worked, finishing the toe area on one foot and then treating the toe area on the other, and so on, going from one foot to the other.

Although it is emphasized that reflexology is to be applied on the feet as a whole, it is important to work specifically on several systems of the body. These specific systems are, for example: the digestive system to increase proper elimination, the lymphatic system to increase the clearance of waste materials, the bladder and kidneys to increase urine and energy flow as the kidneys are one source of Qi, the solar plexus, which is the area around the stomach where feelings and emotions are stored (this is important to know when working on this area to increase relaxation), all internal glands to stimulate their functions, and lungs to increase oxygen consumption. By using reflexology on these body systems, the reflexologist is increasing both circulation and elimination, and is also working on the meridians and affecting the flow of the Qi because all organs are interconnected with each other by meridians.

There are several techniques used, depending on what area of the foot is worked on. One hand is used to support the foot while the fingers and the thumb of the other are used to massage the skin. A period of 45 minutes to 1 hour is estimated to be enough time to perform reflexology on both feet; this will allow for extra time to work on specific areas that need further care. At the end of each session the client is encouraged to relax for several minutes. Reflexology can be used in combination with other complementary therapies such as massage (Long, 1996).

Techniques

There are some standard pressure techniques for working on the reflexes of the feet. The two techniques described here are thumb walking and hook and back up (Kunz & Kunz, 2003). Other grips are used depending on what area one is working on. It is important not to forget any area and to finish one area before starting the next one. See Table 21.1.

Measurement of Outcomes

The philosophy behind reflexology is that it affects the body as a whole, but based on the literature, which will be discussed in detail later, more studies have measured physiological or psychological outcomes of reflexology than its overall effects. It is important to measure the effect of reflexology over a period of sessions to gain insight about its overall benefits.

Precautions

Before beginning treatment the nurse should always be well centered and make sure the patient is relaxed. It must be emphasized that many people do not like to have their feet touched and approval from the patient is needed before starting. The condition of the feet must be examined before massage for swelling, color, ulcerations, toe deformities, and odor (Kunz & Kunz, 2003). The physical condition of the patient is also very important and therefore his or her health history must be reviewed. If patients have a problem regarding the blood flow to the limbs because of diabetes, neurological diseases (Dougans, 1999; Ingham, 1984; Kunz & Kunz, 2003; Vennells, 2001), or arteriosclerosis, the therapist must be careful about the pressure of the massage, as the patient may be more alert to pain. The elderly may have concerns about things such as restricted

TABLE 21.1 Techniques

Thumb walking

The goal of the thumb walking technique is to apply a constant, steady pressure to the surface of the foot or the hand.

1. With the other hand (holding hand) stretch the sole of the foot. Rest your working thumb on the sole and your fingers on the top of the foot. Drop your wrist to create leverage, which exerts pressure with the thumb.
2. Bend and unbend the thumb's first joint, moving it forward a little bit at a time. When your working hand feels stretched, reposition it and continue walking it forward. Take a little step forward with each unbend. The goal is to take small bites to create a feeling of constant, steady pressure. Always walk in a forward direction, not backward. Keep your thumb slightly cocked as you work to prevent overextending it.

Hook and back up

The hook and back up technique is used to work a specific point, rather than to cover a large area. It is a relatively stationary technique, with only small movements of the working thumb involved. To avoid digging your fingernail into the flesh, apply pressure using more of the flat of the thumb.

1. Support and protect the area to be worked with the holding hand. The hand wraps around the area while the thumb and fingers hold it in place. Place the fingers of the working hand over those of the holding hand.
2. Place the working thumb in the center of the area to be worked. Hook and back up, using the edge of the thumb.

Note: Adapted from *Reflexology: Health at your fingertips*, by K. Kunz and B. Kunz, 2003. New York: DK Publishing.

movement, incontinence, arthritis, and aching joints. Under those circumstances it may be better to consider comfort and touch as the primary goal.

USES

Research testing the effects of reflexology is limited and includes many of the approaches and practices of reflexology used in the studies mentioned below. Some conditions for which it has been used are shown in Table 21.2.

Reflexology has been found to significantly reduce the anxiety and pain of patients with lung and breast cancer after one session (Stephenson, Weinrich, & Tavakoli, 2000). In another study, the duration of the effects

TABLE 21.2   Uses of Reflexology

- Decrease pain (Launsö, Brendstrup, & Arnberg, 1999; Stephenson, Dalton, & Carlson, 2003; Stephenson et al., 2000)
- Decrease anxiety (Gambles, Crooke, & Wilkinson, 2002; Stephenson et al., 2000)
- Improve the quality of life (Gambles et al., 2002; Hodgson, 2000; Milligan, Fanning, Hunter, Tadjali, & Stevens, 2002)
- Reduce the symptoms of multiple sclerosis (Joyce & Richardson, 1997; Siev-Ner, Gamus, Lerner-Geva, & Achiron, 2003)
- Promote relaxation (Gambles et al., 2002; Hodgson, 2000; Joyce & Richardson, 1997; Launsö et al., 1999; Milligan et al., 2002; Ross et al., 2002; Trousdell, 1996)
- Improve sleep (Gambles et al., 2002; Joyce & Richardson, 1997; Milligan et al., 2002)

---

of reflexology on pain was tested in patients with various types of cancer. The immediate effects were supported, but the pain-relieving effects were not significant at 3 and at 24 hours after the reflexology session (Stephenson et al., 2003). In a study by Ross and colleagues (2002), the effects of reflexology on anxiety and depression were compared to those of simple foot massage in two groups of cancer patients. These patients received six sessions of intervention, and depression and anxiety were measured at baseline and within 24 hours after each session. No significant differences were found between the groups with respect to anxiety and depression, but both groups indicated deriving relaxing effects from the treatment.

Quality of life (QoL) has been found to be enhanced in cancer patients after reflexology. To examine if reflexology has any impact on QoL, Hodgson (2000) studied 12 cancer patients. They were randomized into two groups to receive either reflexology or placebo for 40 minutes. All of the participants in the reflexology group reported an increase in QoL, compared to 33% in the placebo group. To investigate patient satisfaction with reflexology service and its impact on QoL, an audit was undertaken in a Scottish hospice (Milligan et al., 2002). Twenty cancer patients completed self-report questionnaires after receiving from three to more than five reflexology sessions from a nurse trained in the therapy. The patients reported that reflexology reduced pain, improved sleep, enhanced relaxation, and reduced stress. In England, a similar study took place in which 34 cancer patients under palliative care were asked to comment about reflexology therapy they had received (Gambles et al., 2002). The patients received from four to six individually tailored interventions. They commented on reflexology as being emotionally beneficial in reducing anxiety and tension, improving sleep, and coping with the side effects of medications.

Patients with multiple sclerosis (MS) tend to suffer from a variety of chronic muscular symptoms. In a study by Joyce and Richardson (1997), improvements were found in sleep, balance, pain, and spasms; however, these findings were based only on subjective responses. Siev-Ner and colleagues (2003) conducted a randomized, controlled clinical trial to detect the effects of reflexology on the symptoms of MS. Statistically significant positive differences for the scores of paresthesia, urinary symptoms, and spasticity were found in the group receiving reflexology compared to the control group.

Reflexology has been found to have an impact on migraine headaches (Launsö et al., 1999). Two hundred and twenty patients with migraine headaches receiving reflexology sessions for 6 months reported a decrease in their medication consumption. By the final treatment, 23% of the patients reported being cured, and 55% were completely relieved of their symptoms.

Eleven women with emotional problems received eight reflexology sessions (Trousdell, 1996). In open-ended interviews afterward they all reported increased relaxation, and many of them found improvements in their emotional and mental state such as feeling higher self-esteem and more in control. Furthermore, many of the women reported a number of physical and emotional improvements including reduced irritable bowel syndrome symptoms; alleviation of back problems; reduced premenstrual symptoms; and improvements in headache pain, appetite, and sleep.

Two studies in Denmark were conducted to test the effects of reflexology on symptoms of asthma (Brygge et al., 2001; Petersen, Faurschou, Olsen, & Svendsen, 1992). Neither study found significant effects. Similarly, the symptoms of irritable bowel syndrome were not found to improve significantly in a study by Tovey (2002).

FUTURE RESEARCH

The scientific basis behind reflexology is growing, and promising results of its use for some symptoms are beginning to emerge, but more rigorous research is needed if it is to be used effectively by nurses within health care settings. Although the principle behind reflexology states that it can affect the body as a whole, this phenomenon has not been captured in the studies reviewed. Nurses are in a primary position to conduct research on reflexology because their holistic background is in tune with its philosophies. Some questions for future research are:

1. What are the specifics of reflexology in relation to other complementary therapies? Recommendations from best clinical practice experience and valid research findings should be used in combination to guide the results (Mackereth, Dryden, & Frankel, 2000).

2. What is the mechanism behind reflexology? This needs to be better understood to provide a basis for outcome measures.

3. How do patients experience reflexology, and how do they give meaning to these experiences and the effect of the therapist on the overall outcome? Using qualitative research methods may greatly enhance the understanding and increase the validity of the results (Verhoef, Casebeer, & Hilsden, 2002).

REFLEXOLOGY-SPECIFIC WEB SITES

Kevin and Barbara Kunz hold out two web sites offering the basics on reflexology theory and practice and information on developments in reflexology research.

www.reflexology-reserach.com

www.foot-reflexologist.com

Other web sites offer lists of worldwide reflexology organizations and interactive information on reflexology products and practice.

www.reflexology-usa.net

www.reflexology.org

www.myreflexologist.com

www.aor.org.uk

www.icr-reflexology.org

REFERENCES

Brygge, T., Heinig, J. H., Collins, S., Ronborg, P. M., Gehrchen, P. M., Hilden, J., et al. (2001). Reflexology and bronchial asthma. *Respiratory Medicine*, 95, 173–179.

Byers, D. C. (1983). *Better health with foot reflexology.* St. Petersburg, FL: Ingham.

Dougans, I. (1999). *The complete illustrated guide to reflexology.* Boston: Element Books.

Ehling, D. (2001). Oriental medicine: An introduction. *Alternative Therapies in Health and Medicine, 7*(4), 71–82.

Gambles, M., Crooke, M., & Wilkinson, S. (2002). Evaluation of a hospice based reflexology service: A qualitative audit of patient perceptions. *European Journal of Oncology Nursing, 6*(1), 37–44.

Hodgson, H. (2000). Does reflexology impact on cancer patients' quality of life? *Nursing Standard, 14*(31), 33–38.

Ingham, E. D. (1984). *Stories the feet can tell thru reflexology/Stories the feet have told thru reflexology.* Saint Petersburg, FL: Ingham.

Joyce, M., & Richardson, R. (1997, July). Reflexology can help MS. *International Journal of Alternative and Complementary Medicine, 15*(7), 10–12.

Kaptchuck, T. J. (2000). *The web that has no weaver: Understanding Chinese medicine.* Chicago: Contemporary Books.

Kunz, K., & Kunz, B. (2003). *Reflexology: Health at your fingertips.* New York: DK Publishing.

Launsö, L., Brendstrup, E., & Arnberg, S. (1999). An exploratory study of reflexological treatment for headache. *Alternative Therapies in Health and Medicine, 5*(3), 57–65.

Long, C. K. (1996, Jan/Feb). Reflexology combined with massage to improve treatments and business. *Massage, 59,* 26–33.

Mackereth, P., Dryden, S. L., & Frankel, B. (2000). Reflexology: Recent research approaches. *Complementary Therapies in Nursing and Midwifery, 6,* 66–71.

Milligan, M., Fanning, M., Hunter, S., Tadjali, M., & Stevens, E. (2002). Reflexology audit: Patient satisfaction, impact on quality of life and availability in Scottish hospices. *International Journal of Palliative Nursing, 8,* 489–496.

National Center for Complementary and Alternative Medicine (NCCAM). *About NCCAM.* Retrieved September 11, 2003, from http://altmed.od.nih.gov/health/whatiscam

Omura, Y. (1994). Accurate localization of organ representation areas on the feet & hands using the bi-digital O-ring test resonance: Its clinical implication in diagnosis & treatment—part II. *Acupuncture & Electro-Therapeutics Research, International Journal, 19,* 153–190.

Petersen, L. N., Faurschou, P., Olsen, O. T., & Svendsen, U. G. (1992). Fodzone-therapy og asthma bronchiale. *Ugeskrift for Læger, 154,* 2065–2068.

Ross, C. S. K., Hamilton, J., Macrae, G., Docherty, C., Gould, A., & Cornbleet, M. A. (2002). A pilot study to evaluate the effect of reflexology on mood and symptom rating of advanced cancer patients. *Palliative Medicine, 16,* 544–545.

Siev-Ner, I., Gamus, D., Lerner-Geva, L., & Achiron, A. (2003). Reflexology treatment relieves symptoms of multiple sclerosis: A randomized controlled study. *Multiple Sclerosis, 9,* 356–361.

Stephenson, L. N., Dalton, J. A., & Carlson, J. (2003). The effect of foot reflexology on pain in patients with metastatic cancer. *Applied Nursing Research, 16,* 284–286.

Stephenson, L. N., Weinrich, S. P., & Tavakoli, A. S. (2000). The effects of foot reflexology on anxiety and pain in patients with breast and lung cancer. *Oncology Nursing Forum, 27*(1), 67–72.

Tovey, P. (2002). A single-blind trial of reflexology for irritable bowel syndrome. *British Journal of General Practice, 52*, 19–23.

Trousdell, P. (1996). Reflexology meets emotional needs. *International Journal of Alternative and Complementary Medicine, 14*(11), 9–12.

Vennells, D. F. (2001). *Reflexology for beginners: Healing through foot massage of pressure points.* St. Paul, MN: Llewellyn.

Verhoef, M. J., Casebeer, A. L., & Hilsden, R. J. (2002). Assessing efficacy of complementary medicine: Adding qualitative research methods to the "gold standard." *The Journal of Alternative and Complementary Medicine, 8*, 275–281.

PART IV

Manipulative and Body-Based Therapies

OVERVIEW

This category of the National Center for Complementary/Alternative Medicine (NCCAM) includes therapies that involve the manipulation and movement of body parts. Three large groups of therapies comprise this category: chiropractic, osteopathy, and massage. Other therapies in this category are reflexology, Trager body work, acupuncture, acupressure, and Rolfing. (Acupressure and reflexology were placed in Part III because of their tie with the flow of energy.) Nurses may use some of the other therapies in this group such as hydrotherapy, diathermy, light and color, heat, and alternate nostril breathing.

Massage, in the form of back rubs, is a basic skill that has been included in nursing curricula over the years. In recent years back rubs have been largely abandoned by nurses with "too busy" the reason cited for the decline in use. However, a number of nurses have pursued education to become massage therapists. The practice of massage therapy is often separate from their practice of nursing, although some nurses who are massage therapists use this modality in nursing homes and in independent practice as advanced practice nurses.

Although many of the therapies in this group are routinely administered by other therapists such as chiropractors and massage therapists, a number of them are used by nurses. Exercise is commonly prescribed to promote health and prevent disease. Likewise, Tai Chi can be used to improve health and functioning. Nurses teach and coach patients in techniques of muscle relaxation to achieve benefits such as pain relief, improved sleep, and reduced symptoms of stress. A growing body of research on these therapies supports their use.

CHAPTER 22

Massage

Mariah Snyder

Massage is an ancient therapy that has been used in China for more than 5,000 years (McRee, Noble, & Pasvogel, 2003). It is one of the most widely used complementary therapies and has been part of the nursing armamentarium for centuries. Ironically, however, at a time when massage is increasingly being used by the general public, nurses rarely administer back rubs or other types of massage. Rather, some institutions have massage therapists on staff with patients paying for these services.

Massage is often combined with other therapies such as music, aromatherapy, acupressure, and simple touch, making it hard to differentiate the specific effects of massage from those resulting from a combination of therapies. The results in many studies point to the positive effects of massage in producing relaxation, improving sleep, and reducing pain.

DEFINITION

The term *massage* is derived from the Arabic word *mass'h*, which means to press gently (Furlan, Brosseau, Imamura, & Irvin, 2004). As defined by the American Massage Therapy Association (2004), massage is "the application of manual techniques and adjunctive therapies with the intention of positively affecting the health and well-being of the client." Various strokes are used in applying friction and pressure on cutaneous and subcutaneous tissue. Results depend on a number of factors: type and speed of movements; pressure exerted by the hands, fingers, or thumbs; and area of the body treated.

There are a number of types of massage: Swedish (a more vigorous massage with long, flowing strokes); Esalen (a meditative massage with a light touch, and a highly variable style); deep tissue or neuromuscular (an intense kneading of the body); sports (a vigorous massage to loosen and ease sore muscles); Shiatsu (a Japanese pressure-point technique to relieve stress); and reflexology (a deep foot massage stimulating all parts of the body). The various types of massage incorporate different strokes and procedures. Strokes can be administered to the entire body or to specific areas such as the back, feet, or hands.

SCIENTIFIC BASIS

Massage is a natural healing process that helps to connect the body, mind, and spirit. It produces therapeutic effects on multiple body systems: integumentary, musculoskeletal, cardiovascular, lymph, and nervous. Manipulating the skin and underlying muscle makes the skin more supple. Massage increases or enhances movement in the musculoskeletal system by reducing swelling, loosening and stretching contracted tendons, and aiding in the reduction of soft-tissue adhesions. Friction to the cutaneous and subcutaneous tissues releases histamines that in turn produce vasodilation of vessels and enhance venous return.

Massage has been found to produce a relaxation response (Hattan, King, & Griffiths, 2002; Holland & Pokorny, 2001; McNamara, Burnham, Smith, & Carroll, 2003). Investigators have reported that massage resulted in a decrease in physiological parameters (systolic and diastolic blood pressure, heart rate, and skin temperature) indicative of the relaxation response (Holland & Pokorny; Snyder, Egan, & Burns, 1995a).

Reduction of pain, a frequently desired outcome of massage, is closely related to the production of the relaxation response. Reports from numerous studies have validated that patients were more comfortable after the administration of massage (Chang, Wang, & Chen, 2002; Furlan et al., 2004; Hernandez-Rief et al., 2001; Walach, Guthlin, & Konig, 2003). The positive impact of massage on pain reduction is often posited on the gate control theory with massage stimulating the large diameter nerve fibers that have an inhibitory input on T-cells (Furlan et al.).

Results from some studies on the use of massage have shown that it does not always produce relaxation. One factor that may contribute to the arousal response is that a short duration of massage may initially cause stimulation of the sympathetic nervous system before the relaxation response occurs (Ferrell-Torry & Glick, 1993). Tyler, Winslow, Clark, and White (1990) administered a 1-minute back rub to patients who were critically ill. Findings included increases in the heart rate and decreases in the SVO_2; these gradually returned to baseline after 4 minutes. The investigators suggested that although these changes were statistically significant, they were not clinically significant as the heart rate only increased by four beats per minute. However, in the majority of studies reviewed, subjective indices for relaxation (anxiety inventories and self-reports) suggested that subjects felt relaxed after the massage intervention.

The impact of massage on the psychoneuroimmunological functions of the body and mind is beginning to be explored. Groer and colleagues (1994) reported that administering a 10-minute back massage stimulated the production of antibodies (salivary secretory immunoglobulin A, s-IgA). Anecdotal reports have suggested that massage has produced positive results in persons with HIV infection.

Massage is a holistic therapy and as such promotes overall health. Studies have shown that it also improves psychological well-being (Chang et al., 2002; Hattan et al., 2002), quality of life (Wilkinson, Aldridge, Salmon, Cain, & Wilson, 1999), and self-esteem (Hernandez-Rief, Field, Fielt, & Theakston, 1998). Hanley, Stirling, and Brown (2003) commented that although the patients in a massage group offered no different findings on sleep and well-being than patients who listened to a relaxation tape, patients expressed a strong preference for massage versus the relaxation tape.

INTERVENTION

The techniques for hand and shoulder massage will be presented. The environment in which massage is administered and the oils or lotion used add to the therapeutic effects. Room temperature is very important; the room must be warm enough so that the person is comfortable. Shivering would negate the effects of the massage. In addition, privacy needs to be ensured.

Adding music and aromatherapy to a massage session has been thought to increase its effectiveness. Fellowes, Barnes, and Wilkinson (2004), however, did not find any convincing evidence that aromatherapy contributed to additional improvement in outcomes. Chapter 7 details the intervention of music and aromatherapy is described in chapter 26.

Massage Strokes

The various types of massage involve several stroke techniques. Commonly used strokes include effleurage, friction, pressure, petrissage, vibration, and percussion. Effleurage is a slow, rhythmic stroking with light skin contact. It may be applied with varying degrees of pressure, depending on the part of the body being massaged and the outcome desired. The palmar surface of the hands is used for larger surfaces with the thumbs and fingers used for smaller areas. On large surfaces, long, gliding strokes about 10 to 20 inches in length are applied.

In friction movements, moderate, constant pressure to one area is made with the thumbs or fingers. The fingers may be held in one place or moved in a small circumscribed area. The pressure stroke is similar to the friction stroke, except that pressure strokes are made with the hands.

Petrissage, or kneading, involves lifting a large fold of skin and the underlying muscle and holding the tissues between the thumb and fingers. The tissues are pushed against the bone, then raised and squeezed in circular movements. The grasp on the tissues is alternately loosened and tightened. Tissues are supported by one hand while kneading is done with the other hand. Variations of kneading include pinching, rolling, wringing, and kneading with fists or fingers. Petrissage is limited to tissues having a significant muscle mass.

Vibration strokes can be administered with either the entire hand or with the fingers. Rapid, continuous strokes are used. Because administering vibration strokes requires much energy, mechanical vibrators are often used.

For percussion strokes, the wrist acts as a fulcrum for the hand, with the hand hitting the tissue. Strokes are made with a rapid tempo over a large body area. Tapping and clapping are variants of percussion strokes.

Shoulder Massage

Shoulder massage can be easily implemented by nurses and others. The person receiving the massage sits so that the back is accessible to the person administering it. The massage can be administered with the person's shoulders uncovered or clothed. If clothed, no oil or lotion is used.

The massage begins with some gentle pressure applied on the shoulders using the palm of the hand. Next, attention is given to stretching the trapezius muscles, moving from the center of the back to the insertion in the scapula at the shoulder joint. Fingers can be used to massage the fibers in the muscles of the shoulder. The skin can be lifted and the muscle fibers massaged between the fingers. Attention is given to the attachment of the muscles at the base of the skull by massaging up the neck and cross fibers and stretching the muscles. If the person is unable to hold the head up, a hand can be placed on the forehead to support the head. The massage is concluded with lighter percussion strokes along the top of the shoulder.

Hand Massage

A technique for implementing hand massage is presented in Table 22.1. The technique is easy to implement with many populations including

TABLE 22.1 Technique for Hand Massage

Each hand is massaged for $2^1/2$ minutes. Do not massage if hand is injured, reddened, or swollen.

1. Back of hand
   (a) Short medium-length straight strokes are done from the wrist to the finger tips; moderate pressure is used (effleurage).
   (b) Large half-circle stretching strokes are made from the center to the side of the hand using moderate pressure.
   (c) Small circular strokes are made over the entire hand using light pressure (make small O's with the thumb).
   (d) Featherlike straight strokes are made from the wrist to the fingertips using very light pressure.

2. Palm of hand
   (a) Short, medium-length straight strokes are made from the wrist to the fingertips using moderate pressure (effleurage).
   (b) Gentle milking and lifting of the tissue of the entire palm of the hand is done using moderate pressure.
   (c) Small circular strokes are made over the entire palm using moderate pressure (making little O's with index finger).
   (d) Large half-circle stretching strokes are used from the center of the palm to the sides using moderate pressure.

3. Fingers
   (a) Gently squeeze each finger from the base to the tip on both sides and the front and back using light pressure.
   (b) Gentle range of motion of finger.
   (c) Gentle pressure on nail bed.

4. Completion
   (a) Place client's hand on yours and cover it with your other hand. Gently draw your top hand toward you several times. Turn the client's hand over and gently draw the other hand toward you several times.

older adults (Cho & Snyder, 1996; Snyder et al., 1995a) and infants and children (Field, 2002). The time suggested for administering massage is $2^{1}/_{2}$ minutes per hand. However, the amount of time needed can be individualized for each patient.

Measurement of Outcomes

Both physiological and psychological outcomes have been used to measure the effectiveness of massage. Indices of relaxation (heart rate, blood pressure, skin temperature, and muscle tension) have been measured in many studies. Anxiety inventories and scales to determine pain level, sleep time and quality, and quality of life indices have been used to determine the efficacy of massage. It is important that both short- and long-term effects of massage be measured.

Precautions

Before administering massage, the nurse should explain the intervention and obtain the patient's permission. Also, a history and assessment need to be made to determine if patients have received massage in the past and if they experienced any adverse reactions, and to ascertain their overall response to touch. The area to be massaged is assessed for redness, bruises, edema, or rashes. Some people may be averse to being touched because of past negative experiences. Others may be hypersensitive to touch. One method for overcoming this sensitivity is beginning with light touch and slowly increasing the pressure.

Because blood pressure may be lowered during massage, initial monitoring for light-headedness is suggested following the initial massage sessions, particularly in older adults. Allowing a light-headed person to remain recumbent for several minutes may help to lessen hypotension. Monitoring of blood pressure and pulse rate are needed in persons with cardiac conditions to determine if adverse effects are being experienced.

Ernst (2003) reviewed literature to determine adverse reactions to massage. Although a number of negative reactions were noted, the majority of these were associated with exotic types of massage and not with the Swedish massage technique.

USES

A list of conditions for which massage has been used is found in Table 22.2. Use of massage to produce relaxation and reduce pain will be discussed.

TABLE 22.2   Uses for Massage

Promote relaxation

- Decrease aggressive behaviors (Snyder et al., 1995a, 1995b)
- Produce sleep (Richards, 1998)
- Lessen fatigue (Ahles et al., 1999)

Lessen pain (Chang et al., 2002; Ernst, 2004; Hulme, Waterman, & Hillier, 1999)

Improve mobility (Smith, Stallings, Mariner, & Burrall, 1999)

Increase weight in preterm infants (Field, 2002)

Increase psychological well-being (Hattan et al., 2002)

Lessen depression (Kite et al., 1998)

Lessen anxiety (Fellowes et al., 2004; Johnson, Frederick, Kaufman, & Mount-joy, 1999)

Relaxation

Many people use a massage therapist to ameliorate their stress. Holland and Pokorny (2001) reported a positive response in patients in a rehabilitation setting to a slow stroke back massage. Hattan and colleagues (2002) found that subjects receiving foot massage reported feeling much calmer than before the therapy. In a review of studies on the use of massage in acute and critical care, Richards, Gibson, and Overton-McCoy (2000) found that massage decreased anxiety in 8 of the 10 studies in which it was administered.

In addition to patients, massage can also be used with family members who are experiencing high levels of stress due to the condition of the family member who is a patient. A short hand massage may help to relax a family member who has difficulty resting or sleeping. Lloyd (1995) suggested that nurses could give quick massages to colleagues to promote relaxation.

Pain

Numerous studies have found that massage resulted in reduction of pain. Ernst (2004), in a meta-analysis of seven studies, found that Swedish massage may be effective in lessening pain. However, the investigator also noted that there were many methodological concerns about the studies, such as small sample size, short follow-up, and no funding of investigator to group. In a review of research on the use of massage and aromatherapy in persons with cancer, Fellowes and colleagues (2004) found a reduction in pain in three studies. Hulme et al. (1999) reported that foot massage decreased postoperative pain, with similar findings reported by Nixon, Teschendorff, Finney, and Karnilowicz (1997) and Wang and Keck (2004).

FUTURE RESEARCH

In reviews of the research that have been conducted using massage, a number of methodological issues were identified. One challenge posed in conducting research on massage is having a comparable control group. McNamara and others (2003) compared massage and standard care in patients having a diagnostic test. Others have compared the effects of massage and other therapies such as imagery (Hattan et al., 2002). The following are suggestions for research that will help guide practitioners in using massage.

1. Few studies on massage have investigated the impact it has on psychoneuroimmunologcial functions. Such studies would help validate its effects on health conditions such as HIV infection and cancer.

2. Ernst (2003) examined studies to determine the safety of massage. Studies need to give more attention to determining any adverse effects of the various types of massage and its use with different conditions and populations.

3. As noted earlier, massage has often been combined with other therapies such as aromatherapy and music. Designs are needed that determine differences in outcomes with the combination of therapies. Fellowes and colleagues (2004), in their review of aromatherapy and massage, questioned whether the use of aromatherapy added anything to the outcomes beyond those outcomes that might be attributable to massage.

WEB SITES

The following are web sites that will provide additional information about massage:

http://www.massagenetwork.com

http://www.massagetherapy.com

http://www.massageresource.com

REFERENCES

Ahles, T. A., Tope, D. M., Pinkson, B., Walch, S., Hann, D., Whedon, M., et al. (1999). Massage therapy for patients undergoing autologous bone marrow transplantation. *Journal of Pain and Symptom Management, 18*, 157–163.

American Massage Therapy Association. (2004). Retrieved January 5, 2005, from http://www.amtmassage.org/about/definition/html

Chang, M. Y., Wang, S. Y., & Chen, C. H. (2002). Effects of massage on pain and anxiety during labour: A randomized controlled trial in Taiwan. *Journal of Advanced Nursing, 38*, 68–73.

Cho, K., & Snyder, M. (1996). Use of hand massage with presence to increase relaxation in Korean-American elderly. *The Journal of Academy of Nursing, 26*, 623–626.

Ernst, E. (2003). The safety of massage therapy. *Rheumatology, 42*, 1101–1106.

Ernst, E. (2004). Manual therapies for pain control: Chiropractic and massage. *Clinical Journal of Pain, 20*, 8–12.

Fellowes, D., Barnes, K., & Wilkinson, S. (2004). Aromatherapy and massage for symptom relief in patients with cancer. Retrieved February 26, 2004, from *The Cochrane Database for Systematic Reviews, 2.*

Ferrell-Torry, A. T., & Glick, O. J. (1993). The use of therapeutic massage as a nursing intervention to modify anxiety and the perception of cancer pain. *Cancer Nursing, 16*, 93–101.

Field, T. (2002). Preterm infant massage therapy studies: An American approach. *Seminars in Neonatology, 7*, 487–494.

Furlan, A. D., Brosseau, L., Imamura, M., & Irvin, E. (2004). Massage for low-back pain. Retrieved February 2004, from *The Cochrane Database of Systematic Reviews, 2.*

Groer, M., Mozingo, J., Droppleman, P., Davis, M., Jolley, M., Boynton, M., et al. (1994). Measures of salivary immunoglobulin A and state anxiety after a nursing back rub. *Applied Nursing Research, 7*(1), 2–6.

Hanley, J., Stirling, P., & Brown, C. (2003). Randomised controlled trial of therapeutic massage in the management of stress. *British Journal of General Practice, 53*, 20–25.

Hattan, J., King, L., & Griffiths, P. (2002). The impact of foot massage and guided relaxation following cardiac surgery: A randomized controlled trial. *Journal of Advanced Nursing, 37*, 199–207.

Hernandez-Rief, M., Field, T., Fielt, T., & Theakston, H. (1998). Multiple sclerosis patients benefit from massage therapy. *Journal of Bodywork and Movement Therapies, 2*, 168–174.

Hernandez-Rief, M., Field, T., Largie, S., Hart, S., Redzepi, M., Nierenberg, B., et al. (2001). Children's distress during burn treatment is reduced by massage therapy. *Journal of Burn Care & Rehabilitation, 22*, 191–195.

Holland, B., & Pokorny, M. W. (2001). Slow stroke back massage on patients in a rehabilitation setting. *Rehabilitation Nursing, 26*, 182–186.

Hulme, J., Waterman, H., & Hillier, V. F. (1999). The effect of foot massage on patients' perception of care following laparoscopic sterilization as day case patients. *Journal of Advanced Nursing, 30*, 460–468.

Johnson, S. K., Frederick, J., Kaufman, M., & Mountjoy, B. (1999). A controlled investigation of bodywork in multiple sclerosis. *Journal of Alternative and Complementary Medicine, 5*, 237–243.

Kite, S. M., Maher, E. J., Anderson, K., Young, T., Young, J., Wood, J., et al. (1998). Development of an aromatherapy service at a cancer centre. *Palliative Medicine, 12*, 171–180.

Lloyd, K. (1995). The power to colleagues and clients with a two-minute massage. *The Lamp, 51*(22), 30.

McNamara, M. E., Burnham, D. C., Smith, C., & Carroll, D. L. (2003). The effects of back massage before diagnostic cardiac catheterization. *Alternative Therapies in Health and Medicine 9*(1), 50–57.

McRee, L. S., Noble, S., & Pasvogel, A. (2003). Using massage and music therapy to improve postoperative outcomes. *AORN Journal, 78*, 433–440, 445–447.

Nixon, M., Teschendorff, J., Finney, J., & Karnilowicz, W. (1997). Expanding the nursing repertoire: The effect of massage on post-operative pain. *Australian Journal of Advanced Nursing, 14*(3), 21–26.

Richards, K. C. (1998). Effect of a back massage and relaxation intervention on sleep in critically ill patients. *American Journal of Critical Care, 7*, 288–299.

Richards, K. C., Gibson, R., & Overton-McCoy, A. L. (2000). Effects of massage in acute and critical care. *AACN Clinical Issues, 11*, 77–96.

Smith, M. C., Stallings, M. A., Mariner, S., & Burrall, M. (1999). Benefits of massage therapy for hospitalized patients: A descriptive and qualitative evaluation. *Alternative Therapies in Health and Medicine, 5*(4), 64–71.

Snyder, M., Egan, E. C., & Burns, K. R. (1995a). Efficacy of hand massage in decreasing agitation behaviors associated with care activities in persons with dementia. *Geriatric Nursing, 16*(2), 60–63.

Snyder, M., Egan, E. C., & Burns, K. R. (1995b). Interventions for decreasing agitation behaviors in persons with dementia. *Journal of Gerontological Nursing, 21*(7), 34–40.

Tyler, D. O., Winslow, E. H., Clark, A. P., & White, K. M. (1990). Effects of a 1-minute back rub on mixed venous oxygen saturation and heart rate in critically ill patients. *Heart and Lung, 19*, 562–565.

Walach, H., Guthlin, C., & Konig, M. (2003). Efficacy of massage therapy in chronic pain: A pragmatic randomized trial. *Journal of Alternative and Complementary Medicine, 9*, 837–846.

Wang, H. L., & Keck, J. F. (2004). Foot and hand massage as an intervention for postoperative pain. *Pain Management Nursing, 5*, 59–65.

Wilkinson, S., Aldridge, J., Salmon, I., Cain, E., & Wilson, B. (1999). An evaluation of aromatherapy massage in palliative care. *Palliative Medicine, 13*, 409–417.

CHAPTER 23

Exercise

Diane Treat-Jacobson, Daniel L. Mark, and Ulf Bronäs

BACKGROUND

Exercise is rapidly becoming recognized as a lifelong endeavor essential for energetic, active, and healthy living. Mortality and morbidity are reduced in physically fit individuals compared with sedentary individuals (Kujala, Kapiro, Sarna, & Koskenvuo, 1998; Paffenbarger et al., 1993; Sherman, D'Agostino, Cobb, & Kannel, 1994). The research supporting the benefits of exercise is substantial. Its effects have been linked to many positive physiological and psychological responses, from reduction in the stress response to an increased sense of well-being (Crews & Landers, 1987; Pender, 1996). Surprisingly, despite the tremendous benefits of exercise, it is an activity largely ignored by the general population. Indeed, the U.S. Surgeon General (1996) issued a report identifying millions of inactive Americans as being at risk for a wide range of chronic diseases and ailments including coronary heart disease (CHD), adult onset diabetes, colon cancer, hip fractures, hypertension, and obesity. *Healthy People 2010* (2000) specified several objectives for improving health, including physical activity and exercise. These include reducing the percentage of adults who do not participate in any physical activity, increasing the percentage of adults who engage in moderate physical activity on most days of the week, and increasing the percentage of adults participating in vigorous exercise, as well as exercises to improve strength and flexibility. There are additional objectives related to physical activity and exercise habits of children and adolescents, including goals to increase participation in daily school physical education classes. The alarmingly low (<27%) percentage of children participating in physical activity in school and outside of school is reportedly contributing to the nation's growing childhood obesity problem (Andersen, Crespo, Bartlett, Cheskin, & Pratt, 1998; McKenzie et al., 1996).

It is important to recognize the role of exercise as a component of good health. Exercise *must* be an integral part of personal lifestyle if it is to have optimum effects. Maintaining physical fitness can be enjoyable and rewarding for persons of all ages and can contribute significantly to extending longevity and improving quality of life. Nurses' knowledge of exercise and its application in multiple populations will assist in the delivery of expert nursing care. This chapter discusses the definition, physiological basis, and application of exercise as a nursing intervention.

DEFINITION

Physical activity is defined as "any bodily movement produced by skeletal muscles that results in caloric expenditure" (Pender, 1996, p. 185). Definitions of exercise are complex and vary according to discipline; however, they all incorporate physical activity into their descriptions. Exercise is commonly considered to be a planned, recurring subset of physical activity that results in physical fitness, a term used to describe cardiorespiratory fitness, muscle strength, body composition, and flexibility related to the ability of a person to perform physical activity (Thompson et al., 2003).

Exercise is commonly classified according to the rate of energy expenditure, which is expressed in either absolute terms as metabolic equivalents (MET) or in relative terms according to what percentage of maximal heart rate or maximal oxygen consumption exercise is performed (Astrand, Rodahl, Dahl, & Stromme, 2004; Thompson et al., 2003). Exercise is aerobic when the energy demand by the working muscles is supplied by aerobic ATP production as allowed by inspired oxygen and mitochondrial enzymatic capacity (Astrand et al.). In general, aerobic exercise increases demand on the respiratory, cardiovascular, and musculoskeletal systems. Sustained periods of work require aerobic metabolism of energy at a level compatible with the body's oxygen supply capabilities (i.e., oxygen uptake equals oxygen requirements of the tissues). Anaerobic exercise is exercise during which the energy demand exceeds what the body is able to produce through the aerobic process or when the body is performing short bursts of high intensity exercise (Astrand et al.; Kisner & Colby, 1996).

SCIENTIFIC BASIS

Better understanding of exercise physiology and the body's response to various stages of physical activity will assist in the development of exercise programs appropriate for the individual and the goal of the exercise. The response of the body to exercise occurs in stages. The initial response to acute exercise is a withdrawal of parasympathetic stimulation of the heart through the vagal nerve. This results in a rapid increase in heart rate (HR) and cardiac output (CO). The sympathetic stimulation occurs more slowly and becomes a dominant factor once HR is above approximately 100 beats per minute. Sympathetic stimulation is fully completed after approximately 10 to 20 seconds during which time a large sympathetic outburst occurs and the heart overshoots the rate needed, but then returns to the rate required for increased activity (Rowell, 1993). The brain stimulates the initial cardiovascular response together with impulses from muscles being exercised, which are sent to the brain; an increase in the heart rate is initiated and the blood flow is shunted toward the exercising muscles (Astrand et al., 2004; Fletcher, 1982; Rowell, 1993). During this phase, there is a sluggish adjustment of respiration and circulation, resulting in an O_2 deficit; the initial energy needed by the exercising tissue is mainly fueled by the anaerobic metabolism of creatine phosphate and anaerobic glycolysis (glucose) (Kisner & Colby, 1996).

As exercise continues, oxygen consumption (VO_2) increases in a linear fashion in relation to the intensity of exercise. The increase in VO_2 is caused by an increase in oxygen extraction by the working muscles and an increase in cardiac output (CO). Oxygen extraction by the working muscle tissues is approximately 80% to 85% or a three-fold increase from rest, in sedentary and moderately active individuals. This is caused by an increase in the number of open capillaries, thereby reducing diffusion distances and increasing capillary blood volume (Fletcher et al., 2001; Rowell, 1993). Cardiac output is increased to meet the increased O_2 demands of the working muscle. The increase in CO is due to increased stroke volume (SV) which is due to an increase in ventricular filling pressure brought on by increased venous return and decreased peripheral resistance offered by the exercising muscles. Together with the withdrawal of parasympathetic stimulation and increases in sympathetic stimulation, the increase in heart rate (HR) further accentuates the increase in CO as well as increased myocardial contractibility (from positive inotropic sympathetic impulses to the heart) (Astrand et al., 2004; Fletcher, 1982). In normal individuals, CO can increase 4 to 5 times, allowing for increased delivery of O_2 to exercising muscle beds and facilitating removal of lactate, CO_2, and heat. Respiration increases to deliver O_2 and to allow for elimination of CO_2. Blood pressure increases as a result of increased cardiac output and the sympathetic vasoconstriction of vessels in the non-exercising muscles, viscera, and skin. During this "steady state" exercise phase, O_2 uptake equals O_2 tissue requirement, aerobic metabolism of glucose and fatty acids occurs, and there is no accumulation of lactic acid.

As exercise becomes more strenuous, there is a shift toward anaerobic metabolism of glucose, resulting in increased production of lactic acid (Balady & Weiner, 1992). The anaerobic threshold is a point during exercise at which ventilation abruptly increases despite linear increases in work rate. As exercise goes beyond steady state, the O_2 supply does not meet the oxygen requirement, and energy is provided through anaerobic glycolysis and creatine phosphate breakdown. This increases proton release and phosphate accumulation, increasing acidosis (Robergs, Ghiasvand, & Parker, 2004; Westerblad, Allen, & Lannergren, 2002). Shortly beyond the anaerobic threshold, fatigue and dyspnea ensue and work ceases. This usually coincides with a significant drop in blood glucose levels (Hargraves, 1995). Exercise at a level that allows for aerobic metabolism and reduces the need for anaerobic metabolism and reliance on glucose metabolism as the primary fuel may delay onset of these symptoms.

Following cessation of exercise, there is a period of rapid decline in oxygen uptake followed by a slow decline toward resting levels. This slow phase of oxygen uptake return is termed excess post-exercise oxygen consumption. During this period, the body attempts to resynthesize used creatine phosphate, remove lactate, restore muscle and blood oxygen stores, decrease body temperature, return to resting levels of HR and BP, and lower circulating catecholamines (Astrand et al., 2004; Fleg & Lakatta, 1986). It is important to facilitate this phase of exercise by performing a 5- to 10-minute cool-down, as will be discussed below.

INTERVENTION

Healthy People 2010 is a set of objectives for the nation to try to achieve by 2010 (www.healthypeople.gov). One of these objectives is to improve health, fitness, and quality of life through daily physical activity. According to the NIH consensus statement (1995), exercise is considered to be beneficial to health. In 1996 the U.S. Surgeon General released a report detailing the benefits of physical activity including (1) decreased risk of premature death, (2) decreased risk of premature death from heart disease, (3) decreased risk of acquiring type 2 diabetes, (4) decreased risk of incurring high blood pressure, (5) decreased high blood pressure in hypertensive individuals, (6) decreased risk of acquiring colon cancer, and (7) decreased feelings of uneasiness and despair. According to this report, exercise also (8) aids in weight control, (9) helps in the strengthening and maintenance of muscles, joints, and bones, (10) assists older adults with balance and mobility, and (11) fosters feelings of psychological well-being. In addition to these benefits, the American Heart Association (Thompson et al., 2003) and the American College of Sports Medicine (Mazzeo et al., 1998; Pollock et al., 1998) have published scientific statements summarizing evidence confirming physical activity as a significant factor in both primary and secondary prevention of cardiovascular disease. There is a relationship between lack of physical activity and development of coronary artery disease and increased cardiovascular mortality (Thompson et al.). Further, there is evidence that persons who engage in regular exercise as part of their recovery post myocardial infarction have improved rates of survival (Fletcher et al., 1996).

Given that the benefits apply to all age groups across a broad spectrum of health and disease, it is important for nurses to recognize opportunities to promote exercise as a nursing intervention. There are countless activities included under the umbrella of exercise. Finding the activity that fits an individual's capabilities and that meets the purposes for which exercise is prescribed is key to the success of the intervention (Gavin, 1988). When prescribing an intervention, it is important to take into account the recommended exercise intensity for the patient population being served.

Evidence suggests that exercise is more likely to be initiated if the individual (1) recognizes the need to exercise, (2) perceives the exercise to be beneficial and enjoyable, (3) perceives that the exercise has minimal negative aspects such as expense, time burden, or negative peer pressure, (4) feels capable and safe engaging in the exercise, (5) has ready access to the activity and can easily fit it into the daily schedule (NIH Consensus Statement, 1995).

Technique

An exercise session should involve three phases: warming up, aerobic exercise, and cooling down. These phases are designed to allow the body opportunity to sustain internal equilibrium by gradually adjusting its physiological processes to the stress of exercise and thus maintaining homeostasis.

Warm-Up Phase

The goal of the warm-up is to allow the body time to adapt to the rigors of aerobic exercise. Warming up results in an increase in muscle temperature, a higher need for oxygen in order to meet the increased demands of the exercising muscles, dilatation of capillaries resulting in increased circulation, adjustments within the neural respiratory center to the demands of exercise, and a shifting of blood flow centrally from the periphery, resulting in increased venous return (Kisner & Colby, 1996). In addition, a good warm-up increases flexibility and decreases or prevents arrhythmias and ischemic ECG changes (Kisner & Colby). Warming-up exercises should be done for 10 minutes, involve all major body parts, and achieve a heart rate within 20 beats per minute of the target heart rate for the following aerobic exercise (Kisner & Colby). In addition, a good warm-up should incorporate stretching exercises. Stretching exercises are done at a slow, steady pace and help maintain a full range of motion in body joints while strengthening tendons, ligaments, and muscles.

Aerobic Exercise Phase

The aerobic phase of exercise is also known as the stimulus phase. It consists of four essential components: intensity (which is usually measured as the relative percentage of maximal aerobic capacity), frequency, duration, and mode of exercise. The combination of these components determines the effectiveness of the exercise. The mode of exercise should involve rhythmic, continuous movement of large muscle groups such as walking, jogging, cycling, swimming, or cross-country skiing. The frequency should be most days of the week, with a duration of at least 30 to 60 minutes of cumulative exercise. This could be achieved by exercising 3 times for 10 to 20 minutes. The intensity should be moderate or between 55% and 90% of maximum heart rate as calculated by the method described below. For most individuals physical fitness improvements may be gained with an intensity of 55% to 75% of maximal heart rate.

As physical fitness improves, it may be necessary to increase one of the components to gain additional benefits (Institute of Medicine Report [IOM], 2004; NIH Consensus Statement, 1995; Pollock et al., 1998; U.S. Surgeon General, 1996). It should be emphasized to the patient that it is the accumulated amount of daily moderate physical activity and exercise that is important. Although individuals who perform 30 minutes of accumulated moderate physical activity show significant health benefits compared to sedentary individuals, those who perform 60 minutes show additional health benefits, including prevention of weight gain. A balance needs to be achieved to obtain maximal benefit with the least risk and discomfort. Adjustment of intensity is important not only for safety reasons, but also for comfort and enjoyment of the activity (Foster & Tamboli, 1992). If exercise can be kept at a comfortable level, the individual is more likely to continue to perform the activity. As tolerance develops, any or all of the exercise components can be increased to meet the individual's aerobic capacity. For example, if an individual is comfortable with the intensity of the exercise, the duration and frequency can be increased to further improve training effect.

Cool Down

Immediately following the endurance exercises, the person should engage in a cooling-down period. The cool down allows the body to return to its normal resting state. This allows the HR and BP to return to resting levels and attenuates any post-exercise hypotension by improving venous return. The cool down also improves heat dissipation and elimination of blood lactate, and provides a means to combat any potential post-exercise rise in catecholamines (Fleg & Lakatta, 1986). Five to ten minutes are needed for the body to adjust to a slower pace. Cooling-down exercises may include walking slowly and deep breathing, and stretching.

Maintenance

The maintenance phase begins after 6 months of regular training, with the goal of maintaining achieved improvements in physical fitness (NIH Consensus Statement, 1995). Maintaining the exercise program is the key to the effectiveness of the intervention. Setting both short- and long-term goals helps improve adherence. The individual can experience a sense of accomplishment upon meeting short-term goals while still striving for overall goals. Keeping a record or graph supplies a visual demonstration of progress and may provide insight into adjustments to the exercise program that may assist in achievement of goals.

Reversibility and Detraining

Once participation in exercise has ceased there is a rapid return to pre-exercise levels of physical fitness. Most of the rapid decline occurs during the first 5 weeks following cessation of exercise and is usually complete within 12 weeks (Coyle et al., 1984; Saltin et al., 1968). With disuse, the muscle tissues atrophy. Additionally, the decreased caloric expenditure leads to a positive energy balance, which can result in increased accumulation of adipose tissue.

Specific Technique: Walking

One of the strategies identified by *Healthy People 2010* to improve health and quality of life through daily physical activity is an increase in "trips made by walking." Walking has declined rapidly in the United States and has reached the point at which 75% of all trips 1 mile or less are made by car (U.S. Department of Transportation [DOT], 1994). Walking is an easy and enjoyable activity that has significant health benefits. Moreover, it is an exercise in which persons of all age groups and with varying levels of ability or disability can engage to improve endurance. A major advantage is that walking requires no special equipment, facilities, or new skills. It is also safer and easier to maintain than many other forms of exercise. Intensity, duration, and frequency are easily regulated and adjusted to accommodate a wide range of physical capabilities and limitations. The initial intensity should be outlined at the start of the program and is dependent on baseline level of conditioning, physical or disease-related limitations or precautions, and outcome goals.

A walking program can be approached in two ways. The exercise can be completed in one or more daily sessions. For example, a previously sedentary individual may wish to begin an exercise program consisting of 2-minute brisk walks throughout the day. This could be increased to 5-minute walks, and then 10-minute walks as stamina increases. The more traditional alternative is to engage in one longer session at least three times per week; the recommended frequency for optimal benefits is 60 minutes of enjoyable moderate physical activity most days of the week (Daniels et al., 2005). These sessions would include a warm-up session for 5 to 10 minutes, an aerobic period that could start at 10 to 15 minutes and be gradually increased 30 to 60 minutes, and a cool-down period of 5 to 10 minutes (AHA, 1995). Tips for fitness walking are included in Table 23.1.

Exercising individuals should monitor their body's response to the activity to ensure that the intensity is appropriate. This can be done in several ways:

> *Monitor Target Heart Rate:* The target heart rate for a previously sedentary individual should be between 50% and 75% of the maximal heart rate, which is calculated by subtracting one's age from 220 (AHA, 1995) to gain improvements in physical fitness. The heart rate should be assessed one-third to halfway through the exercise session and immediately after stopping exercise. Exercise intensity can be increased or decreased based on this measurement.
>
> *The Talk Test:* The talk test can replace target heart rate monitoring when an individual is exercising at a moderate intensity. If

TABLE 23.1   Tips for Fitness Walking

- Warm up by performing a few stretches.
- Think tall as you walk. Stand straight with your head level and your shoulders relaxed.
- Your heel will hit the surface first. Use smooth movements rolling from heel to toe.
- Keep your hands free and let your arms swing naturally in opposition to your legs.
- When you're ready to pick up the pace, quicken your step and lengthen your stride, but don't compromise your upright posture or smooth, comfortable movements.
- To increase your intensity, burn more calories, and tone your upper body, bend your arms at the elbows and pump your arms. Keep your elbows close to your body.
- Breathe in and out naturally, rhythmically, and deeply.
- Use the "Talk Test" to check your intensity, or take your pulse to see if you are within your target heart rate.
- Cool down during the last 3 to 5 minutes by gradually slowing your pace to a stroll.

American Heart Association (1995)

the exercise prevents the individual from talking comfortably, the intensity should be decreased. A variation of this technique is to whistle; if the individual is unable to whistle, the intensity is too great and should be decreased.

Rating of Perceived Exertion: This is a scale that describes the sense of effort during the exercise. This scale can be ranked from one to ten with one being no effort and ten being maximal effort (AHA, 1995).

Conditions/Populations in Which the Intervention Has Been Used

Several populations for whom exercise is particularly beneficial include children, the elderly, those with affective disorders, individuals with heart disease, and those with peripheral arterial disease. The application and demonstrated effects of exercise intervention in each of these populations are discussed below.

Overweight Children and Adolescents

The number of overweight children and adolescents is rapidly increasing. Of particular concern are the increasing rates of type 2 diabetes mellitus and metabolic syndrome diagnosed in overweight children and adolescents, problems that used to be primarily limited to adults. Lack of physical activity and excess caloric intake cause central obesity, which, in turn, is believed to promote development of these conditions. Treatment includes dietary modification and initiation of physical activity. Increased physical activity has been shown to improve insulin sensitivity, blood pressure, cholesterol, and vascular function, and prevent further weight gain. The current recommendations are essentially the same as for healthy adults: 60 minutes of enjoyable, moderate physical activity most days of the week. An additional goal is to achieve less than 2 hours per day of consecutive sedentary activity, and at least 90 minutes to achieve weight loss (Andersen et al., 1998; Daniels et al., 2005; Sallis & Patrick, 1994).

The Elderly

The fastest growing segment of the population in the United States is individuals over the age of 65. The benefit of exercise as a therapy to prevent or delay functional decline and disease and improve quality of life is demonstrated by the numerous favorable changes occurring in response to exercise. Improvements in cardiovascular function have been shown to help lower risk factors for disease and reduce the need for assisted living (Mazzeo et al., 1998). The elderly are especially prone to the "hazards of immobility" that affect many of the body's systems. Exercise results in increased bone strength (Smith & Reddan, 1976), and increased total body calcium (Dalsky et al., 1988), as well as improved coordination, which may result in a reduction in falls (Bassett, McClamrock, & Schmelzer, 1982). Exercise has also been shown to improve body functioning and overall well-being. Blumenthal, Schocken, Needles, and Hindle (1982) reported in their study that 40% of the elderly who exercised felt healthier, were more satisfied with life, and had more self-confidence and improved mood.

It is particularly important to tailor exercise programs for the elderly, who may have specific limitations. Exercise needs to be initiated at lower levels and increased gradually. Previously sedentary elderly individuals may be more comfortable initiating an exercise program with some supervision, which allows them to become accustomed to this new level of activity in a safe environment. Group exercise may be especially appealing to older persons.

Affective Disorders

Exercise is an effective although underused intervention for individuals with affective disorders. There is considerable evidence supporting the positive effects of exercise in combating depression and anxiety (Byrne & Byrne, 1993). There are fewer, if any, side effects when compared with pharmacotherapy, and exercise is often more cost effective than psycho-therapy and pharmacotherapy (Yaffe, 1981). Although most studies have evaluated the effects of aerobic activity as the intervention, anaerobic activity has also been shown to be beneficial in alleviating depression. This suggests that improvement in mood is associated with exercise in general, rather than increased aerobic capacity (Doyne et al., 1987).

Heart Disease

Cardiac (exercise) rehabilitation (CR) is a common intervention pre-scribed for those with coronary heart disease (CHD), providing a safe environment for the initiation of an exercise program. Programs usually have several phases and are tailored to the specific needs, limitations, and characteristics of individual patients, helping them resume active and productive lives (Foster & Tamboli, 1992; Hamm & Leon, 1992; Leon et al., 2005). Exercise has multiple protective mechanisms that contribute to reduction of CHD risk, including anti-atherosclerotic, anti-arrhythmic, anti-ischemic, and anti-thrombotic effects (Leon et al.).

Exercise training has been shown to improve symptom-limited exer-cise capacity in CHD patients primarily as a result of peripheral hemody-namic adaptations (Ferguson et al., 1982; Juneau, Geneau, Marchand, & Brosseau, 1991; Wenger, 1993). Patients with CHD have a low skeletal muscle oxidative capacity that is significantly improved with training, despite relatively low workloads and exercise intensities, consistent with other non-heart disease populations (Ferguson et al.). Prior to training, patients with CHD are often unable to perform activities of daily living (ADLs) without symptoms. Exercise-trained CHD patients function fur-ther above the ischemic threshold in performing ADLs and thus require a lower percentage of maximal effort to perform activities. This increases stamina and endurance and helps to maintain independence (Wenger). Even patients with heart failure (HF), who typically have very poor cardiac function, have found that CR improves their exercise tolerance (Koch, Douard, & Broustet, 1992; Sullivan, 1994).

Peripheral Arterial Disease

Peripheral arterial disease (PAD), a prevalent atherosclerotic occlusive disease, limits functional capacity and is related to decreased quality of life. Individuals with PAD typically experience exercise-induced ischemic pain in the lower extremities, known as claudication. Exercise training is one of the most effective interventions available for the treatment of claudication due to PAD (Hiatt, Regensteiner, Hargarten, Wolfel, & Brass, 1990; Regensteiner, Steiner, & Hiatt, 1996). Exercise training has been shown to improve walking distance up to 180% (Regensteiner, 1997; Regensteiner & Hiatt, 1995). Prior to program initiation, an exercise prescription should be generated based on a graded exercise test and patients should start training at 50% of their functional capacity (Ekers & Hirsch, 1999). During a typical session, patients will exercise at a moderate pace until they experience moderate to severe claudication. At that point they will rest until the pain subsides. This exercise/rest pattern is repeated throughout the exercise session (Hiatt et al.). The most effective exercise programs for the treatment of claudication include the following components. The patient should exercise to the point of almost maximal claudication. The exercise session should be at least 30 minutes in length, with at least 3 sessions per week. The exercise program should continue for at least 6 months, with intermittent walking as the most effective mode of exercise (Gardner & Poehlman, 1995).

Measurement of Effectiveness

The appropriate measure of the effectiveness of an exercise intervention depends on the specific exercise prescribed and the goals of the intervention. Changes in atherosclerotic risk factors (i.e., cholesterol levels, triglycerides, insulin sensitivity, waist circumference, BP, and BMI) may be measured if cardiovascular health is the primary outcome of the exercise program. If cardiovascular fitness is the targeted outcome, an aerobic exercise program would be prescribed and improvements in the cardiovascular system such as increased CO, VO_2, and improved local circulation would be used to determine the effectiveness of the intervention (Fletcher et al., 2001; Halfman & Hojnacki, 1981). Cardiovascular response to submaximal exercise may provide further information and may be even more beneficial in assessing the impact on quality of life, as most activities of daily living are performed at submaximal intensity. Exercise prescribed to improve function may use parameters such as improved joint mobility, prevention or reduction of osteoporosis, and improved strength in determining exercise effectiveness (Benison & Hogstel, 1986). Assessment may also include changes in physical functioning and disability, ability to perform ADLs, changes in symptoms and activity tolerance, and other variables that reflect the individual's ability to function in daily life. Lower intensity programs, which may not demonstrate great changes in maximal exercise capacity, might produce sufficient changes in these outcome variables to make a difference in the individual's quality of life. Such programs would be especially appropriate in elderly and very sedentary individuals where low intensity exercise can produce a modest increase in fitness and more significant improvements in function (Belman & Gaesser, 1991; Foster, Hume, Byrnes, Dickenson, & Chatfield, 1989). Development and implementation of programs designed to meet the specific needs of patients can help maximize functional and quality-of-life outcomes.

Precautions

Before initiating an exercise program pre-participation screening procedures are recommended. These include such questionnaires as the Physical Activity Readiness Questionnaire (PAR-Q), designed to identify potential patients in need of medical advice prior to exercising (Canadian Society for Exercise Physiology, 1994). If a patient is identified as having potential or actual medical concerns, it is advisable that a graded exercise test be performed. The American College of Sports Medicine recommends that a graded exercise test be performed for any individual with more than two risk factors for CHD. This is done to rule out any potential contraindications to exercise and to provide a tool for determining initial exercise intensity (ACSM, 1998; Fletcher et al., 2001).

To avoid injury, it is important to begin an exercise program slowly, to follow safety guidelines, and to exercise consistently, several times per week. Potential exercise-related injuries include muscle and joint pain, cramps, blisters, shin splints, low back pain, tendonitis, and other sprains or muscle strains. The most commonly reported adverse event of exercise is musculoskeletal injury; approximately 25% of adults between 20 and 85 years reported an injury occurring at least once during 1 year (Hootman et al., 2002). It is possible that some of these are misclassified as injuries instead of muscle soreness due to a rapid increase in volume or intensity of training without proper knowledge of the principles of training.

The AHA (1995) has listed general guidelines to help ensure exercise safety. These include (1) stretching the muscles and tendons prior to beginning exercise; (2) wearing appropriate footwear; (3) exercising on a surface with some "give" to it, especially during high impact activities; and (4) learning the exercise properly and continuing good form even with increased speed or intensity. Should exercise-related injuries occur, they can usually be treated with one or a combination of therapies including rest, ice, compression, and elevation (AHA).

Previously sedentary elderly individuals and those with chronic disease, especially heart disease, should consult a physician prior to initiating an exercise program to ensure that an appropriate exercise prescription is given. Warning signs of heart disease should be provided prior to initiation of an exercise program, especially to those in high-risk categories.

AREAS IN WHICH FUTURE RESEARCH IS NEEDED

There are many gaps in our knowledge related to exercise, its measurement, the benefits, and methods to improve exercise adherence. Specific research areas needed include:

- development of measures of exercise behavior that are valid and reliable in different populations and with various levels of activity,

- development and testing of specific interventions to increase exercise adherence in multiple populations,

- assessment of the impact of exercise interventions in multiple populations through controlled longitudinal studies, and

- development of strategies to increase lifelong physical activity and exercise.

SELECTED EXERCISE INFORMATION WEB SITES

National Institute on Aging (2004) AgePage: Exercise: Getting fit for life: http:// www.niapublications.org/engagepages/exercise.asp
Physical Activity Task Force Reference List: http://www.patf.dpc.wa.gov.au/ documents/reflist.pdf
Overweight in children and adolescents: Pathophysiology, consequences, prevention, and treatment: http://circ.ahajournals.org/cgi/content/full/111/15/1999 ?ck=nck
Exercise and physical activity in the prevention and treatment of atherosclerotic cardiovascular disease: http://circ.ahajournals.org/cgi/content/full/107/ 24/3109
Resistance exercise in individuals with and without cardiovascular disease: http:// circ.ahajournals.org/cgi/content/full/101/7/828
Exercise and heart failure: http://www.circ.ahajournals.org/cgi/content/full/107/ 8/1210
Physical activity and exercise recommendations for stroke survivors: http:// www.guideline.gov/summary/summary.aspx?view_id=1&doc_id=5358

REFERENCES

American College of Sports Medicine. (2000). *Guidelines for graded exercise testing and exercise prescription* (6th ed.) Baltimore, MD: Lippincott, Williams & Willkins.

American Heart Association. (1995). *Your heart: An owner's manual.* Englewood Cliffs, NJ: Prentice Hall.

Andersen, R. E., Crespo, C. J., Bartlett, S. J., Cheskin, L. J., & Pratt, M. (1998). Relationship of physical activity and television watching with body weight and level of fatness among children: Results from the Third National Health and Nutrition Examination Survey. *Journal of the American Medical Association, 279*, 938–942.

Astrand, P., Rodahl, K., Dahl, K., & Stromme, B. (2004). *Textbook of work physiology* (4th ed.). Champaign IL: Human Kinetics.

Balady, G., & Weiner, D. (1992). Physiology of exercise in normal individuals and patients with coronary heart disease. In N. Wenger and H. Hellerstein (Eds.), *Rehabilitation of the coronary patient* (pp. 103–122). New York: Churchill Livingstone.

Bassett, C., McClamrock, E., & Schmelzer, M. (1982). A 10-week exercise program for senior citizens. *Geriatric Nursing, 3*, 103–105.

Belman, M., & Gaesser, G. (1991). Exercise training below and above the lactate threshold in the elderly. *Medicine and Science in Sports and Exercise, 23*, 562–568.

Benison, B., & Hogstel, M. O. (1986). Aging and movement therapy: Essential interventions for the immobile elderly. *Journal of Gerontological Nursing, 12*(12), 8–16.

Blumenthal, J., Schocken, D., Needles, T., & Hindle, P. (1982). Psychological and physiological effects of physical conditioning on the elderly. *Journal of Psychosomatic Medicine 26, 505–510.*

Byrne, A., & Byrne, D. G. (1993). The effect of exercise on depression, anxiety and other mood states: A review. *Journal of Psychosomatic Research, 37*, 565–574.

Canadian Society for Exercise Physiology. (1994). *PAR-Q and you.* Canadian Society for Exercise Physiology, 1–2.

Coyle, E. F., Martin, W. H., Sincacore, D. R., Joyner, M. J., Hagberg, J. M., & Holloszy, J. O. (1984). Time course of loss of adaptation after stopping prolonged intense endurance training. *Journal of Applied Physiology, 57*, 1857–1864.

Crews, D., & Landers, D. (1987). A meta-analytic review of aerobic fitness and reactivity to psychosocial stressors. *Medicine and Science in Sports and Exercise, 19*(suppl), S114–S120.

Dalsky, O., Stocke, K., Ehsani, A., Slatopolsky, E., Lee, W., & Birge, S. (1988). Weight-bearing exercise training and lumbar bone mineral content in postmenopausal women. *Annals of Internal Medicine, 108*, 824–829.

Daniels, S. R., Arnett, D. K., Eckel, R. H., Gridding, S. S., Hayman, L. L., Kumanyika, S., et al. (2005). Overweight in children and adolescents: Pathophysiology, consequences, prevention, and treatment. *Circulation, 111*, 1999–2012.

Doyne, E. J., Osip-Klein, D. J., Bowman, E. D., Osborn, K. M., McDougall-Wilson, I. B., & Neimeyer, R. A. (1987). Running versus weight-lifting in the treatment of depression. *Journal of Consulting and Clinical Psychology, 55*(5), 748–754.

Ekers, M. A., & Hirsch, A. T. (1999). Vascular medicine and vascular rehabilitation. In V. Fahey (Ed.), *Vascular nursing* (3rd ed., pp. 188–211). Philadelphia: Saunders.

Ferguson, R., Taylor, A., Cote, P., Charlebois, J., Dinelle, Y., Perionnet, F., et al. (1982). Skeletal muscle and cardiac changes with training in patients with angina pectoris. *American Journal of Physiology, 243*, H830–H836.

Fleg, J., & Lakatta, E. (1986). Prevalence and significance of post exercise hypotension in apparently healthy subjects. *American Journal of Cardiology, 57*(15), 1380–1384.

Fletcher, G. (1982). *Exercise in the practice of medicine.* Mount Kisco, NY: Futura.

Fletcher, G. F., Balady, G. J., Amsterdam, E. A., Chaitman, B., Eckel, R., Fleg, J., et al. (2001). Exercise standards for testing and training: A statement for healthcare professionals from the American Heart Association. *Circulation, 104*, 1694–1740.

Fletcher, G. F., Balady, G., Blair, S., Blumenthal, J., Casperson, C., Chairman, B., et al. (1996). Statement on exercise: Benefits and recommendations for physical activity programs for all Americans. *American Heart Association Scientific Statement.* Retrieved from http//www.americanheart.org/Scientific/statements/1996/0815_exp.html

Foster, C., & Tamboli, H. (1992). Exercise prescription in the rehabilitation of patients following coronary artery bypass graft surgery and coronary angioplasty. In R. Shephard & H. Miller (Eds.), *Exercise and the heart in health and disease* (pp. 283–298). New York: Marcel Dekker.

Foster, V., Hume, G., Byrnes, W., Dickenson, A., & Chatfield, S. (1989). Endurance training for elderly women: Moderate vs. low intensity. *Journal of Gerontology, 44*(6), M184–M178.

Gardner, A. W., & Poehlman, E. T. (1995). Exercise rehabilitation programs for the treatment of claudication pain: A meta-analysis. *Journal of the American Medical Association, 274*(12), 975–980.

Gavin, J. (1988). Psychological issues in exercise prescription. *Sports Medicine, 6*, 1–10.

Halfman, M., & Hojnacki, L. (1981). Exercise and the maintenance of health. *Topics in Clinical Nursing, 3*(2), 1–10.

Hamm, L., & Leon, A. (1992). Exercise training for the coronary patient. In N. Wenger & H. Hellerstein (Eds.), *Rehabilitation of the coronary patient* (pp. 367–402). New York: Churchill Livingstone.

Hargraves, M. (1995). Exercise metabolism. In M. Hargraves (Ed.), *Exercise metabolism* (pp. 41–73). Champaign, IL: Human Kinetics.

Healthy people 2010: Understanding and improving public health. (2000). Washington, DC: Department of Health and Human Services, Public Health Service.

Hiatt, W. R., Regensteiner, J. G., Hargarten, M. E., Wolfel, E. E., & Brass, E. P. (1990). Benefit of exercise conditioning for patients with peripheral arterial disease. *Circulation, 81*(2), 602–609.

Hootman, J. M., Macera, C. A., Ainsworth, B. E., Addy, C. L., Martin, M., & Blair, S. N. (2002). Epidemiology of musculoskeletal injuries among sedentary and physically active adults. *Medicine and Science in Sports and Exercise, 34*(5), 838–844.

Institute of Medicine Report. (2004). Retrieved from www.iom.edu/report.asp?id=4340

Juneau, M., Geneau, S., Marchand, C., & Brosseau, R. (1991). Cardiac rehabilitation after coronary artery bypass surgery. *Cardiovascular Clinics, 12*(2), 25–42.

Kisner, C., & Colby, L. (1996). *Therapeutic exercise: Foundations and techniques* (3rd ed.). Philadelphia: Davis.

Koch, M., Douard, H., & Broustet, J-P. (1992). The benefit of graded physical exercise in chronic heart failure. *Chest, 101*(5 suppl), 231S–235S.

Kujala, U. M., Kapiro, J., Sarna, S., & Koskenvuo, M. (1998). Relationship of leisure-time physical activity and mortality: The Finnish twin cohort. *Journal of the American Medical Association, 279*(6), 440–444.

Leon, A. S., Franklin, B. A., Costa, F., Balady, G. J., Berra, K. A., Stewart, K. J., et al. (2005). Cardiac rehabilitation and secondary prevention of coronary heart disease. *Circulation, 111*, 369–376.

Mazzeo, R. S., Cavanagh, P., Evans, W. J., Evans, W. J., Fiatarone, M., Hagberg, J., et al. (1998). Exercise and physical activity for older adults: American College of Sports Medicine position stand. *Medicine and Science in Sports and Exercise, 30*(6), 992–1008.

McKenzie, T. L., Nader, P. R., Strikmiller, P. K., Yang, M., Stone, E. J., Perry, C. L., et al. (1996). School physical education: Effect of the child and adolescent trial for cardiovascular health. *Preventive Medicine, 25*(4), 423–431.

NIH Consensus Statement. Physical Activity and Cardiovascular Health. (1995, December 18–20), 13(3), 1–33.

Paffenbarger, R. S., Hyde, R. T., Wing, A. L., Lee, I. M., Jung, D. L., & Kampert, J. B. (1993). The association of changes in physical activity level and other lifestyle characteristics with mortality among men. *New England Journal of Medicine, 328*(8), 538–545.

Pender, N. (1996). *Health promotion in nursing practice* (3rd ed.). Stamford, CT: Appleton & Lange.

Pollock, M. L., Gaesser, G. A., Butcher, J. D., Despres, J. P., Dishman, R. K., Franklin, B. A., et al. (1998). The recommended quantity and quality of exercise for developing and maintaining cardiorespiratory and muscular fitness and flexibility in healthy adults: American College of Sports Medicine position stand. *Medicine and Science in Sports and Exercise, 30*(6), 975–991.

Regensteiner, J. G. (1997). Exercise in the treatment of claudication: Assessment and treatment of functional impairment. *Vascular Medicine, 2*(3), 238–242.

Regensteiner, J. G., & Hiatt, W. R. (1995). Exercise rehabilitation for patients with peripheral arterial disease. *Exercise and Sport Sciences Reviews, 23*, 1–24.

Regensteiner, J. G., Steiner, J. F., & Hiatt, W. R. (1996). Exercise training improves functional status in patients with peripheral arterial disease. *Journal of Vascular Surgery, 23*(1), 104–115.

Robergs, R., Ghiasvand, F., & Parker D. (2004). Biochemistry of exercise-induced metabolic acidosis. *American Journal of Physiology. Regulatory, Integrative, and Comparative Physiology, 287*, R502–R516.

Rowell, L. (1993). *Human cardiovascular control.* New York: Oxford University Press.

Sallis, J. F., & Patrick, K. (1994). Physical activity guidelines for adolescents: Consensus statement. *Pediatric Exercise Science, 6*(4), 302–314.

Saltin, B., Blomqvist, G., Mitchell, J. H., Johnson, R. L., Wildenthal, K., & Chapman, C. B. (1968). Response to exercise after bed rest and after training. *Circulation, 38*(Suppl 5), VII1–VII78.

Sherman, S. D., D'Agostino, R. B., Cobb, J. L., & Kannel, W. B. (1994). Physical activity and mortality in women in the Framingham Heart Study. *American Heart Journal, 128*(5), 879–884.

Smith, E., & Reddan, W. (1976). Physical activity—a modality for bone accretion in the aged. *American Journal of Roentgenology, 126,* 1297.

Stevenson, J., & Topp, R. (1990). Effects of moderate and low intensity long-term exercise by older adults. *Research in Nursing and Health, 13,* 209–218.

Sullivan, M. (1994). New trends in cardiac rehabilitation in patients with chronic heart failure. *Progress in Cardiovascular Nursing, 9*(1), 13–21.

Thomas, S., Reading, J., & Shephard, R. J. (1992). Revision of the Physical Activity Readiness Questionnaire (PAR-Q). *Canadian Journal of Sports Science, 17,* 338–345.

Thompson. P. D., Buchner, D., Pina, I. L., Balady, G. J., Williams, M. A., Marcus, B. H., et al. (2003). Exercise and physical activity in the prevention and treatment of atherosclerotic cardiovascular disease: American Heart Association scientific statement. *Circulation, 107,* 3109–3116.

U.S. Department of Transportation (DOT). (1994). *National bicycling and walking study: Transportation choices for a changing America* (Pub. FH10A PD 94-023). Washington, DC: DOT, Federal Highway Administration.

U.S. Surgeon General. (1996). *Report on physical activity and health.* Retrieved from http://www.cde.800/nccdphd/sgr/mm.htm

Wenger, N. (1993). Modern coronary rehabilitation: New concepts in care. *Postgraduate Medicine, 94*(2), 131–141.

Westerblad, H., Allen, D., & Lannergren, J. (2002). Muscle fatigue: Lactic acid or inorganic phosphate the major cause? *News in Physiological Science, 17,* 17–21.

Yaffe, M. (1981). Sport and mental health. *Journal of Biosocial Science-Supplement, 7,* 83–95.

CHAPTER 24

Tai Chi

Kuei-Min Chen

Due to the pressures of work, many people do not have proper exercise, which may lead to mental strain, nervous breakdown, or inefficiency in their daily work (Cheng, 1994). Good health is essential, and how to acquire a strong and healthy body is a vital concern. It is commonly recognized that proper physical exercise is the best method of keeping our bodies fit and healthy. However, it is not easy to find an exercise that suits people of all ages (Cheng).

Tai Chi, a manipulative and body-based therapy, is one of the interventions widely recommended across different professions, including nurses, physicians, occupational therapists, physical therapists, and recreational therapists. A manipulative and body-based therapy can heighten individuals' awareness of their bodies and take advantage of their body structure for expressing feelings and ideas. Gradually, individuals become more aware of their total being, which promotes harmony within themselves and leads to enhanced well-being (Lange, 1975). The purpose of this chapter is to introduce and describe Tai Chi.

DEFINITION

Tai Chi, which means "supreme ultimate," is a traditional Chinese martial art (Koh, 1981) and a mind–body exercise (Forge, 1997). It involves a series of fluid, continuous, graceful, dance-like postures, and the performance of movements known as forms (Perry, 1982; Smalheiser, 1984). The graceful body movements are integrated by mind concentration, the balanced shifting of body weight, muscle relaxation, and breath control. They are performed in a slow, rhythmic, and well-controlled manner (Plummer, 1983).

There are several styles of Tai Chi that are currently practiced: Chen (quick and slow large movements), Yang (slow large movements), Wu (mid-paced compact), and Sun (quick compact) (Jou, 1983). Each style has a characteristic protocol that differs from the other styles in the postures or forms included, the order in which they appear, the pace at which movements are executed, and the level of difficulty; yet, the basic principles are the same (Yang, 1991). For example, one significant difference between Chen and Yang styles is that Yang movements are relaxed, evenly paced, and graceful. It is the most popular Tai Chi practiced by older adults (Jou). In comparison, the Chen style is characterized by alternating slow movements with quick and vigorous ones, and restrained and controlled actions, which reflect a more martial origin (Yang).

There are a few simplified, Westernized forms of the ancient Tai Chi. The most common one is called Tai Chi Chih, which was developed by an American, Justin Stone. Tai Chi Chih consists of 20 simple, repetitive, non-strenuous movements and an ending pose. It emphasizes a soft, flowing, continuous motion and is easier for beginners to learn. Most Tai Chi movements were named after animals, such as "white crane spreads its wings" and "grasp the bird's tail" (Koh, 1981).

SCIENTIFIC BASIS

Tai Chi practice is closely linked to Chinese medical theory, in which the vital life energy, chi (or qi), is thought to circulate throughout the body in discrete channels called meridians. Using correct postures and adequate relaxation, the principle of Tai Chi is to promote the free flow of chi throughout the body, which improves the health of an individual. In 1992, Tse and Bailey reported that regular Tai Chi practice significantly improved balance control in three of five tests and advocated the following factors as an explanation for the improvements:

1. All Tai Chi movements are circular, slow, continuous, even, and smooth. Patterns of movement flow from one to the next. The even, slow tempo facilitates a sensory awareness of the speed, force, trajectory, and execution of movement throughout the exercise.

2. Because movements are well controlled, all unnecessary exertion is avoided, and only sufficient effort is used to overcome gravity. Muscle coordination instead of rigid contraction can therefore be promoted.

3. Throughout the exercise, the body is constantly shifted from one foot to the other. This is likely to facilitate improvement of dynamic standing balance.

4. Throughout the exercises, different parts of the body take turns in playing the role of stabilizer and mover, allowing smooth movements to be executed without compromising the balance and stability of the body.

The performance of Tai Chi looks like a classical dance with graceful movements and attentive actions, regulated by the timing of deep breathing and the movement of the diaphragm. It offers a balanced exercise to the muscles and joints of the various parts of the body (Cheng, 1994). In addition, a peaceful state of mind and spiritual dedication to each movement during the exercise ensure that the central nervous system is given sufficient training and is consequently toned up with time as the exercise continues. A strong central nervous system is the basic condition of a healthy body and the various organs depend largely on the soundness of the central nervous system (Cheng).

INTERVENTION

In Eastern countries such as Taiwan, it is common and popular for older adults to practice Tai Chi as a group in parks or on the athletic grounds of elementary schools in the early morning. Tai Chi practice groups are usually led by masters who are pleased to share its essence with others. People who are interested in Tai Chi are welcome to join the groups and learn the movements from these masters. In Western countries, there is a growing interest in the practice of Tai Chi. Various Tai Chi clubs are available to the public through community centers, health clinics, or private organizations. General information is widespread through web sites, books, and videos. Tai Chi is a convenient exercise that can be practiced in any place, at any time, and without any equipment.

Techniques

As mentioned earlier, although various styles of Tai Chi are currently practiced, the underlying practice principles are the same. In Schaller's study (1996), five essential principles of movement were identified:

1. Hand and leg movement should be synchronous.
2. The emphasis should be on a soft, relaxed rather than a hard, tense position.
3. Moves should be practiced with a quiet and open mind.
4. The soles of the feet should be rooted to the ground with the knees bent in a low stance and the primary focus of awareness within the lower abdomen.
5. The physical force should be rooted in the feet, passed up through the legs as weight is shifted, and distributed by the pivoting of the waist.

In the physical performance, an individual must relax and think of nothing else before starting. The movements should be slow and rhythmic with natural breathing. Every action becomes easy and smooth, the waist turns freely, and the feelings of comfort and relaxation are gradually developed (Cheng, 1994). In the spiritual aspect, Tai Chi is an exercise that produces harmony of body and mind. Each movement should be guided by thought instead of physical strength. For instance, to lift up the hands an individual must first have the necessary mental concentration, and then the hands can be raised slowly in a proper manner. Hence, the breathing will become deeper and the body will be strengthened (Cheng).

Guidelines

The prototype for performing the movement called "around the platter" is presented in Table 24.1. Various videotapes on Tai Chi are also available through local video rental stores. Welsch (1998) identified the following books as useful for learning Tai Chi:

- *Tai Chi Chuan for Health and Self-defense* (Liang, 1977) is an introduction and reflection on the art of Tai Chi.
- *The Elements of Tai Chi* (Crompton, 1991) provides a basic introduction to Tai Chi as a martial art and as a way to achieve better health.
- *Tai Chi: Transcendent Art* (Cheng, 1994) demonstrates each Tai Chi movement through pictures and graphs.

Additional information can be found through several useful web links:

- www.supply.com/lee/tcclinks.html, which provides links to more than a hundred other web sites on Tai Chi and related topics;

TABLE 24.1   Prototype for Performing "Around the Platter"

---

1. Hands are held at chest level, wrists slightly bent and elbows close to sides. Fingers are spread apart. Legs are slightly apart and bent with the left in front of the right. Weight is equally distributed between legs.
2. Begin to rock forward, shifting weight to the left leg with hands moving to the left. (Imagine a round platter at the chest level, and the hands circling around the platter from left to right.)
3. As most of the weight shifts to the left leg and the hands are directly in front of the body, the left heel comes off the ground. As the hands move right of midline, the weight begins to shift to the right leg. When the hands have completed a full circle (held at chest level), most of the weight is on the right leg and the right toe is off the ground.
4. This movement can be repeated 6–9 times and then repeated again going from right to left.

Note: Adapted from *Tai Chi Chih: Joy Through Movement*, by J. F. Stone, 1994, Fort Yates, ND, Good Karma.

- http://sunflower.signet.com.sg/~limttk/index.htm, which is a valuable site with complete historical and background information on Tai Chi.

Measurement of Outcomes

According to Plummer (1983), mind concentration and breathing control are two of the major tenets of Tai Chi practice. When practicing Tai Chi with a peaceful, focused mind and incorporating smooth breathing into each movement, a person will experience physical and psychological relaxation, which leads to enhanced well-being, both physically and psychologically (Plummer). With this conceptual framework in mind, the measurement of the effects of Tai Chi could be for both physical and psychological well-being. Based on the literature, which will be discussed in detail later, more studies were done to measure the physical outcomes of Tai Chi practice (such as cardiovascular functioning) with little emphasis on psychological well-being outcomes (such as mood states).

Precautions

Tai Chi is unique for its slow graceful movements with low impact, low velocity, minimal orthopedic complications, and is a suitable conditioning exercise for older adults (Lai, Lan, Wong, & Teng, 1995). Although many research studies have shown the benefits of Tai Chi, there are some contraindications to its practice, such as an acute stage of angina, ventricular arrhythmia, or myocardial ischemia. The instructor and the learner have to be aware of those contraindications and an initial assessment is necessary to determine an individual's exercise tolerance and other limitations (Forge, 1997). While learning Tai Chi, a novice should be periodically evaluated in terms of progress, program adherence, cognitive response, muscular strength, balance, and level of flexibility at fairly regular (e.g., 4-week) intervals for the first 60 to 90 days of participation in such a program, and, if progress is considered satisfactory, at 6-month intervals thereafter (Forge). It is strongly recommended that one learn Tai Chi from an experienced master who is able to teach the movements based on individual needs and physical tolerance. Recommendations for choosing a class are provided in Table 24.2.

USES

Tai Chi is especially appropriate for older adults or for patients with chronic diseases because of its low intensity, steady rhythm, and low physical and mental tension (Xu & Fan, 1988). It has been shown to enhance cardiovascular and respiratory functions, improve health-related fitness, and promote positive health status (Brown, Mucci, Hetzler, & Knowlton, 1989; Lai et al., 1995; Lan, Lai, Chen, & Wong, 1998; Lan, Lai, Wong, & Yu, 1996). In addition, practicing Tai Chi has been effective in lowering blood pressure (Channer, Barrow, Barrow, Osborne, & Ives, 1996; Jin, 1989, 1992; Thornton, Sykes, & Tang, 2004; Tsai et al., 2003; Wolf et al., 1996). However, in a pretest–posttest study on the effects of a 10-week, short-term Tai Chi training program, there were no significant improvements of health status or blood pressure in the community-dwelling elders as compared to their baseline data (Schaller, 1996). Schaller explained that these non-significant results might be attributed to the fact that the health status measures may not have been sensitive or specific enough to detect changes in a short-term exercise program.

TABLE 24.2   Choosing a Tai Chi Class

---

1. If possible find a studio or organization that specializes in tai chi.
2. Find an experienced teacher (6–10 years of experience) who demonstrates and verbally explains the movements. Ask to observe a class before joining.
3. Find a class with fewer than 20 students.
4. Avoid purchasing any special clothing or equipment.

Note: Adapted from "Tai Chi," by L. B. Downs, 1992, *Modern Maturity*, 35, pp. 60–64.

Falls are common in the older population, and they often cause severe physical trauma (Tideiksaar, 1989). Most studies have shown that Tai Chi increases postural stability and enhances balance (Brown et al., 1995; Jacobson, Chen, Cashel, & Guerrero, 1997; Shih, 1997; Thornton et al., 2004; Tsang & Hui-Chan, 2004; Tse & Bailey, 1992; Wolf et al., 1996), which lead to a reduction in the risk of falls (Hainsworth, 2004; Shih, 1997). Furthermore, several studies found that Tai Chi enhanced positive mood states and decreased mood disturbances (Brown et al., 1995; Jin, 1992), and improved quality of sleep (Li et al., 2004). However, one study showed that it had no significant impact on mood states in community-dwelling elders (Schaller, 1996).

Tai Chi also plays an important role in symptom control of chronic illnesses. Chen and Yen (2002) summarized experimental studies on the effects of Tai Chi on symptom control in patients with various chronic illnesses. Most results indicated that it was beneficial to those with cardiovascular diseases, arthritis, chronic obstructive pulmonary disease, and low back pain. Chen, Snyder, and Krichbaum (2001) also found that Tai Chi practitioners had better physical and mental health status, lower systolic and diastolic blood pressure, fewer falls within the past year, less mood disturbance, and better mood states when compared to non-practitioners. Researchers have suggested that Tai Chi could be incorporated into community programs or senior center activities to promote the well-being of community-dwelling elders. It could also be included as one of the activities in nursing homes or in rehabilitation programs in hospital settings.

No studies were found on the use of Tai Chi specifically with children. However, the movements may be enticing to children as many enjoy participating in various martial arts.

FUTURE RESEARCH

Overall, practicing Tai Chi appropriately has various benefits, as evidenced in the literature, and it is highly recommended for the appropriate populations. More studies about the effects of Tai Chi from a nursing perspective are needed in order to provide guidance to nurses in its use with various populations (Chen & Snyder, 1999). Some questions for further research include:

1. What are the possible benefits and harms of practicing Tai Chi?
2. Which populations, especially children, can most benefit from practicing Tai Chi and are there conditions that would preclude its use?

3. What is the nature of stability or change in the well-being status of elders who practice Tai Chi?

4. What are the differences on well-being outcomes of beginners (people who are just starting to learn Tai Chi movements), practitioners (people who have practiced Tai Chi regularly for more than a year), and masters (people who have practiced Tai Chi regularly for more than a decade and are licensed by the National Tai Chi Association to be instructors)?

REFERENCES

Brown, D. D., Mucci, W. G., Hetzler, R. K., & Knowlton, R. G. (1989). Cardiovascular and ventilatory responses during formalized tai chi chuan exercise. *Research Quarterly for Exercise and Sport, 60,* 246–250.

Brown, D. R., Wang, Y., Ward, A., Ebbeling, C. B., Fortlage, L., Puleo, E., et al. (1995). Chronic psychological effects of exercise and exercise plus cognitive strategies. *Medicine and Science in Sports and Exercise, 27,* 765–775.

Channer, K. S., Barrow, D., Barrow, R., Osborne, M., & Ives, G. (1996). Changes in haemodynamic parameters following Tai Chi Chuan and aerobic exercise in patients recovering from acute myocardial infarction. *Postgraduate Medical Journal, 72,* 349–351.

Chen, C. H., & Yen, M. F. (2002). The effects of Tai Chi on symptom control in patients with chronic illness. *The Journal of Nursing, 49*(5), 22–27.

Chen, K. M., & Snyder, M. (1999). A research-based use of Tai Chi/movement therapy as a nursing intervention. *Journal of Holistic Nursing, 17,* 267–279.

Chen, K. M., Snyder, M., & Krichbaum, K. (2001). Tai Chi and well-being of Taiwanese community-dwelling elders. *Clinical Gerontologist, 24*(3/4), 137–156.

Cheng, T. H. (1994). *Tai Chi: Transcendent art.* Hong Kong: The Hong Kong Tai Chi Association.

Crompton, P. (1991). *The elements of Tai Chi.* Boston: Element.

Downs, L. B. (1992). Tai chi. *Modern Maturity, 35*(4), 60–64.

Forge, R. L. (1997). Mind–body fitness: Encouraging prospects for primary and secondary prevention. *Journal of Cardiovascular Nursing, 11*(3), 53–65.

Hainsworth, T. (2004). The role of exercise in falls prevention for older patients. *Nursing Times, 100*(18), 28–29.

Jacobson, B. H., Chen, H. C., Cashel, C., & Guerrero, L. (1997). The effect of tai chi chuan training on balance, kinesthetic sense, and strength. *Perceptual and Motor Skills, 84,* 27–33.

Jin, P. (1989). Changes in heart rate, noradrenaline, cortisol and mood during tai chi. *Journal of Psychosomatic Research, 33,* 197–206.

Jin, P. (1992). Efficacy of tai chi, brisk walking, meditation, and reading in reducing mental and emotional stress. *Journal of Psychosomatic Research, 36,* 361–370.

Jou, T. H. (1983). *The tao of tai chi chuan: Way to rejuvenation* (3rd ed.). Piscataway, NJ: Tai Chi Foundation.

Koh, T. C. (1981). Tai chi chuan. *American Journal of Chinese Medicine, 9,* 15–22.

Lai, J. S., Lan, C., Wong, M. K., & Teng, S. H. (1995). Two-year trends in cardiorespiratory function among older tai chi chuan practitioners and sedentary subjects. *Journal of the American Geriatrics Society, 43,* 1222–1227.

Lan, C., Lai, J. S., Chen, S. Y., & Wong, M. K. (1998). 12-month tai chi training in the elderly: Its effect on health fitness. *Medicine and Science in Sports and Exercise, 30,* 345–351.

Lan, C., Lai, J. S., Wong, M. K., & Yu, M. L. (1996). Cardiorespiratory function, flexibility, and body composition among geriatric tai chi chuan practitioners. *Archives of Physical Medicine and Rehabilitation, 77,* 612–616.

Lange, R. (1975). *The nature of dance.* London: Macdonald & Evans.

Li, F., Fisher, K. J., Harmer, P., Irbe, D., Tearse, R. G., & Weimer, C. (2004). Tai chi and self-rated quality of sleep and daytime sleepiness in older adults: A randomized controlled trial. *Journal of the American Geriatrics Society, 52,* 892–900.

Liang, T. T. (1977). *Tai Chi Chuan for health and self-defense.* Boston: Redwing.

Perry, P. (1982). Sports medicine in China: A group philosophy of fitness. *The Physician and Sports Medicine, 10,* 177–178.

Plummer, J. P. (1983). Acupuncture and tai chi chuan (Chinese shadow boxing): Body/mind therapies affecting homeostasis. In Y. Lau & J. P. Fowler (Eds.), *The scientific basis of traditional Chinese medicine: Selected papers* (pp. 22–36). Hong Kong: Medical Society.

Schaller, K. J. (1996). Tai chi chih: An exercise option for older adults. *Journal of Gerontological Nursing, 22*(10), 12–17.

Shih, J. (1997). Basic Beijing twenty-four forms of tai chi exercise and average velocity of sway. *Perceptual and Motor Skills, 84,* 287–290.

Smalheiser, M. (1984). Tai chi chuan in China today. *Tai Chi Chuan: Perspectives of the Way and Its Movement, 1,* 3–5.

Stone, J. F. (1994). *Tai chi chih: Joy through movement.* Fort Yates, ND: Good Karma.

Thornton, E. W., Sykes, K. S., & Tang, W. K. (2004). Health benefits of Tai Chi exercise: Improved balance and blood pressure in middle-aged women. *Health Promotion International, 19,* 33–38.

Tideiksaar, R. (1989). *Falling in old age: Its prevention and treatment* (Springer series on adulthood and aging, Vol. 22). New York: Springer Publishing.

Tsai, J. C., Wang, W. H., Chan, P., Lin, L. J., Wang, C. H., Tomlinson, B., et al. (2003). The beneficial effects of Tai Chi Chuan on blood pressure and lipid profile and anxiety status in a randomized controlled trial. *Journal of Alternative & Complementary Medicine, 9,* 747–754.

Tsang, W. W., & Hui-Chan, C. W. (2004). Effects of exercise on joint sense and balance in elderly men: Tai chi versus golf. *Medicine & Science in Sports & Exercise, 36,* 658–667.

Tse, S., & Bailey, D. M. (1992). Tai chi and postural control in the well elderly. *American Journal of Occupational Therapy, 46,* 295–300.

Welsch, C. (1998, January 25). Tai chi. *Star Tribune*, pp. G6, G7, Minneapolis, MN.

Wolf, S. L., Barnhart, H. X., Kutner, N. G., McNeely, E., Coogler, C., & Xu, T. (1996). Reducing frailty and falls in older persons: An investigation of Tai chi and computerized balance training. *Journal of American Geriatrics Society, 44*, 489–497.

Xu, S. W., & Fan, Z. H. (1988). Physiological studies of tai ji quan in China. *Medicine Sport Science, 28*, 70–80.

Yang, Z. (1991). *Yang style Taijiquan* (2nd ed.). Beijing: Morning Glory.

CHAPTER 25

Muscle Relaxation Techniques

Mariah Snyder, Elizabeth Pestka, and Catherine Bly

Relaxation techniques have been used for millennia. Ancient religions such as Hinduism and Buddhism document the use of yoga and breathing exercises as relaxation techniques. Reducing muscle tension is a component of many complementary therapies used in decreasing anxiety and promoting comfort. For example, muscle relaxation is often a part of guided imagery. Many techniques exist to promote muscle relaxation. Progressive muscle relaxation (PMR), developed by Edmund Jacobson (1938), serves as the basis for many of these techniques.

DEFINITION

Muscle relaxation is bringing awareness to muscles in the body and the tension that exists in them, and reducing this tension. Awareness can be achieved either by tensing the muscles even more and then releasing the tension or by focusing attention on the muscles and imaging them being free of tension.

Progressive muscle relaxation is the tensing and relaxing of successive muscle groups. A person's attention is drawn to discriminating between the feelings experienced when the muscle group is relaxed and when it was tensed. With continued use of PMR, an individual can sense muscle tension without having to go through the tensing and relaxing of specific muscle groups.

The relaxation response proposed by Benson (1975) directs attention to muscle relaxation and incorporates meditative techniques. The relaxation response consists of a mental device, a passive attitude, and decreased muscle tone. (The relaxation response is described in Chapter 11.) A quiet environment is recommended for achieving relaxation using this technique.

SCIENTIFIC BASIS

When people perceive an actual or potential event as a threat to their well-being, a sympathetic nervous system response occurs, which is often referred to as the fight–flight response. It includes dilation of the pupils, shallowness of respiration, increased heart rate, and tensing of muscles. This response assists humans in handling short-term stressful situations such as moving quickly to avoid a car that appears suddenly. However, if the perceived stressor persists over time or the person perceives it as such, the repeated psychophysiological stress response can have deleterious effects on the body. The desired outcome of relaxation strategies is the mitigation of persisting high levels of stress or their avoidance.

Brown (1977) noted that the stress response is part of a closed feedback loop between the muscles and the brain. Appraisal of stressors results in a tensing of the muscles that send stimuli to the brain, establishing a feedback loop. The brain alerts the entire body that a stressor, real or imagined, is being encountered and then sends signals to the muscles to prepare to handle the stressor. This results in increased tension in the muscles. Relaxing the muscles interrupts the feedback loop.

Jacobson (1938) reported that PMR decreased the body's oxygen consumption, metabolic rate, respiratory rate, muscle tension, premature ventricular contractions, and systolic and diastolic blood pressure, and increased alpha brain waves. Subsequent studies have validated Jacobson's findings. Additionally, Teshima, Sogawa, and Mizobe (1991) proposed that relaxation could enhance B-endorphins and potentially enhance cellular immune function.

Although findings from many studies have shown positive outcomes from the use of muscle relaxation techniques, positive results have not been reported in all of the studies in which they were explored. Reasons for the differences in outcomes may relate to the wide variation in the types of relaxation techniques, the length and type of instruction, the degree of mastery of the technique, and irregular or sporadic use of the technique.

INTERVENTION

Numerous techniques for muscle relaxation have been developed since Jacobson publicized his technique in 1938. Some of the techniques focus on active tensing and relaxing of the muscles whereas others direct the person to "just relax" the muscles without first tensing them. Often the techniques include attention to breathing (Schaffer & Yucha, 2004). Two web sites that provide helpful information and products for muscle relaxation are http://www.HealthyPlace.com and http://www.healthstore.com/.

Technique

Some general guidelines apply to the use of any muscle relaxation technique. A quiet environment is needed so that the person can concentrate on relaxing the muscles. This includes eliminating interruptions, reducing noises, and dimming the lighting. The instructor assists the individual to identify a place in the home that is quiet and restful in which to practice relaxation. A comfortable chair that provides support for the body is ideal. A bed or couch may be used, but the horizontal position may result in the person's falling asleep. Clothing should be loose and not restrictive; shoes, glasses, and contact lenses should be removed. The person may wish to use the bathroom before practicing muscle relaxation.

Progressive Muscle Relaxation (PMR) Technique

The PMR technique developed by Bernstein and Borkovec (1973) is widely used. They combined the 108 muscles and muscle groups of Jacobson's original technique into the initial tensing and relaxing of 16 muscle groups. Subsequently the number of groups is reduced to 7 and then 4 (Table 25.1). Although Bernstein and Borkovec included instructions for tensing muscles of the feet, these are not included in Table 25.1 because spasms in the foot may result when tensing these muscles. The ultimate goal is to achieve muscle relaxation throughout the body without initially having to tense the muscles. Through practice the person acquires a mental image of how the muscles feel when they are relaxed and is able to relax them using this image.

TABLE 25.1   Guidelines for 14-Muscle Group Progressive Muscle Relaxation

---

General Information:

Instruct persons to tense a specific muscle group when they hear "tense," and to release the tension when they hear "relax." Tension is held for 7 seconds. Conversation is used to draw attention to the feelings of tension and relaxation. When muscles are relaxed, attention is drawn to the differences between the two states.

Tensing Specific Muscle Groups:

Dominant hand and forearm: Make a tight fist and hold it.

Dominant upper arm: Push elbow down against the arm of the chair.

Repeat instructions for the non-dominant arm.

Forehead: Lift eyebrows as high as possible.

Central face (cheeks, nose, eyes): Squint eyes and wrinkle nose.

Lower face and jaw: Clench teeth and widen mouth.

Neck: Pull chin down toward chest but do not touch chest.

Chest, shoulders, and upper back: Take deep breath and hold it, pull shoulder blades back.

Abdomen: Pull stomach in and try to protect it.

Dominant thigh: Lift leg and hold it straight out.

Dominant calf: Point toes toward ceiling.

Repeat instructions for non-dominant side.

Note: Adapted from Progressive Relaxation Training, by D. Bernstein and T. Borkovec, 1973, Champaign, IL: Research Press.

The scientific basis for the use of PMR is provided during the first session. Stressors, the impact of stress on the body, and the signs and symptoms of high levels of stress are discussed. Descriptions and demonstrations for achieving tension of each muscle group are given, and persons then practice tensing each of the muscle groups. If difficulty is encountered in achieving tension with the demonstrated method, an alternate method can be tried.

After progressing through all the muscle groups, the instructor asks the patient to identify whether tension remains in any of them. The instructor observes the patient to assess if general relaxation has occurred. Indicators of relaxation are slowed, deeper breathing; arms relaxed and shoulders forward; and feet apart with toes pointing out. Two or three minutes are provided at the conclusion of the session for the patient to enjoy the feelings associated with relaxation.

Terminating relaxation is done gradually. The instructor counts backward from four to one. On the count of four, the patient is instructed to move the hands and feet; on three, the arms and legs; on two, the head and neck; and on one, to open the eyes. An opportunity is provided for the patient to ask questions or discuss the feelings experienced.

Bernstein and Borkovec proposed using 10 sessions to teach PMR. However, in many studies instruction has been limited to fewer sessions with positive results (Peck, 1997; Sloman, Brown, Aldana, & Chu, 1994). A critical factor in determining the number of teaching sessions needed is ensuring that persons have mastered relaxing the muscle groups and have integrated PMR into their lifestyles.

An essential factor in the effectiveness of PMR and other relaxation techniques is daily practice. At least one 15-minute practice session a day is recommended. Schaffer and Yucha (2004) suggest two 10-minute sessions. Helping patients find a time of day to practice relaxation is an important component of instruction. The particular time of day PMR is practiced is not what matters, but it must become a part of the person's daily routine. Often an audiotape of the instructions is provided for home practice. Persons are also instructed to use the relaxation technique anytime they feel tense or before an event that may cause them to become anxious and tense.

Posture Relaxation Technique

Schaffer and Yucha (2004) provide guidelines for achieving muscle relaxation by giving attention to posture. This is a passive form of muscle relaxation as the person does not tense muscle groups, but rather concentrates on relaxing the body. The patient should be sitting or reclining, but not lying flat. The following components are included:

Head is motionless with the nose in the mid-line of the body.

Lips and teeth are slightly parted.

Shoulders are dropped and even in height.

Torso, hips, and legs are kept quiet and positioned in symmetry with the center of the body.

Palms of hands are facing down and fingers are slightly curled.

Feet are held at a 60 to 90 degree angle and pointed away from each other.

Breathing is slow, deep, and quiet.

A modification could be to have the person use this technique in bed when attempting to get to sleep.

Measurement of Outcomes

A variety of outcomes have been used to measure the efficacy of muscle relaxation techniques. Physiological measurements that are often used include blood pressure and heart rate, body posture, and respiratory rate. Electromyogram readings are occasionally taken to determine the degree of tension in the specific muscle groups. Practitioners need to be alert to underlying pathology or medications that may interfere with reduction in physiological parameters. Also, if a patient does not have an elevated blood pressure or heart rate, few changes will occur with the use of muscle relaxation techniques.

Anxiety is the most frequently used subjective measure. The State-Trait Anxiety Inventory (STAI) of Spielberger, Gorsuch, Luschene, Vagg, and Jacobs (1983) has been widely used. Persons' self-report about feelings of relaxation have been included in many studies because satisfaction is a good indicator of whether a person will continue to use an intervention. Reports of comfort, reduction of pain, and improved sleep are other results that have been used to measure the effects of muscle relaxation techniques.

Precautions

Although muscle relaxation techniques have been used with multiple populations and have been proven to be an effective therapy for nurses to use, some cautions should be observed. It is important for practitioners to know if patients practice the relaxation techniques on a regular basis as this may affect the pharmacokinetics of medications. Adjustment in doses may be indicated.

Relaxation of muscles may produce a hypotensive state. People are instructed to remain seated for a few minutes after practice. Movement in place and gradual resumption of activities helps in raising the blood pressure. Taking a person's blood pressure at the conclusion of teaching sessions helps in identifying those who are prone to hypotensive states after muscle relaxation.

Some persons with chronic pain have reported a heightened awareness of pain following the tensing and relaxing of muscles. Concentrating on tensing and relaxing of muscles may draw attention to the pain rather than to the muscle sensation. A good assessment of individuals is needed to determine whether negative outcomes are occurring.

USES

Muscle relaxation techniques have been used to achieve a variety of outcomes in diverse populations. Table 25.2 lists conditions and popula-

TABLE 25.2 Conditions for Which Muscle Relaxation Techniques Have Been Used

Stress Reduction

Chronic obstructive pulmonary disease (Chang et al., 2004)

Depression and anxiety in patients with advanced cancer (Sloman, 2002)

Hypertension (Sheu, Irvin, Lin, & Mar, 2003)

Insomnia (Richardson, 2003; Simeit, Deck, & Conta-Marx, 2004)

Reduction of seizures (Whitman, Dell, Legion, Eibhlyn, & Staatsinger, 1990)

Pain Reduction

Cancer (Sloman, 1995)

Headache (Fichtel & Larrson, 2001)

Postoperative (dePaula, deCarvalho, & dos Santos, 2002; Good, Anderson, Stanton-Hicks, Grass, & Makii, 2002)

Health Promotion

Cardiac rehabilitation (Wilk & Turkoski, 2001)

Decrease of nausea and vomiting (Molassiotis, Yung, Yam, Chan, & Mok, 2002)

Tinnitus (Weber, Arck, Mazurek, & Klapp, 2002)

tions in which these techniques have been used. Their use in health promotion, relief of pain, and reduction of stress in specific conditions will be discussed.

Health Promotion

Nursing has been at the forefront in teaching patients about health promotion practices. Although muscle relaxation techniques may not reduce heart rate and blood pressure in those who have readings within the normal range, use of these techniques on a regular basis by healthy persons may help to prevent the development of hypertension. Progressive muscle relaxation was found to decrease both systolic and diastolic blood pressure and heart rate in those with essential hypertension; these indices decreased more as they continued to practice (Sheu et al., 2003; Yung, French, & Leung, 2001). Thus, muscle relaxation techniques can be used in conjunction with hypertensive medications in persons with high blood pressure.

Pain

Muscle relaxation techniques have been used extensively in the management of many types of pain. Muscle tension increases the perception of pain, so lessening anxiety and tension may help in reducing it. Use of these techniques may provide people with a sense of control over their pain. Carroll and Seers (1998) reviewed studies that had used relaxation for the relief of chronic pain. In the nine studies that met the investigators' inclusion criteria, positive findings were found in only four; however, positive results have been reported in numerous other studies (dePaula et al., 2002; Good et al., 2002). Gay, Philippot, and Luminet (2002) reported that persons using the Jacobson relaxation technique required less medication for managing osteoarthritis pain than subjects in the control group.

Muscle relaxation techniques have been used as an adjunct or complementary therapy in the management of pain, particularly with patients who have cancer. Sloman's study (1995) found that 92% of the patients with cancer who were taught PMR reported that relaxation occurred, and 90% noted that they would continue to use the therapy. In a subsequent study, Sloman (2002) reported a reduction in depression and anxiety in patients with advanced stages of cancer.

Reduction of Stress

As noted in Table 25.2, muscle relaxation techniques have been effective in reducing the stress associated with a number of conditions. Wilk and Turkoski (2001) reported that using progressive muscle relaxation as an adjunct therapy helped to reduce blood pressure, heart rate, and state anxiety on patients in a cardiac rehabilitation program. Persons with epilepsy often have high levels of stress because of their fear of having a seizure even though they are on anticonvulsants. Whitman et al. (1990) found a 54% decrease in seizures in persons who practiced progressive muscle relaxation as an adjunct to their anticonvulsant medications. Patients with cancer undergoing chemotherapy had a reduction in nausea and vomiting symptoms with the use of progressive muscle relaxation (Molassiotis et al., 2002). Muscle relaxation techniques can be used both to prevent and decrease stress.

FUTURE RESEARCH

Muscle relaxation techniques, particularly progressive muscle relaxation, have been used singly and in combination with other therapies. A scientific body of knowledge is emerging to guide the use of these therapies in practice, but considerably more research is necessary. The following are several areas in which studies are needed:

1. There is beginning research on the effect that muscle relaxation techniques have on immune function (Gruzelier, 2002; Weber et al., 2002). Further studies about the effect muscle relaxation techniques have on immune function are needed, particularly in conditions such as HIV infection.

2. A combination of therapies has been used in a number of studies. Some studies have used excellent designs to compare the efficacy of each technique. However, numerous other studies fail to differentiate the effects from each therapy. Attention to study design in muscle relaxation studies is needed.

3. Sheu and colleagues (2003) found continuing improvement over a month's period of practice. In the majority of studies, however, the effects of muscle relaxation techniques have been evaluated immediately following administration of the intervention. Longitudinal studies are needed to determine long-term effects.

REFERENCES

Benson, H. (1975). *The relaxation response.* New York: Avon.

Bernstein, D., & Borkovec, T. (1973). *Progressive relaxation training.* Champaign, IL: Research Press.

Brown, B. (1977). *Stress and the art of biofeedback.* New York: Bantam.

Carroll, D., & Seers, K. (1998). Relaxation for the relief of chronic pain: A systematic review. *Journal of Advanced Nursing, 27*, 476–487.

Chang, B. H., Jones, D., Hendricks, A., Boehmer, U., Locastro, J. S., & Slawsky, M. (2004). Relaxation response for Veterans Affairs patients with congestive heart failure: Results from a qualitative study within a clinical trial. *Preventive Cardiology, 7*(2), 64–70.

dePaula, A. A., deCarvalho, E. C., & dos Santos, C. B. (2002). The use of the "progressive relaxation" technique for pain relief in gynecology and obstetrics. *Revista Latino-Americana de Enfermagem, 10*, 654–659.

Fichtel, A., & Larsson, B. (2001). Does relaxation treatment have differential effects on migraine and tension-type headache in adolescents? *Headache, 41*, 290–296.

Gay, M. C., Philippot, P., & Luminet, O. (2002). Differential effectiveness of psychological interventions for reducing osteoarthritis pain: A comparison of Erikson hypnosis and Jacobson relaxation. *European Journal of Pain, 6*, 1–16.

Good, M., Anderson, G. C., Stanton-Hicks, M., Grass, J. A., & Makii, M. (2002). Relaxation and music reduce pain after gynecologic surgery. *Pain Management Nursing, 3*, 61–70.

Gruzelier, J. H. (2002). A review of the impact of hypnosis, relaxation, guided imagery, and individual differences on aspects of immunity and health. *Stress, 5*, 147–163.

Jacobson, E. (1938). *Progressive relaxation*. Chicago: University of Chicago Press.

Molassiotis, A., Yung, H. P., Yam, B. M., Chan, F. Y., & Mok, T. S. (2002). The effectiveness of progressive muscle relaxation training in managing chemotherapy-induced nausea and vomiting in Chinese breast cancer patients: A randomized controlled trial. *Supportive Care in Cancer, 10,* 237–246.

Peck, S. (1997). The effectiveness of therapeutic touch for decreasing pain in elders with degenerative arthritis. *Journal of Holistic Nursing, 15*(2), 13–26.

Richardson, S. (2003). Effects of relaxation and imagery on the sleep of critically ill adults. *Dimensions of Critical Care Nursing, 22,* 182–190.

Schaffer, S. D., & Yucha, C. B. (2004). Relaxation & pain management: The relaxation response can play a role in managing chronic and acute pain. *American Journal of Nursing, 104*(8), 75–82.

Sheu, S., Irvin, B. L., Lin, H. S., & Mar, C. L. (2003). Effects of progressive muscle relaxation on blood pressure and psychosocial status of clients with essential hypertension. *Holistic Nursing Practice, 17*(1), 41–47.

Simeit, R., Deck, R., & Conta-Marx, B. (2004). Sleep management training for cancer patients with insomnia. *Supportive Care in Cancer, 12,* 176–183.

Sloman, R. (1995). Relaxation and the relief of cancer pain. *Nursing Clinics of North America, 30,* 697–709.

Sloman, R. (2002). Relaxation and imagery for anxiety and depression control in community patients with advanced cancer. *Cancer Nursing, 25,* 432–435.

Sloman, R., Brown, R., Aldana, E., & Chu, E. (1994). The use of relaxation for promotion of comfort and pain relief in persons with advanced cancer. *Contemporary Nurse, 3*(1), 6–12.

Spielberger, C., Gorsuch, R., Luschene, R., Vagg, P., & Jacobs, G. (1983). *Manual for STAI*. Palo Alto, CA: Consulting Psychological Press.

Teshima, H., Sogawa, H., & Mizobe, K. (1991). Application of psychoimmunotherapy in patients with alopecia universalis. *Psychotherapy and Psychosomatics, 56,* 235–241.

Weber, C., Arck, P., Mazurek, B., & Klapp, B. F. (2002). Impact of a relaxation training on psychometric and immunologic parameters in tinnitus sufferers. *Journal of Psychosomatic Research, 52,* 29–33.

Whitman, S., Dell, J., Legion, V., Eibhlyn, A., & Staatsinger, J. (1990). Progressive relaxation for seizure reduction. *Journal of Epilepsy, 3,* 17–22.

Wilk, C., & Turkoski, B. (2001). Progressive muscle relaxation in cardiac rehabilitation: A pilot study. *Rehabilitation Nursing, 26,* 238–242.

Yung, P., French, P., & Leung, B. (2001). Relaxation training as complementary therapy for mild hypertension control and the implications of evidence-based medicine. *Complementary Therapies in Nursing & Midwifery, 7,* 59–65.

PART V

Biologically Based Therapies

OVERVIEW

Biologically based therapies are the most popular of the complementary therapies. More than 90 million Americans use at least one herbal preparation and many also use nutraceuticals (additives, vitamins, and special diets). It is difficult to page through a magazine or watch television without encountering a reference to nutraceuticals or dietary supplements. The authors have placed aromatherapy in the biologically based category because it uses essential oils, which are naturally occurring plant substances. The National Center for Complementary/Alternative Medicine also places therapies such as laetrile and shark cartilage in this category.

Whereas research on herbs is relatively sparse in the United States, a significant amount has been conducted in other countries, particularly Germany. The chapter on herbal preparations details concerns about their use in the United States, but suggestions are given to increase the safety in the use of herbs. Because of the growing percentage of Americans who use herbal preparations, it is incumbent on nurses to know about common preparations and to assess for a patient's use of herbs.

Although nurses ordinarily will not be in a position to prescribe or recommend specific nutraceuticals to patients, the wide use of this group of biologically based therapies requires that nurses be knowledgeable about them. Much information is available to the public about food additives, vitamins, and special diets; knowing about a patient's use of these products will assist the health care team in devising a safe and more optimal plan of care. Additionally, knowledge of the patients' use of these preparations allows the nurse the opportunity to determine whether the substances contribute to patients' symptoms or illness.

As with many of the other biologically based therapies, the essential oils found in aromatherapy have a much wider use in other countries than in the United States. Much of the research on essential oils has been conducted in France and England, and it is only within recent years that aromatherapy has been introduced into health facilities in the United States.

Many lists of herbal preparations and other biologically based therapies refer to products common in the Western world. Little attention has been given to those therapies used in other health systems such as Traditional Chinese Medicine and health care systems of indigenous cultures. The increasing number of first-generation Americans from countries that have traditionally used indigenous herbal preparations requires that health professionals expand their knowledge about herbs and other biologically based therapies to avoid drug interactions and other complications.

CHAPTER 26

Aromatherapy

Linda L. Halcón and Jane Buckle*

Aromatherapy is a recent addition to nursing care in the United States, although it has been accepted as part of nursing in Switzerland, Germany, Australia, Canada, and the United Kingdom for many years. It is particularly well suited to nursing because it takes into account the therapeutic value of sensory experience such as smell and touch in care delivery.

Aromatherapy is an offshoot of herbal or botanical medicine that dates back 6,000 years and was used throughout the world. The renaissance of modern Western clinical aromatherapy occurred in France just prior to World War II; physician Jean Valnet, chemist Maurice Gattefosse, and nurse Marguerite Maury were key figures. The use of synthetic scents in the last few decades is not part of aromatherapy. Eisenberg and colleagues (1998) reported that 5.6% of the 2,055 adults surveyed indicated that they used aromatherapy. Aromatherapy in nursing can be considered part of our botantial heritage (Libster, 2002).

DEFINITION

There are many operant definitions of aromatherapy, some of which contribute to common misconceptions. The word *aromatherapy* can lead

---

*(Parts of this chapter authored by Jane Buckle appeared in the fourth edition of *Complementary/Alternative Therapies in Nursing.*)

people to believe it simply involves smelling scents (Schnaubelt, 1999), but this is incorrect. Styles (1997) defined aromatherapy as the use of essential oils for therapeutic purposes that encompass mind, body, and spirit, a broad definition consistent with holistic nursing practice. Although there are many facets of aromatherapy, when nurses use it clinically its purposes should be explicit and its targeted outcomes should be measurable. Clinical aromatherapy in nursing is defined as the use of essential oils for expected and measurable health outcomes (Buckle, 2000).

The definition of essential oils is also very specific. According to Tisserand and Balacs (1995), essential oils are the steam distillates of aromatic plants. Citrus peel oils are usually obtained by expression, however, and carbon dioxide extraction of some essential oils is gaining the acceptance of reputable aromatherapy practitioners and scientists. Essential oils are found in the flowers, leaves, bark, wood, roots, seeds, and peels of many plants. They are highly volatile, complex mixtures of organic chemicals consisting of terpenes and terpenic alcohols, esters, aldehydes, oxides, ketones, phenols, and lactones. There are 100 to 300 separate chemicals in each essential oil, with the proportions of these constituents varying according to plant species, climate, and the extraction process used. The chemistry of an essential oil determines its therapeutic properties; therefore, knowing the part of the plant, the country of origin, and the method of extraction can provide an indication of the essential oil's chemical constituents using readily accessible reference books. Essential oils do not necessarily have the same medicinal properties as the plants from which they are derived because they are more concentrated and contain only the lipophilic and lighter weight molecules present in the plants.

SCIENTIFIC BASIS

The pharmacologic activity of essential oils occurs through the olfactory, respiratory, and integumentary systems; however, all body systems can be affected once essential oils reach the circulatory and nervous systems. The many different molecules in each essential oil act as olfactory stimulants that travel via the nose to the olfactory bulb, and from there nerve impulses travel to the limbic system of the brain. Of the limbic system regions, the amygdala and the hippocampus are of particular importance in the processing of aromas. The amygdala governs emotional responses. Similar to diazepam (Valium), *Lavandula angustifolia* (true lavender) is thought to reduce the effect of external emotional stimuli by increasing gamma aminobutyric acid (GABA) that inhibits neurons in the amygdala, producing a sedative effect similar to diazepam (Tisserand, 1988). The hippocampus is involved in the formation and retrieval of explicit memories. This is where the chemicals in an aroma or an essential oil trigger learned memory. Inhaled essential oils also reach the lungs and enter the bloodstream through the respiratory system.

Topically applied essential oil preparations are absorbed rapidly through the skin; some have been used to enhance the dermal penetration of pharmaceuticals (Williams & Barry, 1989). Massage can enhance dermal penetration through heat and friction. Essential oils are lipotrophic (fat soluble) and are excreted from the body through respiration, kidneys, and insensate loss.

INTERVENTION

Essential oils can be applied to the body through inhalation, topical methods, or ingestion. Nursing scope of practice does not include ingestion. The compounds within an essential oil find their way into the bloodstream however they are applied (Tisserand & Balacs, 1995). Inhaled aromas have the fastest effect, although compounds absorbed through massage can be detected in the blood within 20 minutes (Jager, Bauchbauer, Jirovetz, & Fritzer, 1979). The choice of application method depends on the nurse's knowledge and practice parameters, the available or desired time for the action to occur, the targeted outcome, the chemical components of the essential oil, and the preferences and psychological needs of the patient. It would appear that the effects of inhaled essential oils do not last as long as topically applied essential oils; however, it is difficult to analyze exactly what impact touch has in outcomes of aromatherapy.

Inhalation

When people are ill the sense of smell can be heightened or altered and familiar pleasant aromas can make a person feel more secure. Although essential oils are not always pleasant smelling, direct inhalation through the olfactory system is one of the simplest and most direct application methods. With this method, one to five drops of an essential oil can be placed on a tissue or floated on hot water in a bowl and then inhaled for 5 to 10 minutes. More indirect inhalation techniques include the use of burners, nebulizers, and vaporizers that can be operated by heat, battery, or electricity and may or may not include the use of water.

Larger, portable aroma systems are available commercially to provide controlled release of essential oils into rooms of any size.

Inhalation effects are also experienced when essential oils are used in a bath. Four to six drops of the essential oil are dissolved first in a teaspoon of milk, rubbing alcohol, or carrier oil (cold-pressed) and then placed in the bath water. Because essential oils are not soluble in water, they would float on the top of the water if used undiluted, giving an uneven and possibly too concentrated treatment. Before a person relaxes in the bath for approximately 10 minutes, the water should be vigorously agitated. Essential oils can also be dissolved in salts, such as Epsom salts, which can be soothing to muscles and joints. One such recipe consists of one tablespoon of baking soda, two tablespoons of Epsom salts, and three tablespoons of sea salt with four to six drops of essential oils mixed throughout. The salts should be added to the bath water just before immersion.

Topical Applications

Essential oils are absorbed through the skin by diffusion, with the epidermis and fat layer acting as a reservoir before the components of the essential oils reach the dermis and the bloodstream. Compresses are a useful method for applying essential oils to treat skin conditions or injuries topically. To prepare a compress, add four to six drops of essential oil to warm water. Soak a soft cotton cloth in the mixture, wring it out, and apply the cloth to the affected area, contusion, or abrasion. Cover the compress with plastic wrap to retain moisture, place a towel over the plastic wrap, and keep it in place for up to 4 hours. The use of hot or very warm water can enhance the absorption of at least some of the components of essential oils.

Massage also can facilitate absorption of essential oils. Aromatherapy using touch can enhance communication with patients. To create a mixture for massage, dilute one to two drops of an essential oil in a teaspoon (5 ml) of cold-pressed vegetable oil, cream, or gel. The amount of essential oil absorbed from a full body massage using a 1% to 5% dilution will normally be 0.002 ml to 0.3 ml (Tisserand & Balacs, 1995).

Essential oils should not be used undiluted on mucous membranes; even on intact skin they are generally used in concentrations of only one to five percent, seldom exceeding 10%. They can be used diluted in pessaries and suppositories to treat conditions such as vaginal infections. For yeast infections (candidiasis), a 5% solution in carrier oil can be applied to a tampon and inserted in the vagina. Only essential oils high in alcohols, such as tea tree, are appropriate in pessaries as alcohols are unlikely to cause skin irritation. Tampons should be changed regularly.

General Guidelines for Use of Essential Oils

There are some general guidelines for use of essential oils that nurses can use for patient education and in practice. These include:

- Store essential oils away from open flames; they are volatile and highly flammable.

- Store essential oils in a cool place away from sunlight; use amber or blue colored glass containers. Essential oils can oxidize in the presence of heat, light, and oxygen, changing their chemistry and their actions.

- Essential oils can stain clothing—beware!

- Keep essential oils away from children and pets.

- Use essential oils from reputable suppliers.

- Close the container immediately after use.

- Care is needed when using essential oils with persons who have a history of severe asthma or multiple allergies.

Despite the relative safety of essential oils when used properly, sensitization and skin irritation can occur. Inform patients what to do in the case of a reaction.

Measurement of Outcomes

The methods for measuring aromatherapy treatment effects will depend on the problem for which essential oils are used. For example, if lavender is used to promote sleep, outcomes would be chosen to determine if insomnia decreased. For psychological conditions such as depression or anxiety, a variety of validated questionnaire measures are available and can be correlated with physiological measures such as cortisol levels or skin temperature. For infectious disease outcomes, standard laboratory tests can be used to measure the effect of treatment on microbial load. Digital photography provides an easily accessible way to measure wound or lesion size changes. Other useful measures could include pain scales, quality of life scales, or tests of cognitive performance. Using established measurement tools where possible is helpful in facilitating interpretation and comparing the effects of essential oils with those of other approaches.

Precautions

Aromatherapy is a very safe complementary therapy if it is used with knowledge and within accepted guidelines. Nurses should not administer essential oils orally as this is outside a nurse's scope of practice, and poisonings have been documented (Jacobs & Hornfeldt, 1994). If an essential oil gets into the eyes, rinse it out with milk or carrier oil first and then with water. A list of contraindicated essential oils can be found in training manuals; both novices and more experienced practitioners should consult these lists. Essential oils that are high in phenols tend to be aggressive and should not be used undiluted on the skin or for long periods of time. Some essential oils should not be used during early pregnancy and should be used cautiously in later pregnancy. Nurses need to be aware of essential oils that can cause photosensitivity, such as bergamot (*Citrus bergamia*) (Clark & Wilkinson, 1998), and should provide appropriate patient education and protection when they are used.

Many essential oils have been tested by the food and beverage industry for use as flavorings (Opdyke, 1977), and other research has been carried out by the perfume industry. Most of the essential oils commonly used in clinical aromatherapy have been given GRAS (generally regarded as safe) status. They are very concentrated and potent compounds, however, and in most cases must be diluted in carrier oils for topical use. Tea tree (*Melaleuca alternifolia*) and lavender (*Lavandula angustifolia*) are among the few exceptions to this rule. These essential oils can be used (100%) on minor cuts, abrasions, and burns.

Some essential oils are contraindicated in persons with estrogen-dependent tumors, hypertension, seizures, or pregnancy. Extra care is needed when using essential oils with patients receiving chemotherapy because they may affect the absorption rate of certain chemotherapeutic drugs (Williams & Barry, 1989). Other essential oils can potentiate (or decrease) the effects of barbiturates or antibiotics, may cause dermal irritation, or are contraindicated in the presence of ultraviolet light. Some components of essential oils have been found to be carcinogenic or teratogenic (Tisserand & Balacs, 1995). It cannot be assumed that all essential oils are safe because they are "natural."

Product identity confusion is another potential threat to safety. Essential oils should not be confused with herbal extracts, which are completely different chemical mixtures and cannot be used interchangeably. Besides their chemical dissimilarities, herbal extracts and teas are usually taken internally whereas essential oils are not. Also, essential oils are volatile and herbal extracts are not. Nurses share responsibility for ensuring product integrity when essential oils are used in clinical practice. Chemical testing of those used in patient care should be incorporated into ongoing institutional quality assurance/quality control programs.

Perhaps one of the greatest risks in aromatherapy is using an incorrect essential oil for a particular health outcome. This could stem from a nurse's lack of knowledge about plant taxonomy, a system that classifies plants according to their similarities. Many essential oils have familiar common names such as lavender, rose, and rosemary, but it is important to know the full botanical name. For example, lavender is a common name that covers three different kinds of lavender and a number of hybrid plants. The botanical name will give the genus and the species (rather like a surname and a first name, respectively). The genus of lavender is *Lavandula*, and all lavenders begin with this word. *Lavandula angusti-folia* is possibly the most widely used and researched essential oil and is recognized as a relaxant. The other two species used in aromatherapy have very different properties. *Lavandula latifolia* (spike lavender) is a stimulant and expectorant; *Lavandula stoechas* is antimicrobial and not safe to use for long periods of time because it contains a large percentage of ketones that can build up and produce toxicity. Another example of a common herb with potential for confusion is marjoram, which is the common name for *Thymus mastichina* (actually a thyme) and *Origanum marjoranum* (the "real" marjoram). Nurses who use aromatherapy clinically must know the full botanical name of an essential oil (Table 26.1) and must understand the basics of plant taxonomy (Table 26.2).

Credentialing

Currently there is no recognized national certification exam for aroma-therapists and no governing body. The Aromatherapy Registration Council, a nonprofit entity that was established in 2000, administers a national exam and can provide the public with a list of registered practitioners. Nurses and health professionals wishing to use aromatherapy in their practice should check with their licensing bodies and their state board of nursing. There are many different courses available and health professionals should choose one that is relevant to their clinical practice. The largest professional organization is the National Association of Holistic Aromatherapy (NAHA). There are no requirements at this time for a person administering aromatherapy to be certified or accredited. The length of training in aromatherapy ranges from one weekend to several years. Any person, not necessarily just health professionals, can enroll in

TABLE 26.1   Common and Botanical Names of Essential Oils Commonly Used
in Aromatherapy

Common Name	Botanical Name
Basil	*Ocimum basilicum*
Chamomile, German	*Matricaria recutita*
Chamomile, Roman	*Chamaemelum nobile*
Clary sage	*Salvia sclarea*
Eucalyptus	*Eucalyptus globulus*
Fennel	*Foeniculum vulgare*
Geranium	*Pelargonium graveolens*
Ginger	*Zingiber officinale*
Lavender, true	*Lavandula officinalis*
Lemongrass	*Cymbopogon citratus*
Neroli	*Citrus aurantium var. amara*
Palmarosa	*Cymbopogon martinii*
Peppermint	*Mentha piperita*
Rose	*Rosa damascena*
Rosewood	*Aniba rosaeodora*
Sage	*Salvia officinalis*
Sandalwood	*Santalum album*
Ylang-ylang	*Cananga odorata*

TABLE 26.2   Examples of Plant Taxonomy for Two Common Essential Oils

Example 1:	Common name	neroli
	Botanical name	*Citrus aurantium var. amara flos*
	Family	Rutaceae
	Genus	*Citrus*
	Species	*aurantium*
	Variety	amara
	Part	flos (flower)
Example 2:	Common name	lavender
	Botanical name	*Lavandula angustifolia*
	Family	Lamiaceae (was Labiatae)
	Genus	*Lavandula*
	Species	*angustifolia*
	Part	flowering plant

the educational programs. The American Holistic Nurses Association can provide a list of accredited courses.

USES

Many health outcomes that fall within the domain of nursing practice can be addressed with essential oils, either alone or combined with other approaches (Table 26.3). The pharmacologically active components in essential oils work at psychological and physical levels. Essential oils can increase or decrease sympathetic activity in humans, affecting blood pressure, plasma adrenaline, and plasma catecholamine levels (Haze, Sakai, & Gozu, 2002). The effect of odor can be relaxing or stimulating, depending on the individual's previous experiences in addition to the chemistry of the essential oil used; therefore, it is important to explore patient preference when selecting essential oils for therapeutic purposes.

Nurse midwives have long incorporated essential oils into their practice, notably to reduce pain and aid relaxation during and after childbirth (Burns, Blamey, Ersser, Barnetson, & Lloyd, 2000). In long-term care and hospital settings, essential oils are increasingly used to help reduce agitation in patients with dementia (Bowles, Griffiths, Quirk, & Croot, 2002; Gray & Clair, 2002), promote sleep and reduce nighttime sedation (Hardy, Kirk-Smith, & Stretch, 1995), and promote wound healing (Kerr, 2002). Other patient conditions for which aromatherapy has been used include acute or chronic pain (Buckle, 1999), fatigue and nausea (Tate, 1997), infection control (Gravett, 2001), and mood and cognition (Ilmberger et al., 2002; Morris, 2002). Public health nursing topics addressed in the literature include using essential oils in the treatment of head lice (Veal, 1996) and as an aid to smoking cessation (Rose & Behm, 1994).

There is also considerable and growing international literature on the use of plant essential oils against pathogenic microorganisms (Table 26.4). The role of essential oils in the treatment and prevention of infectious diseases has begun to be explored in the United States, with important implications for patient health as well as institutional disinfection and hygiene (Harkenthal, Reichling, Geiss, & Saller, 1999). Methicillin-resistant *Staphylococcus aureus* (MRSA) and other microorganisms have been found to be sensitive to tea tree oil (*Melaleuca alternifolia*) (Caelli, Porteous, Carson, Heller, & Riley, 2000), and preliminary work suggests that essential oils may be effective in other difficult to treat infections (Sherry & Warnke, 2002).

Aromatherapy and Children

Aromatherapy is one of the complementary therapies most used for children and adolescents (Simpson & Roman, 2001). The use of aromather-

TABLE 26.3   Essential Oils Used for Health Problems and Application Methods

Pain Relief

Migraine: peppermint, lavender (T)

Osteoarthritis: eucalyptus, black pepper, ginger, spike lavender, Roman chamomile, rosemary, myrrh (T)

Rheumatoid arthritis: German chamomile, lavender, peppermint, frankincense (T)

Low back pain: lemongrass, rosemary, lavender, sweet marjoram (T)

Cramps: Roman chamomile, clary sage, lavender, sweet marjoram (T)

General aches and pains: rosemary, lavender, lemongrass, clary sage, black pepper, lemon eucalyptus, spike lavender

Gynecological

Menopausal symptoms: clary sage, sage, fennel, aniseed, geranium, rose, cypress

Menstrual cramping: Roman chamomile, lavender, clary sage (T)

Premenstrual syndrome: clary sage, geranium, rose (T)

Infertility with no physiological cause: clary sage, sage, fennel, aniseed, geranium, rose (T)

Cardiovascular

Borderline hypertension: ylang-ylang, lavender

Transient hypotension caused by some antidepressants: rosemary, spike lavender

Urinary

Cystitis: tea tree, palma rosa (T especially sitz bath)

Water retention: juniper, cypress, fennel (T)

Gastrointestinal

Irritable bowel syndrome: Roman chamomile, clary sage, mandarin, cardamom, peppermint, mandarin, fennel, lavender

Constipation: fennel, black pepper (T)

Indigestion: peppermint, ginger (I)

Infection

Bacteria including MRSA, VRSA: tea tree, lavender, peppermint

Other bacteria: eucalyptus, naiouli, sweet marjoram, oregano, tarragon, savory, German chamomile, thyme, manuka

Viral: ravansara, palma rosa, lemon, eucalyptus smithii, melissa, rose, bergamot

Fungal: lemongrass, black pepper, clove, caraway (T); geranium, tea tree (particularly good for toenail fungus; apply undiluted daily to nailbed for several months)

Pediatrics

Behavioral problems: mandarin, lavender, Roman chamomile, rose (I, T)

Colic: Roman chamomile, mandarin (T)

Diaper rash: lavender

Sleep problems: lavender, rose, mandarin

Autism: rose can help multihandicapped children interact socially

TABLE 26.3 *(continued)*

Respiratory

Bronchitis: ravansara, eucalyptus globulus, eucalyptus smithii, tea tree, spike lavender (I)

Sinusitis: eucalyptus globulus, lavender, spike lavender, rosemary (I)

Mild asthma: lavender, clary sage, Roman chamomile (I)

Dermatology

Mild acne: tea tree, juniper, cypress, naiouli (T)

Mild psoriasis: lavender, German chamomile (T)

Diabetic ulcers: lavender, frankincense, myrrh (T)

Oncology

Nausea: peppermint, ginger, mandarin

Post-radiation burns: lavender, German chamomile, Tamanu carrier oil

Older Adults

Memory loss: rosemary, rose, peppermint, basil

Dry flaky skin: geranium, frankincense

Alzheimer's disease: rosemary, lavender, pine, frankincense

Palliative Care

Spiritual: rose, angelica, frankincense

Physical: lavender, peppermint, lemongrass, rosemary

Emotional: geranium, pine, sandalwood

Relaxation: lavender, clary sage, mandarin, frankincense, ylang-ylang

Pressure ulcers: lavender, tea tree, sweet marjoram, frankincense

Care of the Dying

Rites of passage: choose selection of patient's favorite aromas or frankincense, rose

Bereavement: rose, sandalwood, patchouli, angelica, frankincense, myrrh

---

T = topical application

I = inhalation

No designation = can be administered either topically or by inhalation

apy with babies and children presents unique risks and opportunities. We recommend a conservative approach in light of the heightened sensitivity of the very young. Despite the plethora of aromatherapy products on the market for babies, it is recommended that essential oils be used cautiously, if at all, in infants except for specific purposes. Some aroma therapists recommend using hydrolats, the alternate distillation product containing the water-soluble plant components, with infants. As with essential oils, however, it is important to consider the chemistry of the

TABLE 26.4 The Antimicrobial Action of Essential Oils: Selected Examples from the Literature

Microorganism	Essential Oil(s)	Research Studies
Staphylococcus aureus	tea tree, true lavender, peppermint, thyme	Hammer, Carson, & Rileyl (1999) Halcón & Milkus (2004) Caelli et al. (2000)
E. coli 0157:H7	oregano, thyme	Burt & Reinders (2003)
Pseudomonas aeruginosa	lemon, melissa	Larrondo, Agut, & Calco-Torras (1995)
Ringworm	lemongrass	Wannisorm, Jarikasem, & Soontormtanasart (1996)
Candida albicans	tea tree	Jandourek, Vaishampayan, & Vazquez (1998)
HIV	rose, hyssop	Mahmood et al. (1996)
Herpes simplex viruses	sandalwood	Benencia & Courreges (1999)
Haemophilus influenza	thyme, lemongrass	Inouye, Takizawa, & Yamaguchi (2001)

hydrolat and its likely effect on the body of an infant. If dermal applications are used, they should not exceed concentrations of 1% for infants up to 6 months and 2% percent up to 2 years. Oral applications or instillations in the nose are contraindicated for young children and have resulted in serious complications, including coma (Tisserand & Balacs, 1995). Peppermint and some eucalyptus oils should not be used in children under 6 years of age. Menthol, a major constituent of peppermint oil, has been found to produce severe neonatal jaundice in babies with G6PD deficiency (Olowe & Ransome-Kuti, 1980), and peppermint oil has provoked life-threatening glottal spasms in children (Melis, Janssens, & Bochner, 1990). Many accidental poisonings of children have been reported, illustrating the importance of keeping essential oils out of reach in bottles with integral drop dispensers (less than 5 cc of some oils can be fatal) and of knowing their safety profiles.

Despite cautions, essential oils have been used to treat infants and children successfully and safely. Alexandrovich, Rakovitskaya, Kolmo,

Sidorova, and Shushunov (2003) found that a fennel seed oil emulsion worked well in treating infantile colic without apparent side effects. Buckle (2003) recommends true lavender (*Lavandula angustifolia*) as the safest essential oil for children. A few other essential oils considered safe for children include Roman chamomile (*Chamaemelum nobile*), rose otto (*Rosa damascena*), ginger (*Zinziber officinali*), ylang-ylang (*Cananga odorata*), *Eucalyptus smithii*, mandarin (*Citrus reticulata*), and melissa (*Melissa officinalis*). Although little research has been published, essential oils are being used in pediatric oncology settings for nausea and fatigue (spearmint, ginger, mandarin). They have also been used in community settings to treat head lice (tea tree) and to help with ADHD (melissa). Much more research is needed, but nurses who are knowledgeable about essential oils can introduce them in pediatric practice and remain within safety guidelines.

FUTURE RESEARCH

There is a large body of unpublished research on the therapeutic effects of essential oils, much of it proprietary studies conducted by the food, cosmetics, and flavoring industries. There is also a large volume of scientific research published in languages other than English, notably from Japan, China, and European countries. Despite a growing body of research in English-speaking countries, there remains a dearth of studies in English. As with herbal medicine, investigations of aromatherapy are fraught with unanswered methodological questions. Some questions unique to aromatherapy include:

1. What is a good control condition for aroma?
2. Should aroma and touch be evaluated separately when both are used?
3. Should only single essential oils be used and not blends?
4. Can research methods be designed to accommodate adaptogens such as essential oils?

WEB SITE

National Association of Holistic Aromatherapists: www.naha.org

REFERENCES

Alexandrovich, I., Rakovitskaya, O., Kolmo, E., Sidorova, T., & Shushunov, S. (2003). The effect of fennel (Foeniculum Vulgare) seek oil emulsion in infantile colic: A randomized, placebo-controlled study. *Alternative Therapies, 9*(4), 58–61.

Benencia, F., & Courreges, M. (1999). Antiviral activity of sandalwood oil against *Herpes simplex* viruses-1 and -2. *Phytomedicine, 6*(2), 119–123.

Bowles, E. J., Griffiths, M., Quirk, L., & Croot, K. (2002). Effects of essential oils and touch on resistance to nursing care procedures and other dementia-related behaviours in a residential care facility. *The International Journal of Aromatherapy, 12*(1), 22–29.

Buckle, J. (1999). Use of aromatherapy as a complementary treatment for chronic pain. *Alternative Therapies, 5*(5), 42–51.

Buckle, J. (2000). The "m" technique. *Massage and Bodywork*, 52–64.

Buckle, J. (2003). *Clinical aromatherapy: Essential oils in practice* (2nd ed.). New York: Churchill Livingstone.

Burns, E. E., Blamey, C., Ersser, S. J., Barnetson, L., & Lloyd, A. J. (2000). An investigation into the use of aromatherapy in intrapartum midwifery practice. *The Journal of Alternative and Complementary Therapies, 6*(2), 141–147.

Burt, S. A., & Reinders, R. D. (2003). Antibacterial activity of selected plant essential oils against *Escherichia coli* 0157:H7. *Applied Microbiology, 36*, 162–167.

Caelli, M., Porteous, J., Carson, C., Heller, R., & Riley, T. (2000). Tea tree oil as an alternative topical decolonization agent for methicillin-resistant *Staphylococcus aureus*. *Journal of Hospital Infection, 46*(3), 236–237.

Clark, S., & Wilkinson, S. (1998). Phototoxic contact dermatitis from 5-methoxypsoralen in aromatherapy oil. *Contact Dermatitis, 38*, 289.

Eisenberg, D. M., Davis, R. B., Ettner, S. L., Appel, S., Wilkey, S., Van Rompay, M. I., et al. (1998). Trends in alternative medicine in the USA, 1990–1997: Results of a follow-up national survey. *Journal of the American Medical Association, 280*, 784–787.

Gravett, P. (2001). Aromatherapy treatment for patients with Hickman Line infection following high-dose chemotherapy. *The International Journal of Aromatherapy, 11*(1), 18–19.

Gray, S., & Clair, A. (2002). Influence of aromatherapy on medication administration to residential-care residents with dementia and behavioral challenges. *American Journal of Alzheimer's Disease and Other Dementias, 17*(3), 169–173.

Halcon, L., & Milkus, K. (2004). *Staphylococcus aureus* and wounds: A review of tea tree oil (*Melalueca alternifolia*) as a promising antibiotic. *American Journal of Infection Control, 3*, 402–408.

Hammer, K. A., Carson, C. F., & Riley, T. V. (1999). Antimicrobial activity of essential oils and other plant extracts. *Journal of Applied Microbiology, 86*, 985–990.

Hardy, M., Kirk-Smith, M., & Stretch, D. (1995). Replacement of drug treatment for insomnia by ambient odor. *The Lancet, 346*, 701.

Harkenthal, M., Reichling, J., Geiss, H., & Saller, R. (1999). Comparative study on the *in vitro* antibacterial activity of Australian tea tree oil, cajuput oil, niaouli oil, manuka oil, kanuka oil, and eucalyptus oil. *Pharmazie, 54*(6), 460–463.

Haze, S., Sakai, K., & Gozu, Y. (2002). Effects of fragrance inhalation on sympathetic activity in normal adults. *Japanese Journal of Pharmacology, 90,* 247–253.

Ilmberger, J., Heuberger, E., Mahrhofer, C., Dessovic, H., Kowarik, D., & Buchbauer, G. (2001). The influence of essential oils on human attention. I. Alertness. *Chemical Senses, 26,* 239–245.

Inouye, S., Takizawa, T., & Yamaguchi, H. (2001). Antibacterial activity of essential oils and their major constituents against respiratory tract pathogens by gaseous contact. *Journal of Antimicrobial Chemotherapy, 47,* 565–573.

Jacobs, M., & Hornfeldt, C. (1994). Melaleuca oil poisoning. *Clinical Toxicology, 32*(4), 461–464.

Jager, W., Bauchbauer, G., Jirovetz, L., & Fritzer, M. (1979). Percutaneous absorption of lavender oil from a massage oil. *Journal of Social Cosmetology Chemistry, 43*(1), 49–54.

Jandourek, A., Vaishampayan, J., & Vazquez, J. (1998). Efficacy of melaleuca oral solution for the treatment of fluconazole refractory oral candidiasis in AIDS patients. *AIDS, 12*(9), 1033–1037.

Kerr, J. (2002). Research project—using essential oils in wound care for the elderly. *Aromatherapy Today, 23,* 14–19.

Larrondo, J., Agut, M., & Calco-Torras, M. (1995). Antimicrobial activity of essences of labiates. *Microbios (Cambridge), 82,* 171–172.

Libster, M. (2002). *Delmar's integrative herb guide for nurses.* Australia: Delmar, Thompson Learning.

Mahmood, N., Piacente, S., Pizza, C., Burke, A., Khan, A. I., & Hay, A. J. (1996). The anti-HIV activity and mechanisms of action of pure compounds isolated from *Rosa damascena. Biochemical and Biophysical Research Communications, 229,* 73–79.

Melis, K., Janssens, G., & Bochner, A. (1990). Accidental nasal eucalyptol and menthol instillation. *Acta Clinica Belgium Supplement, 13,* 101–102.

Morris, N. (2002). The effects of lavender (*Lavandula angustifolium*) baths on psychological well-being: Two exploratory randomized control trials. *Complementary Therapies in Medicine, 10,* 223–228.

Olowe, S. A., & Ransome-Kuti, O. (1980). The risk of jaundice in glucose-6-phosphate dehydrogenase deficient babies exposed to menthol. *Acta Paediatrica Scandinavica, 69,* 341–345.

Opdyke, D. L. J. (1977). Safety testing of fragrances: Problems and implications. *Clinical Toxicology, 19*(1), 61–67.

Rose, J., & Behm, F. (1994). Inhalation of vapor from black pepper extract reduces smoking withdrawal symptoms. *Drug and Alcohol Dependence, 34,* 225–229.

Schnaubelt, K. (1999). *Medical aromatherapy.* Berkeley, CA: Frog Ltd.

Sherry, E., & Warnke, P. (2002). *Alternative for MRSA and tuberculosis (TB): Eucalyptus and tea-tree oils as new topical antibacterials.* Paper presented at American Academy of Orthopaedic Surgeons, Dallas, TX.

Simpson, N., & Roman, K. (2001). Complementary medicine use in children: Extent and reasons. A population based study. *British Journal of General Practice, 51*(472), 914–916.

Styles, J. (1997). The use of aromatherapy in hospitalized children with HIV. *Complementary Therapies in Nursing, 3,* 16–20.

Tate, S. (1997). Peppermint oil, a treatment for postoperative nausea. *Journal of Advanced Nursing, 26,* 543–549.

Tisserand, R. (1988). Lavender beats benzodiazepines. *International Journal of Aromatherapy, 1*(2), 1–2.

Tisserand, R., & Balacs, T. (1995). *Essential oil safety.* London: Churchill Livingstone.

Veal, L. (1996). The potential effectiveness of essential oils as a treatment for head lice, *Pediculus humanis capitus. Complementary Therapies in Nursing and Midwifery, 2*(4), 97–101.

Wannisorm, B., Jarikasem, S., & Soontormtanasart, T. (1996). Antifungal activity of lemongrass oil and lemongrass oil cream. *Phytotherapy Research, 10,* 551–554.

Williams, A., & Barry, B. (1989). Essential oils as novel skin penetration enhancers. *International Journal of Pharmaceutics, 57,* R7–R9.

CHAPTER 27

Herbal Medicines

Gregory A. Plotnikoff with Yun Lu

Herbs and related natural products such as spices are the oldest and most widely used form of medicine in the world. The use of herbs for the treatment of disease and the promotion of well-being can be traced back in many cultures at least 2,500 years. However, herbal medicines are not restricted to historical use. Today, in addition to aspirin, digoxin, and antibiotics, numerous plant-derived medications are available including anticholinergic agents, anticoagulants, antihypertensives, and antineoplastic agents. In fact, of the top 150 pharmaceuticals in 1995, 86 contained at least one major active compound from natural sources. These represented only 35 of the estimated 2,000,000 extant plant species (Grifo, 1997).

The most comprehensive and reliable data on the use of herbal medicine comes from the 2002 National Institutes of Health (NIH) survey of 31,044 adults. Use of natural products, including herbs, for medicinal purposes was documented in 19% of the American population and 55% believed that use of complementary and alternative medicines would support health when used with conventional medical treatments (Barnes, Powell-Griner, McFann, & Nahin, 2004). This is significant as in 1999, 36% of people using herbal medicines did so in lieu of prescription medications and 31% used herbal medicines in combination with prescription medications (Johnson, 2000). The 2004 Council for Responsible

Nutrition survey of 1,000 randomly selected U.S. adults documented that 90% looked to health care professionals, including nurses, for guidance in herbal medicine use (Ward, 2005). Thus, herbal medicine warrants significant attention by all nurses.

DEFINITION

Herbal medicines, or plant-based therapies, continue to occupy a place of central importance in the world's many healing traditions. These include the use of single herbs in many Western traditions and multiple-herb combinations in traditional Asian medical systems. Frequently herbs are part of an overarching belief system that may involve spiritual or metaphysical components. Herbal medicines are often included in the work of shamans and other traditional healers who serve as intermediaries with the spirit world. Herbal medicines are also a tool in traditional Asian medicine and are used like acupuncture to open blocked channels (meridians) for the free flow of qi (life spirit or force).

Herbal medicines, also known as botanicals or phytotherapies, are one component of the range of natural products sold in the United States as dietary supplements. These include fungi-based products (mycotherapies); essential oils (aromatherapies); and vitamin, mineral, and nutritional therapies (nutraceuticals). Since the passage of the Dietary Supplement Health and Education Act of 1994 (DSHEA), these biological modifiers have been available over the counter as dietary supplements. Though neither food nor drug, these substances are still regulated by the Food and Drug Administration (FDA) but with less stringent requirements. Unlike food and drugs, dietary supplements can be sold based on evidence of safety in the possession of the manufacturer and can only be removed from the market if the FDA can prove them unsafe under ordinary conditions of use.

Under DSHEA, herbal medicines can be sold for "stimulating, maintaining, supporting, regulating and promoting health" rather than for treating disease. As dietary supplements rather than drugs, herbal medicines cannot claim to restore normal or correct abnormal function. Additionally, herbs cannot claim to "diagnose, treat, prevent, cure, or mitigate" (DSHEA, 1994). Herbal medicine companies can assert that their product supports cardiovascular health but not that it lowers cholesterol. To do so would suggest that the product is intended for treating a disease (hypercholesterolemia) and is therefore subject to FDA pharmaceutical regulations.

This has raised questions about what constitutes a disease. The FDA originally suggested that a disease is any deviation, impairment, or interruption of the normal structure or function of any part, organ, or system of the body that is manifested by a characteristic set of one or more signs and symptoms. This definition generated many concerns. "Normal structure" appeared to be normed to a 30-year-old male and therefore did not account for gender or aging. For example, are menopause and menstrual cramps diseases? With no signs or symptoms, is hypercholesterolemia a disease or a risk factor? After significant public outcry, the FDA adopted the definition of disease found in the Nutrition Labeling and Health Act of 1990. Disease is currently considered damage to an organ, part, structure, or system of the body such that it does not function properly (e.g., cardiovascular disease) or a state of health leading to such (e.g., hypertension).

SCIENTIFIC BASIS

Significant research has been done using Western biomedical/scientific models on numerous single herbal agents. Beginning in 1978, the German government's *Bundesgesunheitsamt* (Federal Health Agency) began evaluating the safety and efficacy of phytomedicines. The health professionals charged with doing so, known as the Commission E, met until 1994 and evaluated 300 herbal medicines. They recognized 190 as suitable for medicinal use. The complete reports have been translated and are available from the American Botanical Council (2000).

Beginning in 1996, significant meta-analyses and review articles of single herb products began appearing on a regular basis in leading Western medical journals. These are readily accessible via the National Library of Medicine's PubMed web site (http://www.ncbi.nlm.nih.gov/PubMed/). Compiling data from similar studies for analysis (meta-analysis) is complicated by the fact that many studies published to date have left out important information including naming the specific plant species studied (e.g., echinacea versus *Echinacea purpurea, E. pallida*, or *E. augustofolia*), the parts used (stems, leaves, or roots), the form (pressed juice, powdered whole extract, aqueous extract, ethanol extract, or aqueous-ethanol extract), and the formulation (stated proportions of water to alcohol or specifically extracted fractions and concentrations).

Standardization of herbal medicines is crucial both for scientific study and consumer protection. Standardization is equated with reproducibility, guaranteed potency, quality of active ingredients, and documentable effectiveness. However, with herbal medicines, standardization presents several problems. First, the active ingredient may not be known. Second, there may be more than one active ingredient, and third, both content

and activity of an herbal medicine may be related to the means of extraction and processing. This significantly complicates both research and
counseling for health professionals and consumers.

An increasing number of health care professionals are studying the
effects of these substances. With an increase in the FDA's involvement,
we can look forward to a more reliable herb market. Increased knowledge
of herbal indications may increase the safety and efficacy of herbal therapies for patients.

INTERVENTION

Technique

Herbal medicines and dietary supplements need to be addressed in clinical
settings in the same manner one addresses pharmaceutical agents. Every
health professional needs to be aware of the wide use of herbal medicines
and other dietary supplements. Efficient and effective patient advocacy
means including questions on alternative therapies as a standard part of
each patient interview. Reasonable questions include: Are you using any
herbs? Vitamins? Dietary supplements? Follow-up questions include:
What dose? What source? What directions are you following? Why are
you taking it? Asking about the source of information can be quite helpful
as in, "Are you working with any other health professionals?" As with
all good interviewing, listening for understanding rather than agreement
or disagreement enhances the therapeutic alliance. In addition to knowing
the type of herb used, the dose of each herb, and the intended purpose
for each herb, gathering information regarding the duration of herb use
will also be helpful in assessing patients and providing safe and effective care.

Unfortunately, professionals often do not ask such questions and
patients do not volunteer such information. This "don't ask, don't tell"
policy makes no sense in patient care. All health professionals need to
create a safe environment that is conducive to patients' open sharing of
important information such as herbal use or use of other complementary/
alternative therapies without fear of ridicule or other negative responses.
"Ask, then ask again" is a practice policy foundational to safe and effective patient care.

Precautions

A common misconception regarding herbal medicines is that herbs have
no side effects because they are "natural." However, herbs do indeed

have side effects and may be toxic or poisonous if not used appropriately. Consider the toxicity of such widely used natural products as coffee, cocaine, and tobacco. Another dilemma is patient use of herbs in lieu of their prescribed medications. Although herbs may be a good option in particular cases and conditions, the decision to decline medications should be based upon fully informed judgments in partnership with a health professional.

Interviewing for herbal medicine use is crucial for identifying those patients at risk for interactions with prescription medications or for excessive bleeding in surgery. Patients with special risks of drug interactions include those taking the following pharmaceutical agents: anticoagulants, hypoglycemics, antidepressants, sedative-hypnotics, antihypertensives, and medications with narrow therapeutic windows such as digoxin and theophylline.

Pregnancy, lactation, breastfeeding, and child care are special topics in herbal medicine use. For these situations, the most authoritative references are cited in Table 27.1. In the absence of clinical trial data, use is guided by historical experience or breast milk analysis. Herbs that increase breast milk production, such as fenugreek, are frequently recommended by International Board Certified Lactation Consultants (IBCLC).

Nursing skills include the ability to counsel. Table 27.2 lists key teaching points regarding herbal medicines. Herbal therapies are only safe if herbs are prepared in the right way, used for the right indication, in the right amounts, for the right duration, and with appropriate monitoring. Potential herb-herb and herb-drug interactions should be considered when patients are using herbal products. The lack of national standards in the collection and preparation of herbal products complicates this field in the United States. Because many herbs have theoretical or

TABLE 27.1   References for Pregnancy, Breastfeeding, Lactation, and Children

Romm, Aviva Jill. *The Natural Pregnancy Book*. Berkeley, CA: Ten Speed Press, 2003.

Hale, Thomas W. *Medications and Mother's Milk: A Manual of Lactational Pharmacology* 11th Edition. Amarillo, TX: Pharmasoft Medical Publishers, 2004.

Humphrey, Sheila. *The Nursing Mother's Herbal*. Minneapolis, MN: Fairview Press, 2004.

Kemper, Kathi J. *The Holistic Pediatrician* 2nd Edition. New York: Perennial Currents, 2002.

TABLE 27.2   Five Key Patient Learning Points

Just because it is natural does not mean it is safe.

Just because it is safe does not mean it is effective.

Labels may not equal contents.

Self-diagnosis and self-treatment can result in self-malpractice.

Herbs are never a replacement for an emergency room.

actual risks that need to be recognized, it is important for health providers to have reliable and accessible sources of information to prevent adverse herb-related reactions and also to identify and manage complications of herbal therapies; Table 27.3 cites selected reputable herbal references.

All serious adverse reactions should be reported to the FDA through the MedWatch program at 1-800-332-1088 or at http://www.fda.gov/medwatch. An example of a complication associated with herbal therapy

TABLE 27.3   Herbal References and Resources

American Botanical Council: www.herbalgram.org

American Nutraceutical Association: www.americanutra.com

The U.S. FDA center for Food Safety and Applied Nutrition—a link to report adverse events: www.cfsan.fda.gov/~dms/aems.html

National Center for Complementary and Alternative Medicine: www.nccam.nih.gov

Herb Research Foundation: www.herbs.org

Herbal Medicine—The Expanded Commission E Monographs edited by Blumenthal, Goldberg, and Brinckmann. Austin, TX: American Botanical Council, 2000.

Nurses Herbal Medicine Handbook. Published by Lippincott Williams & Wilkins, 2001.

HerbalGram magazine. Published quarterly by the American Botanical Council and the Herb Research Foundation: www.herbalgram.org

Tarascon Pocket Pharmacopoeia. Contains a section on herbal and alternative therapies and has a PDA version that may be downloaded for a free trial: www.tarascon.com

Micromedex Alternative Medicine Database. An authoritative, full-text drug information resource; includes alternative medicine and is one of the most comprehensive resources for herbal medicine: www.library.ucsf.edu/db/micromedex.html

is illustrated in the case of the use of *Ma huang* (Ephedra), marketed in the United States until recently as a major ingredient in formulations for weight reduction. Because use of this herb had been linked to numerous adverse cardiovascular events including stroke, myocardial infarction, and sudden death (Haller & Benowitz, 2000), the U.S. Food and Drug Administration banned sales of this herb in April of 2004.

USES

Given the volume and variety of products, herbal medicine knowledge relevant for nursing practice cannot be summarized quickly. This chapter will now address three leading herbs from an evidence-based perspective. The reader will note that there is a significant range in scientific data available on each and the theoretical risks should be acknowledged and carefully considered both by patients and health professionals. Further, the clinical knowledge related to combining herbal products with prescription and nonprescription drugs is only in the developmental stages; much remains to be known about interactions and side effects.

Chronic illness, surgery, and use of prescription medications are three situations in which herbal medicine reviews by nurses are important. Echinacea does stimulate the immune system, but this is not necessarily a positive effect. Gingko biloba's pharmacologic activity places people at risk in surgery. Saint John's wort is effective for mild to moderate depression but can render many prescription medications ineffective or even toxic. Readers should be aware that many herbs have a sufficient evidence base and potential as alternatives to Western medicine. However, herbal medicine in the United States is a very broad and multicultural phenomenon; it is difficult to know all products used by or all products of potential benefit to patients. Readers should be aware that there are reputable clinical resources readily available for informed decision making (see Table 27.3).

Echinacea (*Echinacea augustofolia, E. pallida, E. purpurea*)

Echinacea is the leading herbal medicine used in the United States. North American gardens commonly contain Echinacea, also known as the purple coneflower. It was traditionally used by Native Americans and early settlers as a remedy for infections and for healing wounds. In vitro research suggests an immunostimulatory effect principally by macrophage, polymorphonuclear leukocyte and natural killer cell activation (Barrett, 2003).

Monocyte secretion of tumor-necrosis factor-alpha (TNF-α) is particularly stimulated (Senchina et al., 2005).

Echinacea is promoted in the United States for the prevention and treatment of the common cold. In Europe, it is used topically for wound healing and intravenously for immunostimulation. Several methodologically valid clinical studies have been published in recent years with unimpressive results, suggesting that Echinacea is not effective for the treatment or prevention of upper respiratory illness for adults (Melchart, Walther, Linde, Brandmaier, & Lersch, 1998; Yale & Liu, 2004) and for children (Taylor et al., 2003). However, three other clinical studies have shown positive results in adults (Dorn, Knick, & Lewith, 1997; Goel et al., 2004; Yale & Liu, 2004).

Echinacea has a good safety profile but has been associated (very infrequently) with gastric upset, rashes, and severe allergic reactions. Echinacea is not recommended for persons with allergies to members of the *Asteraceae* family (formerly termed *Compositae*), which includes ragweed, daisies, thistles, and chamomile. More importantly, nonspecific immunostimulation may exacerbate preexisting autoimmune disease or precipitate autoimmune disease in genetically predisposed persons (Lee & Werth, 2004). Tumor necrosis factor-alpha and interleukin-1 are pro-inflammatory cytokines, and recent evidence demonstrates that anti-TNF and anti-interleukin-1 therapies are effective for autoimmune diseases including Crohn's disease and rheumatoid arthritis. Echinacea cannot be recommended for people with other chronic immunologic diseases, including multiple sclerosis, lupus, and HIV.

The LD_{50} of intravenously administered echinacea juice is 50 ml/kg in mice and rats. Regular oral administration to mice at levels greater than proposed human therapeutic doses has failed to demonstrate toxic effects (Mengs, Clare, & Poiley, 1991). However, one study has suggested that repeated daily doses suppress the immune response (Coeugniet & Elek, 1987). The German government's Commission E recommends that use be limited to 8 weeks. Use of Echinacea for more than 8 weeks is associated with higher risk of neutropenia (Blumenthal et al., 1998).

Gingko (*Gingko biloba*)

Ginkgo is the number one selling herb in Europe for improvement of blood eheology and enhancement of cognition. Clinically, gingko is used for circulatory problems such as peripheral artery disease (Pittler & Ernst, 2005), impotence (Sikora, 1989), and "cerebral insufficiency" (Kleijnen & Knipschild, 1992a). Commission E also approves its use for dementia syndromes with memory deficits, disturbances in concentration, depressive emotional conditions, dizziness, tinnitus, and headaches. European studies published in 1994 and 1996 demonstrated its effectiveness in slowing or reversing dementia (Hofferberth, 1994; Kanowski, Herrmann, Stephan, Wierich, & Horr, 1996). A study published in 1997 confirmed these findings for patients with Alzheimer's disease and multi-infarct dementia in an American trial with 309 subjects (LeBars et al., 1997).

Recently, intriguing data have been published that suggest possible use in Parkinson's disease (Ahmad et al., 2005; Kim, Lee, Lee, & Kim, 2004) and diabetic retinopathy (Huang, Jeng, Kao, Yu, & Liu, 2004). Additionally, there is interest in its use for cognitively intact seniors (Mix & Crews, 2002), cell phone users (Ilhan et al., 2004), and stressed adults (Walesiuk, Trofimuk, & Braszko, 2005). However, larger trials are still needed to confirm such therapeutic benefit.

Ginkgo's leaf extracts are used in Europe both orally and intravenously for treatment of Alzheimer's dementia, multi-infarct dementia, peripheral vascular disease, and vertigo (Kaufmann, 2002; Li, Ma, Scherban, & Tam, 2002). Ginkgo's mechanism of action is believed to be its in vitro antioxidative, vasodilatory, antiplatelet, and neuromodulatory properties (Watanabe et al., 2001). It is more effective than beta-carotene and vitamin E as an oxidative scavenger and inhibitor of lipid peroxidation of cellular membranes (Pietschmann, Kuklinski, & Otterstein, 1992) and stimulates the release of nitric oxide (Chen, Salwinski, & Lee, 1997). Ginkgo is also a potent antagonist of platelet activating factor (Engelsen, Nielson, & Winther, 2002) and thus inhibits platelet aggregation and promotes clot breakdown. Gingko in the CNS inhibits production of pro-inflammatory cytokines and upregulates anti-inflammatory cytokines (Jiao, Rui, Li, Yang, & Qiu, 2005). These properties may result in neuroprotective and ischemia re-perfusion protective effects (Oyama, Chikahisa, Ueha, Kanemaru, & Noda, 1996; Sener et al., 2005; Shen & Zhou, 1995).

Side effects with ginkgo are uncommon. They include gastrointestinal discomfort, headache, and dizziness. Because of its anti-platelet effect, however, there is a risk of significant bleeding when ginkgo is used with anticoagulants and other antiplatelet agents (Bebbington, Kulkarni, & Roberts, 2005; Matthews, 1998; Rosenblatt & Mindel, 1997; Rowin & Lewis, 1996). Gingko should be discontinued 10 days prior to surgery and not restarted until the surgical wound has healed sufficiently to allow for aspirin use.

Saint John's Wort (*Hypericum perforatum*)

Saint John's wort, one of the world's top selling herbs, has been used for centuries in Europe as a sedative and as a balm for skin injuries. Since

1996, it has been widely promoted in the United States as a wonder drug for depression or as "nature's Prozac." Today, it is often used to treat mild to moderate depression, anxiety, and sleep disorders.

In vitro studies have shown that *Hypericum* extract inhibits the neuronal uptake of the neurotransmitters serotonin, noradrenaline, dopamine, gamma-aminobutyric acid (GABA), and L-glutamate (Muller, Rolli, Schafer, & Hafner, 1997). No in vivo MAO-inhibiting activity has been demonstrated with *Hypericum*.

A 1996 review of 23 randomized trials involving 1,757 patients with mild to moderate depression documented that *Hypericum* extracts are significantly better than placebo and similarly effective as tricyclic antidepressants. Overall, 55.1% of subjects responded to Saint John's wort and 22.3% responded to placebo (Linde et al., 1996). These studies have been criticized for not standardizing the diagnosis of depression or the dose of the herb's presumed active ingredient, hypericin. Additionally, the studies were short in duration and enrolled small numbers of subjects. It should be noted, however, that hypericin may not be the active ingredient in Saint John's wort; several constituents such as pseudohypericin and hyperforin have pharmacologic effects.

In a review of 35 double-blind, randomized trials, Saint John's wort demonstrated a much more favorable side-effect profile than tricyclic antidepressants and a slightly better profile than selective serotonin re-uptake inhibitors in patients with mild to moderate depression. Dropout rates are quite low: among 17 observational studies of 35,562 subjects, the rate ranged from 0% to 5.7% (Knuppel & Linde, 2004).

One 6-week randomized, double-blind comparison study of fluoxetine and Saint John's wort in 161 geriatric patients demonstrated nearly identical response rates and declines in the Hamilton Depression Scale scores (Harrer, Schmidt, Kuhn, & Biller, 1999). The Institute of Clinical Pharmacology in Berlin noted that even in high doses, Saint John's wort was well tolerated (Kerb et al., 1996).

The most serious toxicity associated with St. John's wort is the negative interactions with prescription drugs. Saint John's wort is a potent ligand for the nuclear receptor that regulates the expression of cytochrome P450 (CYP) 3A4, the hepatic enzyme involved in the metabolism of more than 50% of all prescription drugs (Moore et al., 2000). These include oral contraceptives, idinavir, cyclosporine, theophylline, digoxin, and warfarin. Hence, the use of Saint John's wort can be life threatening for people requiring prescription medications. Because of its long half-life, the herb should be discontinued at least 5 days prior to initiation of the above medications, and close monitoring of drug levels may be indicated. Additional theoretical concerns include the risk of photosensitivity or the precipitation of a serotonergic crisis with other prescription antidepressants.

FUTURE RESEARCH

Before herbal medicines are more widely accepted by the conventional allopathic medical system, more randomized, double-blind, placebo-controlled trials are needed in the United States. The NIH National Center for Complementary and Alternative Medicine (NCCAM) has funded and will continue to fund such clinical trials of herbal therapies. Promising understudied areas for herbal therapies include the following:

1. numerous herbs for peri-menopausal hot flash management,
2. milk thistle for hepatoprotection in the setting of hepatotoxic agents,
3. feverfew to augment breast milk production,
4. numerous medicinal mushrooms for adjunctive cancer therapy.

Additionally, significant efforts are needed to identify the most promising herbal supports for chemotherapy and radiation therapy as well as for asthma and heart disease.

Western medicine has yet to explore the potential benefits from the world's many healing traditions that use customized combinations of herbs. To research these will require a new paradigm, one that accounts for potential synergy and counterbalancing activities of multiple ingredients. Although intriguing preliminary data exist for many dietary supplements, the historic paucity of funding mechanisms in these areas has meant that scientific support for the use of many commercial products lags significantly behind consumer marketing efforts.

REFERENCES

Ahmad, M., Saleem, S., Ahmad, A., Yousuf, S., Ansari, M. A., Khan, M. B., et al. (2005). Gingko biloba affords dose-dependent protection against 6-hydroxydopamine-induced parkinsonism in rats: Neurobehavioral, neurochemical and immunohistochemical evidence. *Journal of Neurochemistry, 93,* 94–104.

American Botanical Council. (2000). *Herbal medicine: Expanded Commission E Monographs.* Austin, TX: American Botanical Council.

Barnes, P. M., Powell-Griner, E., McFann, K., & Nahin, R. I. (2004). Complementary and alternative medicine use among adults: United States, 2002. *Advances Data, 343,* 1–19.

Barrett, B. (2003). Medicinal properties of Echinacea: A critical review. *Phytomedicine, 10,* 66–86.

Bebbington, A., Kulkarni, R., & Roberts, P. (2005). Ginkgo biloba: Persistent bleeding after total hip arthroplasty caused by herbal self-medication. *Journal of Arthroplasty, 20,* 125–126.

Blumenthal, M., Busse, W. R, Goldberg, A., et al. (1998). The Complete German Commission E Monographs. American Botanical Council, Austin, TX.

Braquet, P. (1987). The gingkolides: Potent platelet activating factor antagonists isolated from Gingko biloba L: Chemistry, pharmacology and clinical applications. *Drug Future, 12,* 643–699.

Chen, X., Salwinski, S., & Lee, T. J. (1997). Extracts of Gingko biloba and ginsenosides exert cerebral vasorelaxation via a nitric oxide pathway. *Clinical Experimental Pharmacology and Physiology, 24,* 958–959.

Coeugniet, E. G., & Elek, E. (1987). Immunomodulation with Viscum album and Echinacea purpurea extracts. *Onkologie, 10*(Suppl. 3), 27.

Dietary Supplement Health & Education Act of 1994, Public Law 103-417, 103rd Congress of the United States of America.

Dorn, M., Knick, E., & Lewith, G. (1997). Placebo-controlled, double-blind study of Echinacea pallidae radix in upper respiratory tract infections. *Complementary Therapies Medicine, 5,* 40–42.

Engelsen, J., Nielson, J. D., & Winther, K. (2002). Effect of coenzyme Q10 and Gingko Biloba on warfarin dosage in stable, long-term warfarin treated outpatients: A randomized double blind placebo-crossover trial. *Thrombosis & Haemostatis, 87*(6), 1075–1076.

Goel, V., Lovlin, R., Barton, R., Lyon, M. R., Bauer, R., Lee, T. D., et al. (2004). Efficacy of a standardized Echinacea preparation (Echinilin) for the treatment of the common cold: A randomized, double-blind, placebo-controlled trial. *Journal of Clinical Pharmacy and Therapeutics, 29,* 75–83.

Grifo, F. (1997). *Biodiversity and human health.* Washington, DC: Island Press.

Haller, C. A., & Benowitz, N. L. (2000). Adverse cardiovascular and central nervous system events associated with dietary supplements containing ephedra alkaloids. *New England Journal of Medicine, 343*(25), 1833–1838.

Harrer, G., Schmidt, U., Kuhn, U., & Biller, A. (1999). Comparison and equivalence between the Saint John's wart extract LoHyp-57 and fluoxetine. *Arzneimittelforschung, 49,* 289–296.

Hofferberth, B. (1994). The efficacy of Egb 761 in patients with senile dementia of the Alzheimer's type: A double-blind, placebo-controlled study on different levels of investigation. *Human Psychopharmacology, 9,* 215–222.

Huang, S. Y., Jeng, C., Kao, S. C., Yu, J. J., & Liu, D. Z. (2004). Improved haemorrheological properties by Gingko biloba extract EGb 761 in type 2 diabetes mellitus complicated with retinopathy. *Clinical Nutrition, 23,* 615–621.

Ilhan, A., Gurel, A., Armutcu, F., Kamisli, S., Iraz, M., Akyol, O., et al. (2004). Gingko biloba prevents mobile phone-induced oxidative stress in rat brain. *Clinical Chim Acta, 340,* 153–162.

International Board Certified Lactation Consultant (IBCLC). Raleigh, North Carolina.

Jiao, Y. B., Rui, Y. C., Li, T. J., Yang, P. Y., & Qiu, Y. (2005). Expression of pro-inflammatory and anti-inflammatory cytokines in brain of atherosclerotic rats and effects of Gingko biloba extract. *Acta Pharmacology Sinica, 26,* 835–839.

Johnson, B. A. (2000). Prevention magazine assesses use of dietary supplements. *HerbalGram, 48,* 65.

Kanowski, S., Herrmann, W. M., Stephan, K., Wierich, W., & Horr, R. (1996). Proof of efficacy of the Gingko biloba extract Egb 761 in outpatients suffering from mild to moderate primary degenerative dementia of the Alzheimer's type of multi-infarct dementia. *Pharmacopsychiatry, 29,* 47–56.

Kaufmann, H. (2002). Treatment of patients with orthostatic hypotension and syncope. *Clinical Neuropharmacology, 25*(3), 133–141.

Kerb, R., Brockmoller, J., Staffeldt, B., Ploch, & Roots, I. (1996). Single-dose and steady state pharmacokinetics of hypercin and pseudohypercin. *Antimicrobial Agents Chemotherapy, 40,* 2087–2093.

Kim, M. S., Lee, J. I., Lee, W. Y., & Kim, S. E. (2004). Neuroprotective effect of Gingko biloba L. extract in a rat model of Parkinson's disease. *Phytotherapy Research, 18,* 663–666.

Kleijnen, J., & Knipschild, P. (1992a). Gingko biloba for cerebral insufficiency. *British Journal of Pharmacology, 34,* 352.

Kleijnen, J., & Knipschild, P. (1992b). Gingko biloba. *Lancet, 340,* 1136–1139.

Knuppel, L., & Linde, K. (2004). Adverse effects of St. John's Wort: A systematic review. *Journal of Clinical Psychiatry, 11,* 1470–1479.

LeBars, P. L., Katz, M. M., Berman, N., Itil, T. M., Freedman, A. M., & Schatzberg, A. F. (1997). A placebo-controlled, double-blind, randomized trial of an extract of Gingko biloba for dementia. *Journal of the American Medical Association, 278,* 1327–1332.

Lee, A. N., & Werth, V. P. (2004). Activation of autoimmunity following use of immunostimulatory herbal supplements. *Archives of Dermatology, 140,* 723–772.

Li, X. F., Ma, M., Scherban, K., & Tam, Y. K. (2002). Liquid chromatography-electrospray mass spectrometric studies of ginkgolides and bilobalide using simultaneous monitoring of proton, ammonium, and sodium adducts. *Analyst, 127,* 641–646.

Linde, K., Ramirez, G., Mulrow, C. D., Pauls, A., Weidenhammer, W., & Melchart, D. (1996, August 3). St John's wort for depression—an overview and meta-analysis of randomised clinical trials. *British Medical Journal, 313*(7052), 253–258.

Matthews, M. K., Jr. (1998). Association of Gingko biloba with intracerebral hemorrhage. *Neurology, 50,* 1933–1934.

Melchart, D., Walther, E., Linde, K., Brandmaier, R., & Lersch, C. (1998). Echinacea root extracts for the prevention of upper respiratory tract infections. *Archives of Family Medicine, 7,* 541–545.

Mengs, U., Clare, C. B., & Poiley, J. A. (1991). Toxicity of Echinacea purpurea. Acute, subacute and genotoxicity studies. *Arzneimittel-Frosch, 41,* 1076–1081.

Mix, J. A., & Crews, W. D., Jr. (2002). A double-blind, placebo-controlled, randomized trial of Gingko biloba extract EGb761 in a sample of cognitively intact older adults: Neuropsychological findings. *Human Psychopharmacology, 17,* 267–277.

Moore, L. B., Goodwin, B., Jones, S. A., Wiselg, C. B., Serabjit-Singh, C. J., Wilson, T. M., Collins, J. L., & Kiewer, S. A. (2000). Saint John's wort induces hepatic metabolism through activation of the pregnane x receptor. *Proceedings of the National Academy of Science, 97,* 7500–7502.

Muller, W. E., Rolli, M., Schafer, C., & Hafner, U. (1997). Effects of Hypericum extract (L160) in biochemical models of antidepressant activity. *Pharmopsychiatry, 30*(Suppl. 2), 102–107.

National Library of Medicine. Retrieved 2005, from http://www.ncbi.nlm.nih.gov/Pubmed

Oyama, Y., Chikahisa, L., Ueha, T., Kanemaru, K., & Noda, K. (1996). Gingko biloba extract protects brain neurons against oxidative stress induced by hydrogen peroxide. *Brain Research, 712,* 349–352.

Pietschmann, A., Kuklinski, B., & Otterstein, A. (1992). Protection from uv-light-induced oxidative stress by nutritional radical scavengers. *Zeitschrift fur die Gesamte Innere Medizin und Ihre Grenzgebite, 47*(11), 518–522.

Pittler, M. H., & Ernst, E. (2005). Complementary therapies for peripheral artery disease: Systematic review. *Atherosclerosis, 18,* 1–7.

Rosenblatt, M., & Mindel, J. (1997). Spontaneous hyphema associated with ingestion of Gingko biloba extract. *New England Journal of Medicine, 336,* 1108.

Rowin, J., & Lewis, S. L. (1996). Spontaneous bilateral subdural hematomas associated with chronic Gingko biloba ingestion have also occurred. *Neurology, 46,* 1775–1776.

Senchina, D. S., McDann, D. A., Asp, J. M., Johnson, J. A., Cunnick, J. E., Kaiser, M. S., et al. (2005). Changes in immunomodulatory properties of Echinacea spp. Root infusions and tinctures stored at 4 degrees C for four days. *Clinical Chim Ada, 355,* 67–82.

Sener, G., Sener, E., Sehirli, O., Ogune, A. V., Cetinel, S., Gedik, N., et al. (2005). Gingko biloba extract ameliorates ischemia reperfusion-induced renal injury in rats. *Pharmacology Research,* Epub May 13.

Shen, J. G., & Zhou, D. Y. (1995). Efficiency of Gingko biloba extract (Egb 761) in antioxidant protection against myocardial ischemia and re-perfusion injury. *Biochemical Molecular Biological Institute, 35,* 125–134.

Sikora, K. (1989). Complementary medicine and cancer treatment. *Practitioner, 233*(1476), 1285–1286.

Taylor, J. A., Weber, W., Standish, L., Quinn, H., Goesling, J., McGann, M., et al. (2003). Efficacy and safety of Echinacea in treating upper respiratory tract infections in children: A randomized controlled trial. *Journal of the American Medical Association, 290,* 2824–2830.

U.S. Government Printing Office. (1990). *Nutrition Labeling and Education Act of 1989.* Washington, DC: Author.

U.S. Government Printing Office. (1999). *Dietary Supplement Health and Education Act: Is the FDA trying to change the intent of Congress.* Washington, DC: Author.

Walesiuk, A., Trofimiuk, E., & Braszko, J. J. (2005). Gingko biloba extract diminishes stress-induced memory deficits in rats. *Pharmacology Reporter, 57,* 176–187.

Ward, E., & Blumenthal, M. (2005). Americans confident in dietary supplements according to CRN survey. *HerbalGram, 66,* 64–65.

Wantanabe, C. M., Wolffram, S., Ader, P., Rimbach, G., Packer, L., Maguire, J. J., Schultz, P. G., & Gohil, K. (2001, June 5). The in vivo neuromodulatory effects of the herbal medicine giko biloba. *Proceedings of the National Academy of Sciences USA, 98*(12), 6577–6580.

Yale, S. H., & Liu, K. (2004). Echinacea purpurea therapy for the treatment of the common cold: A randomized, double-blind, placebo-controlled clinical trial. *Archives of Internal Medicine, 164,* 1237–1241.

CHAPTER 28

Functional Foods and Nutraceuticals

Bridget Doyle and Melissa Frisvold

In the 21st century the focus of the relationship between eating habits and health is changing from an emphasis on health maintenance through recommended dietary allowances of nutrients, vitamins, and minerals to an emphasis on the use of foods to provide better health, increase vitality, and aid in preventing disease and many chronic illnesses. The connection between food and health is not new. Indeed, the adage "Let food be your medicine and medicine your food" was supported by Hippocrates (trans. 1932). Today, the philosophy that supports the paradigm of nutraceuticals as functional foods is once again at the forefront.

Despite this ancient wisdom, the use of nutraceuticals and functional foods remains in its infancy in the Western world. It was not until the late 1970s that the trend toward improved physical fitness and overall well-being began. At that time, scientific evidence began to stress the importance of a balanced diet low in saturated fat, sodium, and cholesterol and higher in fiber. Currently, the use of nutraceuticals, including additives to certain conventional foods, phytochemicals, functional foods, dietary foods and supplements, and medical foods is growing at an astronomical rate. In the past several years, the Food and Drug Administration has worked to examine the possible connections between nutritional products and disease states, including calcium and osteoporosis, sodium and hypertension, lipids and cardiovascular disease, lipids and cancer, and dietary fiber and cardiovascular disease (Gardner, 1994).

With the developing market of functional foods, it is estimated that consumers in the United States spent over $18.7 billion on dietary supplements (Nutrition Business Journal, 2003). One can find calcium added to juices, pasta, rice, dry cereals, and chocolate and caramel candy products. Many companies are using soy protein isolates in foods ranging from candy bars and salad dressings to infant formulas. Plant stanols and sterols are being added to margarine-like spreads in an effort to reduce total cholesterol and LDL levels. Common nutraceuticals receiving broad attention include calcium-fortified fruit drinks and candy; soy protein bars fortified with whey protein; soy protein products and high-fiber cereals; and bars providing L-arginine, which may improve vascular functioning. Coverage of all nutraceuticals is beyond the scope of this chapter; however, several selected products are covered in depth. Because the use of nutraceuticals is so prevalent and because their use may impact health and wellness, it is important that nurses know about nutraceuticals and the potential benefits and risks.

DEFINITIONS

To understand the terms *functional food* and *nutraceuticals*, one must understand the definition of foods. The Food and Drug Administration (FDA) defines foods as "articles used primarily for taste, aroma, or nutritive value" (Federal Food, Drug and Cosmetic Act, 1938, § 210). Historically, the FDA has made several attempts to regulate these products and remove some of them from the market (Kottke, 1998). Functional foods are defined as manufactured foods for which scientifically valid claims can be made. They may be produced by food-processing technologies, traditional breeding, or genetic engineering. Functional foods should safely deliver a long-term health benefit. Accordingly, a functional food may be one of the following:

- A known food to which a functional ingredient from another food is added

- A known food to which a functional ingredient new to the food supply is added

- An entirely new food that contains one or more functional ingredients (Pariza, 1999)

Nutraceutical has been defined as "a blend word of nutrition and pharmaceutical, for a substance that may be considered a food or part of a food and that provides medical or health benefits, including the prevention or treatment of disease" (Marshall, 1994, p. 243). These substances pose problems for official medicine regulators. The Japanese, who were among the first to utilize functional foods, have highlighted three conditions that define a functional food:

- It is a food (not a capsule, tablet, or powder) derived from naturally occurring ingredients.

- It can and should be consumed as part of a daily diet.

- It has a particular function when ingested, serving to regulate a particular body process, such as enhancement of the biological defense mechanism, prevention of a specific disease, recovery from a specific disease, control of physical and mental conditions, and slowing of the aging process (PA Consulting Group, 1990).

According to these definitions, unmodified whole foods such as fruits and vegetables represent the simplest form of a functional food. For example, broccoli, carrots, or tomatoes would be considered functional foods because they contain high levels of physiologically active components such as beta-carotene, lycopene, and sulforaphane. Modified foods, including those that have been fortified with nutrients or enhanced with phytochemicals, are also within the realm of functional foods.

SCIENTIFIC BASIS

During the past century there have been many changes in the types of foods people eat. This reflects the application of scientific findings and technological innovations in the food industry. Although much research has been conducted on nutrition and health and disease, scientific research on the use of nutraceuticals is more limited.

Interest in foodstuffs has generated research to link nutrient and food intake with improvements in health or prevention of disease. More than 200 studies in the epidemiological literature have been reviewed and consistently show an association between a low consumption of fruits and vegetables and the incidence of cancer. The quarter of the population with the lowest dietary intake of fruits and vegetables has roughly twice the rate of cancer compared to those with the highest intake (Shibamoto, Terao, & Osawa, 1997).

Hasler (2002) suggests that claims about the health benefits of functional foods should be based on sound scientific evidence. For example, resveratrol, which is found in red wine and grape juice, appears to benefit health by causing platelet aggregation reduction, with strong evidence to support this assertion. Conversely, the evidence that catechins (found in green tea) reduce the risk of certain types of cancer is moderate. It would indeed be helpful if reliable, evidence-based sources of information were available to the consumer on all nutraceuticals.

Much scientific research has been conducted on the role of the various products added to normal foods to enhance their ability to inhibit or prevent diseases. Many regard dietary intake as the best means of acquiring necessary nutrients (Kottke, 1998). However, supplementation of nutrients is common. The findings of selected scientific research focused on selected nutraceuticals are summarized below.

Dietary Plant Stanols and Sterols

The cholesterol-lowering potential of dietary plant stanols and sterols has been known for many years. Modifying plant stanols and sterols structurally makes them easily incorporated into fat-containing foods without losing their effectiveness in lowering cholesterol (Cater & Grundy, 1998). Dietary plant stanols and sterols inhibit the absorption of cholesterol in the small intestine, which in turn can lower LDL blood cholesterol. Patients using statin drug therapy may see further decreases in their blood cholesterol levels when using plant sterol and stanol esters (Blair et al., 2000). Recent studies of plant sterol and stanol esters in humans have demonstrated, however, that maximum cholesterol lowering benefits are achieved at doses of 2–3 grams per day (Hendriks, Weststrate, van Vliet, & Meijer, 1999; Jones, Ntanios, Raeini-Sarjaz, & Vanstone, 1999; Jones et al., 2000; Maki et al., 2001).

Plant sterols and their esters are Generally Recognized As Safe (GRAS) food-grade substances, indicating there has been a history of safe intake of these products with no demonstrated harmful health effects found in the research (International Food Information Council, 2003). Overall, the Nutrition Committee of the American Heart Association advises that stanols and sterol esters not be used as a preventive measure in the general population with normal cholesterol levels, in light of limited data regarding any potential risks. They may be used, however, for adults with hypercholesterolemia or adults requiring secondary prevention after an atherosclerotic event (Lichtenstein & Deckelbaum, 2001).

Glucosamine, Chondroitin Sulfate, and Collagen Hydrolysate

This combination of nutraceuticals is receiving a great deal of scientific review, particularly their use in the symptomatic treatment of osteoarthritis. Meta-analyses by McAlindon, LaValley, Gulin, and Felson (2000) and Towheed and Hochberg (1997) reviewed clinical trials of glucosamine and chondroitin in the treatment of osteoarthritis. McAlindon and colleagues included 13 double-blind, placebo-controlled trials of greater than 4 weeks' duration, testing oral or parenteral glucosamine or chondroitin for treatment of hip or knee arthritis. All 13 studies were classified as positive, demonstrating substantial benefits in treating arthritis when compared with placebo. Towheed and Hochberg reviewed nine randomized, controlled studies of glucosamine sulfate in osteoarthritis. Glucosamine was superior when compared to placebo in seven random trials. Two of the random trials compared glucosamine sulfate to ibuprofen. In these two trials, glucosamine was superior in one and equivalent in the other.

The literature reflects concern about these specific products. Deal and Moskowitz (1999) underscore that investigators utilizing glucosamine and chondroitin carefully monitor the product manufacturing process because some of the preparations claiming to contain certain doses of these nutraceuticals have significantly less (or none) of the dosages described.

Cost is a factor in the use of these nutraceuticals. The average cost ranges from $35 to $60 per month (Deal & Moskowitz, 1999). In their reviews, the authors emphasize that these agents are not FDA-evaluated or recommended for the treatment of osteoarthritis.

Coenzyme Q10

Coenzyme Q10 (CoQ10) is a compound made naturally in the body. It is used by cells to produce energy needed for cell growth and maintenance. It is also used by the body as an antioxidant. Tissue levels of CoQ10 decrease with age. Some studies have suggested that CoQ10 stimulates the immune system and increases resistance to disease (National Cancer Institute, 2002). Several controlled trials of CoQ10 have been performed for the indication of congestive heart failure (CHF), and the results have varied (Khatta et al., 2000). Other therapeutic claims attributed to CoQ10 involve hypertension, impaired immune status, adjuvant therapy for breast cancer, and various neurologic disorders including Huntington's disease and Parkinson's disease. No outcome data describing clinical benefits from CoQ10 could be found in the literature for these conditions.

Probiotics

Probiotics are microorganism supplements intended to improve health or treat a certain disease. Yogurt is an example of a probiotic food source. The organism must have scientifically proven beneficial physiological effects, be safe for human consumption, remain stable in bile and acid, and be able to adhere to the intestinal mucosa. Probiotics protect the intestinal mucosa by competing with pathogens for attachment sites (Salminen, 1998).

Two controlled studies were completed by Malin, Suomalainen, Saxelin, and Isolauri (1996) with 9 children with juvenile diabetes and 14 children with Crohn's disease. Use of Lactobacillus GG therapy for 10 days demonstrated an increased gut IgA immune response. In a double-blind, randomized, placebo-controlled study of 40 individuals with ulcerative colitis, a mixed-organism probiotic prevented flare-ups of chronic pouchitis (Gionchetti et al., 2000). A meta-review of 143 clinical trials involving 7,500+ subjects revealed no adverse events associated with probiotic use (Naidu, Bidlack, & Clemens, 1999).

INTERVENTION

Many people are using nutraceuticals. Therefore, it is important that nurses include them when they obtain the health history of the patient. Table 28.1 presents guidelines for nurses to use in assessing patients. In addition, Table 28.2 lists reputable sites for information pertaining to nutraceuticals.

Measurement of Outcomes

Outcomes of therapy can be assessed in a number of ways, depending on the nutraceutical and the intent of the therapy. For example, blood levels of the nutrient or effect on the target organ (e.g., bone with the use of calcium) could be monitored over time. Also, it is important that potential side effects of the therapy be evaluated in periodic physical assessments and comprehensive histories. Positive or negative changes in subjective health, energy, and symptoms, or those subsequent to changes in nutraceutical use, can also be assessed in individuals as data for toler-

TABLE 28.1   Guideline: Nutraceutical Assessment Guide for Nurses

- Screen for nutraceutical use as a routine part of the health assessment interview process. Because surgical complications can arise from nutritional supplement use, their use is often discontinued a few weeks before surgery.
- Acquire a working knowledge of functional foods and nutraceuticals, which includes benefits/risks, costs, and possible drug interactions.
- Develop effective communication strategies to ensure that all members of a patient's health care team are aware of nutraceutical use.
- Explore the reasons for the use of nutritional supplements and functional foods. Can the same benefits be achieved by using another product that is safer or less expensive?
- Consider the unique health care needs of various populations. It is important that pregnant women, children, the elderly, and populations with certain medical conditions discuss any nutritional supplementation use with their health care provider.
- Provide educational resources for patients that are easy to access, timely, evidence based, and easy to understand.
- Remember to consult with and refer patients to nutritionists, a very knowledge-able and accessible resource in this promising and rapidly changing area of health and wellness.

ance as part of cost–benefit evaluation. Good teaching of nutraceutical principles, intended purpose, and dose and effects of functional foods will result in informed use by clients and greater awareness of intended and adverse effects.

Precautions

As stated previously, it is of paramount importance that nutraceutical use be assessed as part of the health history and nutritional assessment. Safe use must be carefully considered (Zeisel, 1999); safe dosage, drug interaction, toxic side effects due to overdose, or ineffective clearance should be determined.

A consistent concern expressed in the literature is the lack of regulation of nutraceuticals. Dietary supplements are not formally reviewed for consistency in the manufacturing process and there may be variation in the composition of one supplement batch to another (National Cancer Institute, 2002). Hasler (2002) raises concerns about the plethora of "functional" bars, beverages, cereals, and soups enhanced with botanicals that may pose a health risk to certain consumers. Consistent with these concerns, the General Accounting Office (GAO) in 2000 released a report

TABLE 28.2 Nutraceutical Internet Sites

American Dietetic Association
www.eatright.org

Mayo Clinic
www.mayoclinic.org

National Institutes of Health—National Center for Complementary and Alternative Medicine
http://nccam.nih.gov/

National Institutes of Health—National Library of Medicine
www.ncbi.nlm.nih.gov

National Institutes of Health—Office of Dietary Supplements
http://dietary-supplements.info.nih.gov/

Natural Medicines Comprehensive Database
www.naturaldatabase.com

U.S. Department of Agriculture—Food and Nutrition Information Center
www.nal.usda.gov

U.S. Department of Health and Human Services—Office of Disease Prevention and Health Promotion
www.healthfinder.gov

U.S. Food and Drug Administration—Center for Food Safety and Applied Nutrition
www.cfsan.fda.gov/~dms/supplmnt.html

---

that raised concerns about the safety of certain foods and the lack of guidance from the FDA to companies on safety information labeling for consumers (Hasler, 2002). Finally, the American consumer often receives information on these products through less than reliable resources such as friends, Internet marketing sites, or vitamin store clerks (Morris & Avorn, 2003). When all of these factors are taken into consideration, a situation with inherent potential risks is created.

USES

Nutraceuticals have been used to promote health and to prevent and treat illness. Nutraceuticals can be used to target deficiencies, establish optimal nutritional balance, or treat diseases. Because heart disease, cancer, and stroke are leading causes of death in the United States, nutraceuticals that have been shown to improve risk-factor profiles would be desirable. Furthermore, people in the United States and worldwide could benefit from nutraceuticals when there are deficiencies of specific nutrients.

Children/Adolescents

There is a paucity in the literature about nutraceutical use in the child/adolescent population. This is a population with unique nutritional needs because this is the time when growth and development occur at a rapid pace. Not only can nutrition during this time impact current health status, it may have implications for life-long health as well. Consistent with the need for research in this arena, the National Institutes of Health (NIH) currently is conducting a pilot study on probiotics in the prevention and treatment of pediatric illness. Further information on this exciting research initiative can be assessed at the NIH web site listed in Table 28.2.

The American Academy of Pediatrics (2001) conducted a survey of its members to determine attitudes, knowledge, and behaviors about complementary and alternative therapies (CAM) in their clinical practice. Analysis was done based on the response from 745 pediatricians. Few asked their patients or parents about CAM use. Approximately 1 in 5 pediatricians asked specifically about the use of dietary supplements. The findings from this survey will be used to guide the development of educational programs in this area for its members.

Women's Health and Nutritional Needs

Throughout their life span, women have unique nutritional needs that place them at risk for nutrition-related diseases and conditions. Nutrition has been shown to have a significant influence on the risk of chronic disease and on the maintenance of optimal health status. Although food should be the first choice in meeting needs, nutritional supplementation may be necessary (American Dietetic Association, 2001). The following are some examples of increased nutritional needs across the life span:

- An increase in calcium during pregnancy and menopause is necessary.

- Folic acid requirements increase during pregnancy to prevent neural tube defects.

- Iron needs increase during times of menstruation and pregnancy.

Although acquiring these nutrients through food sources would be ideal, supplementation is often necessary. It is also important to remember that intake of certain nutrients over a certain level can be teratogenic. For example, too much Vitamin A in the first trimester of pregnancy can be teratogenic and because many foods are often enriched with vitamins and minerals, it is possible to consume too much.

FUTURE RESEARCH

Although nutraceuticals have long-standing historical usage, increased interest in these substances to promote health, prevent disease, and treat specific medical conditions is reflected in heightened attention to nutritional science and increased consumption. A consistent theme throughout this chapter has been the need for more research in this area. The following quote from the book, *Complementary and Alternative Medicine in the United States* (Institute of Medicine, 2005), summarizes succinctly what the goal for research in this arena should be: "In terms of medical therapies, a commitment to public welfare is the obligation to generate and provide to health care practitioners, policy makers, and the public access to the best information available on the efficacy of CAM therapies" (p. 169). Consistent with this sentiment and because there is so much interest and hope in this area, interdisciplinary research teams may explore the following questions:

1. Which of the current nutraceuticals should be incorporated on a regular basis to promote health?
2. Are nutraceuticals cost effective?
3. What are the side effects associated with short- and long-term use of specific nutraceuticals?
4. Can we increase research in the use of nutraceuticals in the pediatric population?
5. What are innovative ways to educate health care providers about nutraceuticals?
6. Can we discover more effective methods to educate the American health care consumer about the benefits/risks of nutraceuticals?

REFERENCES

American Academy of Pediatrics. (2001). *Periodic Survey #49: Complementary and alternative medicine (CAM) therapies in pediatric practices.* Retrieved May 25, 2005, from http://www.aap.org/research/periodicsurvey/ps49bex.htm

American Dietetic Association. (2001). *Position paper: Nutrition and women's health*. Retrieved May 31, 2005, from http://www.eatright.org/Member/Policy Initiatives/index_21017.cfm

Blair, S. N., Capuzzi, D. M., Gottlieb, S. O., Nguyen, T., Morgan, J. M., & Cater, N. B. (2000). Incremental reduction of serum total cholesterol and low-density lipoprotein cholesterol with the addition of plant stanol ester-containing spread to statin therapy. *American Journal of Cardiology, 86*(1), 46–52.

Cater, N., & Grundy, S. (1998, November). *Postgraduate medicine* (special report), 6–14.

Deal, C. L., & Moskowitz, R. W. (1999). Nutraceuticals as therapeutic agents in osteoarthritis: The role of glucosamine, chondroidin sulfate, and collagen hydrolysate. *Rheumatic Disease Clinics of North America, 25*(2), 379–953.

Federal Food, Drug and Cosmetic Act. (1938). 52 Stat. 111. 21 U.S.C. § 210 et seq.

Gardner, J. (1994). The development of the functional food business. In I. Goldberg (Ed.), *Functional foods: Designer foods, pharmafoods, and nutraceuticals* (pp. 472–473). New York: Chapman & Hall.

Gionchetti, P., Rizzello, F., Venturi, A., Brigidi, P., Matteuzzi, D., Bazzocchi, G., et al. (2000). Oral bacteriotherapy as maintenance treatment in patients with chronic pouchitis: A double-blind, placebo-controlled trial. *Gastroenterology, 119*(2), 305–309.

Hasler, C. M. (2002). Functional foods: Benefits, concerns and challenges—a position paper from the American council on science and health. *Journal of Nutrition, 132*, 3772–3781.

Hendriks, J. F., Weststrate, J. A., van Vliet, T., & Meijer, G. W. (1999). Spreads enriched with three different levels of vegetable oil sterols and the degree of cholesterol lowering in normocholesterolaemic and mildly hypercholesterolaemic subjects. *European Journal of Clinical Nutrition, 53*(4), 319–327.

Hippocrates. (1932). *Hippocrates* (W. H. S. Jones, Trans.). Cambridge, MA: Harvard University Press.

Institute of Medicine. (2005). *Complementary and alternative medicine in the United States*. Washington, DC: National Academies Press.

International Food Information Council. (2003). *Functional foods fact sheet: Plant stanols and sterols*. Retrieved May 31, 2005, from http://ific.org

Jones, P. J., Ntanios, F. Y., Raeini-Sarjaz, M., & Vanstone, C. A. (1999). Cholesterol-lowering efficacy of a sitostanol-containing phytosterol mixture with a prudent diet in hyperlipidemic men. *American Journal of Clinical Nutrition, 69*(6), 1144–1150.

Jones, P. J., Raeini-Sarjaz, M., Ntanios, F. Y., Vanstone, C. A., Feng, J. Y., & Parsons, W. E. (2000). Modulation of plasma lipid levels and cholesterol kinetics by phytosterol versus phytostanol esters. *Journal of Lipid Research, 41*(5), 697–705.

Khatta, M., Alexander, B. S., Krichten, C. M., Fisher, M. L., Freudenberger, R., Robinson, S. W., et. al. (2000). The effect of coenzyme Q10 in patients with congestive heart failure. *Annals of Internal Medicine, 132*(8), 636–640.

Kottke, M. K. (1998). Scientific and regulatory aspects of nutraceutical products in the United States. *Drug Development and Industrial Pharmacy, 24*(12), 1177–1195.

Kurtzweil, P. (1999). *An FDA guide to dietary supplements*. Retrieved from http://vm.cfsan.fda.gov/~dms/fdsupp.html

Lichtenstein, A. H., & Deckelbaum, R. J. (2001). AHA Science Advisory: stanol/sterol ester-containing foods and blood control levels: A statement for health-care professionals from the Nutrition Committee of the Council on Nutrition, Physical Activity, and Metabolism of the American Heart Association. *Circulation, 103*, 1177.

Maki, K. C., Davidson, M. H., Umporowicz, D. M., Schaefer, E. J., Dicklin, M. R., & Ingram, K. A. (2001). Lipid responses to plant-sterol-enriched reduced-fat spreads incorporated into a national cholesterol education program step I diet. *American Journal of Clinical Nutrition, 74*(1), 33–43.

Malin, M., Suomalainen, H., Saxelin, N., & Isolauri, E. (1996). Promotion of IgA immune response in patients with Crohn's disease by oral bacteriotherapy with lactobacillus GG. *Annals of Nutritional Metabolism, 40*, 137–145.

Marshall, W. E. (1994). Amino acids, peptides and proteins. In I. Goldberg (Ed.), *Functional foods: Designer foods, pharmafoods, and nutraceuticals* (pp. 242–260). New York: Chapman & Hall.

McAlindon, T. E., LaValley, M. P., Gulin, J. P., & Felson, D. T. (2000). Glucosamine and chondroitin for treatment of osteoarthritis: A systematic quality assessment and meta-analysis. *Journal of the American Medical Association, 283*(11), 1483–1484.

Morris, C. A., & Avorn, J. (2003). Internet marketing of herbal products. *Journal of the American Medical Association, 290*(11), 1519–1520.

Naidu, A. S., Bidlack, W. R., & Clemens, R. A. (1999). Probiotic spectra of lactic and bacteria. *Critical Reviews in Food Sciences & Nutrition, 39*(1), 13–126.

National Academy of Sciences. (2005). *Complementary and alternative medicine in the United States*. Retrieved May 31, 2005, from http://www.books.nap.edu/catalog/11182.html

National Cancer Institute. (2002). *Coenzyme Q10: Questions and answers, cancer facts*. Retrieved May 31, 2005, from http://cis.nci.nih.gov/fact/9-16.htm

National Institutes of Health. (n.d.). *Probiotics for pediatric illnesses*. Retrieved May 31, 2005, from http://grants2.nih.gov/grants/guide/pa-files/PA-05-035.html

Nelson, N. J. (1999). Purple carrots, margarine laced with wood pulp? Nutraceuticals move into the supermarket. *Journal of the National Cancer Institute, 91*(9), 755–757.

Nutrition Business Journal. (2003). NBJ's annual industry overview VIII. *Nutrition Business Journal, VIII*(5/6), 2–9.

PA Consulting Group. (1990). *Functional foods: A new global added value market?* London: Author.

Pariza, M. (1999). Functional foods: Technology, functionality and health benefits. *Nutrition Today, 34*, 150–151.

Salminen, S., Bouley, C., Boutron-Ruault, M. C., Cummings, J. H., Franck, A., & Gibson, G. R., et al. (1998). Functional food science and gastrointestinal physiology and function. *British Journal of Nutrition, 80*(Suppl. 1), S147–171.

Shibamoto, T., Terao, J., & Osawa, T. (1997). ACS Symposium Series 701. *Functional foods for disease prevention I: Fruits, vegetables, and trees*. Washington, DC: American Chemical Society.

Towheed, T. E., & Hochberg, M. C. (1997). A systematic review of randomized controlled trials of pharmacological therapy in osteoarthritis of the hip. *Journal of Rheumatology, 24,* 349–357.

Zeisel, S. H. (1999). Regulation of "nutraceuticals." *Science, 285*(5435), 1853–1855.

PART VI

Perspectives on Future Research and Practice

CHAPTER 29

Perspectives on Future Research and Practice

Ruth Lindquist and Mariah Snyder

Nursing's commitment to the generation of high quality, cost-effective patient outcomes requires that a sound scientific basis for practice be established. Previous chapters have identified existing research related to the therapies reviewed. However, most chapters end with statements that more research is needed. The need for more evidence related to the safety, efficacy, timing, "dose," and specific indications for most therapies is clearly evident. As previously noted, there is a large and growing interest in and use of complementary therapies by the public. In fact, the number of annual visits to providers of complementary and alternative therapies now outnumbers visits to primary care physicians (Institute of Medicine [IOM], 2002). Interest in complementary therapies is encountered in a broad range of health care practice settings. Along with public and patient interest, there is a concomitant increased interest on the part of providers who want to deliver these therapies to patients and who also have an interest in therapies for their own personal use (Lindquist, Tracy, & Savik, 2003). As a result of the growing demand and use of therapies, there is a heightened urgency to expand the evidence base to support their use.

Health providers and researchers are challenged to provide care in the emerging context of an increasing volume and broader range in the exploration and use of complementary therapies. There is an acute need to know and understand benefits of therapies, as well as a need to ensure the safety and efficacy of complementary therapies and to understand their effects and interactions when used in combination with other complementary and allopathic therapies. In this chapter the need for more evidence for the expanding use of complementary therapies in practice will be discussed; research designs appropriate for the study of complementary therapies will be explored; the overall state of research on complementary therapies will be described; and implications that the state of evidence and expanded use of complementary therapies have for future nursing research, education, and practice will be identified.

NEED TO EXPAND THE EVIDENCE BASE

The documented growing interest in and use of alternative and complementary therapies and alternative systems of care have caused health care providers to consider the appeal of these therapies to consumers as well as the consideration of their safety and efficacy. With their growing use, there are increases in concern regarding the safety and/or interactions of therapies (for example, the interaction of herbal remedies with prescribed pharmacologic agents), the regulation of these therapies, and the quality of the products and therapies delivered. Scientific data as well as other forms of knowledge are needed by providers to inform their practice; accurate and reliable knowledge is also needed by consumers who wish to make informed decisions regarding their own health practices.

There is a rising interest and indeed a mandate for evidence-based practice. Evidence-based practice integrates the best scientific evidence with clinical expertise and patient preferences. Evidence-based practice (EBP) has been defined by McKibbon (1998) as

> an approach to health care wherein health professionals use the best evidence possible, i.e. the most appropriate information available, to make clinical decisions for individual patients. EBP values, enhances and builds on clinical expertise, knowledge of disease mechanisms, and pathophysiology. It involves complex and conscientious decision-making based not only on the available evidence but also on patient characteristics, situations, and preferences. It recognizes that health care is individualized and ever changing and involves uncertainties and probabilities. Ultimately EBP is the formalization of the care process that the best clinicians have practiced for generations. [p. 396]

Nurses and other providers practicing in the context of allopathic care rely on an evidence base. So, too, nurses and other health professionals are relying on or requiring similar evidence in their use of complementary therapies (IOM, 2002).

It is important that resources to access knowledge be identified, made available, and used by providers. Research findings must be disseminated broadly to practitioners, who need to be informed so that the safety of patients can be protected and the potential benefits of therapies realized. A number of personal data assistants (PDA)-based resources provide access to authoritative information as a resource to professional practice. Databases of research findings (e.g., the Cochrane Database of Systematic Reviews) provide a good resource for synthesized research findings (www.cochrane.org/reviews/). As of 2004, this online source contained 145 reviews related to complementary and alternative therapies. Web sites of government agencies such as the National Center for Complementary and Alternative Medicine (NCCAM) of the National Institutes of Health (NIH) provide other sources of information on a wide range of complementary and alternative therapies (http://nccam.nih.gov/health/bytreatment.htm). Its funding of investigator-initiated research and other programmatic initiatives has begun building a solid foundation from which therapies can be delivered with growing confidence in their safety and efficacy (http://nccam.nih.gov/research/nccamfunds.htm). However, there is much work to be done. The ideal evidence base for complementary therapies would support decision making in a broad range of complex patient situations. It would differentiate effects on persons with diverse characteristics and from various cultures, and would outline the potential differing effects and indications for persons suffering the full range of pathologies and medical conditions.

There are legitimate safety concerns related to therapy selection, quality of the product (the purity or technique of delivery), amount administered, dose, timing, duration, and other considerations related to specific therapies such as herbal therapies, nutraceuticals, and supplements. For example, research is needed to identify potentially adverse drug-herb interactions. Research is also needed to provide data to document the relative risks and benefits for therapies such as the use of diet therapy for hypertension (as opposed to standard allopathic pharmacologic therapies), or to consider benefits of the potential reduction of allopathic agents with side effects when used in combination with a complementary therapy.

The growing evidence base can provide much of the needed information for the consumer and provider. However, additional research is needed to determine the beneficial outcomes of complementary therapies. Alternatively, studies are needed to generate findings that protect the public from harm or from needless, costly therapies that have no evidence to support them, or evidence that clearly shows no benefit. For example, therapies such as the use of laetril to combat cancer caused concern among allopathic providers who feared that the false hope of cure would dissuade patients from seeking legitimate forms of cancer therapy while bleeding fortunes from desperate families, despite the fact that there was no basis for its claims of beneficial effects (Pinn, 2001). Extramural funding opportunities and the peer review system of NIH ensure the continued accumulation of high quality evidence and encourages investigators with ideas, curiosity, and scientific expertise to explore potential therapies for human use.

RESEARCH DESIGNS FOR COMPLEMENTARY THERAPIES

Most theorists would agree that the most rigorous design to test complementary and alternative therapies is the randomized, placebo-controlled, double-blind design that has long been the standard for testing therapies and advancing fields of inquiry (Duley & Farrell, 2002; Fogg & Gross, 2000; IOM, 2002). However, it is not the only type of design that provides useful information, nor are data generated from research the only available evidence base for practice. Other sources of evidence are also important and contribute to our knowledge and understanding of patients' responses to therapies, both allopathic and non-allopathic.

Consumers may be increasingly reluctant to enroll in clinical trials; therefore alternative study designs and strategies for the conduct of clinical research to advance the field may be necessary (Gross & Fogg, 2001). The Committee on the Use of Complementary and Alternative Medicine by the American Public was commissioned by the Institute of Medicine, the Agency for Health Care Quality & Research, NCCAM, and 15 other agencies and institutes of NIH to study and provide specific recommendations regarding complementary and alternative therapies. As part of their report (IOM, 2002), innovative designs that could be used to provide information about the effectiveness of therapies were identified, including

- *Preference RCTs:* trials that include randomized and non-randomized arms, which then permit comparisons between patients who chose a particular treatment and those who were randomly assigned to it

- *Observational and cohort studies:* studies that involve the identification of patients who are eligible for study and who may receive a specified treatment as part of the study

- *Case-control studies*: studies that involve identifying patients who have good or bad outcomes, then "working back" to find aspects of treatment associated with those differing outcomes

- *Studies of bundles of therapies:* analyses of the effectiveness, as a whole, of particular packages of treatments

- *Studies that specifically incorporate, measure, or account for placebo or expectation effects:* patients' hopes, emotional states, energies, and other self-healing processes are not considered extraneous but are included as part of the therapy's main "mechanism of action"

- *Attribute-treatment interaction analyses:* a way of accounting for differences in effectiveness outcomes among patients within a study and among different studies of varying design (p. 3).

Another important area that continues to challenge investigators involves the placebo effect and placebo/attention control groups (Gross, 2005). The placebo effect has been studied in areas of pain and analgesia, neuroimmunology, fear, anxiety, and pharmacotherapy and may have the capacity to stimulate dramatic healing (Harrington, 1997). The power of placebos should not be underestimated (Turner, Deyo, Loesser, Von Korff, & Fordyce, 1994). Placebo effects may lead to improvements in well over 50% of subjects in trials of medical therapies. Methods to manage placebo effects must be carefully considered in research on complementary therapies. In addition, when assessing the overall effects of a therapy, the impact of the healer him- or herself must be considered in terms of what the healer or the therapeutic relationship adds to the outcome (Quinn, Smith, Ritenbaugh, Swanson, & Watson, 2003).

Complementary therapies are often administered in the context of other therapies. This makes it challenging to differentiate the effects of the complementary therapies from those of other therapies simultaneously given, at the same time dissecting out effects of other concomitant disease processes and their treatments. There is a need for studies on the cost effectiveness of complementary therapies, and for research that compares complementary therapies with each other and with other conventional therapies (IOM, 2002). Studies of therapies relevant to aging populations, populations at varied developmental stages, and those having varied cultural backgrounds are also needed. These populations present challenges for the design, recruitment, and implementation of studies. Elderly subjects often have multiple comorbidities and may be taking multiple medications. Language and lack of cultural understanding may post barriers to the inclusion of new immigrants. Access to young children, adolescents, vulnerable adults, and their unique ethical issues may also be perceived as barriers to the inclusion of these groups.

There are other outcomes sought by health care consumers. That a therapy is shown to have beneficial health effects is not the only legitimate reason for its use. Therapies may have cultural significance or be intricately tied with healing traditions; therapies may lead to patients' peace of mind; they may meet patient and family expectations, or lead to their increased satisfaction. In considering the use of complementary therapies, the costs, risks, and value to recipients must be carefully weighed.

CURRENT STATE OF RESEARCH ON COMPLEMENTARY THERAPIES

As previously noted, chapter authors have identified the need to generate more research in order to provide more knowledge to guide practice. Specific research challenges include the need for data-based decision support resources for the combination of therapies. There is a need for research to be conducted with special populations including children, frail elders, and the critically ill. Research is needed to study the effects of complementary therapies in specific health conditions or disease states. Clearly, research lags behind the public's appetite for the therapies; knowledge of the putative mechanisms of action, the qualities of therapies, and the predictability of outcomes is uneven across therapies. The IOM report, *Complementary and Alternative Therapies in the United States* (IOM, 2004), provides perhaps the most comprehensive, authoritative, and up-to-date summary of the research and knowledge base in the field. The report provides an assessment of what is known about complementary and alternative therapies and their use; it also proposes research methods and priorities for research and product evaluation.

Insistence on the use of standard conventions of scientific inquiry has been helpful in increasing the amount of evidence that has been systematically obtained to provide information for decision making in complementary therapies. However, there is a lack of information on the appropriate dose and timing of interventions and for whom the interventions may have the most beneficial effects. A solid evidence base for complementary therapies would support decision making in broad and complex patient situations. Complementary therapies may have different effects on people of diverse ethnic backgrounds and demographic characteristics. So, too, they may have potentially different indications and effects in persons suffering differing pathologies or medical conditions. The lack of such information is limiting to practitioners who rely on a more fully developed evidence base and may hinder the full integration of the use of complementary therapies in practice.

The National Center for Complementary and Alternative Medicine (NCCAM), established by Congress in 1999, has as its mission the exploration of "complementary and alternative healing practices in the context of rigorous science, training CAM researchers, and disseminating authoritative information to the public and professional community" (NCCAM, 2005, p. 2). As previously mentioned, the NCCAM site (http://nccam.nih .gov) provides updated online information about the research conducted in the area of these therapies. It also provides a listing of clinical trials, alphabetized by the name of the therapies, further organized by the five domains of complementary and alternative therapies (the same NCCAM domains that organize the chapters in the five sections of this book). The work of this Center promises to increase the scientific evidence base and improve the context and delivery of therapies in years to come.

Studies have been done that have small sample sizes; meta-analyses can be conducted on such studies to synthesize findings to estimate effect-size of therapies when examined across studies. More of this type of work is also needed in addition to basic research.

IMPLICATIONS FOR NURSING RESEARCH, EDUCATION, AND PRACTICE

There is a great need for nurses and scientists in other disciplines to develop ongoing programs of research related to complementary therapies. As primary care providers, nurses are in a good position to address patients' requests and the need for complementary therapies. Nurses have a vested interest in generating information that can be used to build the knowledge database underlying the use of therapies that may benefit patients. They may also generate data that refute the use of therapies or reveal adverse risk/benefit ratios. Nurses have conducted research on a number of complementary therapies. Most doctorally prepared nurses are schooled in both qualitative and quantitative designs. This gives them an understanding of multiple ways to approach designs of complementary therapies. The need for the expansion and dissemination of evidence and access to it has particular significance for the discipline of nursing and underlies recommendations for future directions in nursing research, education, and practice.

Implications for Nursing Research

The need to generate information that can be used to provide complementary therapies in an informed manner is compelling for nurse scientists.

Specialized clinical expertise of nurse researchers can be used to select therapies to test and to target outcomes of importance to their patient populations. Specialized clinical knowledge has the potential to enhance the identification of instruments that are sensitive enough to assess potential effects of therapies (subjective, objective, or behavioral).

The *Research Teams of the Future* program of the National Institutes of Health (NIH) is an initiative to harness and extend advances in science through interdisciplinary research (NIH, 2004). In keeping with this program, interdisciplinary collaborations between nurse investigators and investigators from other disciplines who bring strengths from basic science, genetics, complementary therapies, or clinical practice may lead to growth of the knowledge base and its breadth, depth, and relevance, which should ultimately improve the quality of care for patients.

Broadening frames of references to include global perspectives and information from around the world will ensure an appropriate and comprehensive view of the field. The World Health Organization (2002) has launched a global strategic initiative to assist countries in blending complementary therapies with the countries' established health care systems. Such global initiatives should serve as catalysts in making information available to practitioners worldwide, and should move the field of complementary/alternative medicine forward. New, emerging, and continually refined technologies aid in the dissemination of information. Electronic means of posting new knowledge, warnings, or updated information on clinical trials speeds the availability of information and literally has the potential to bring a world of information to bear on practice—but only if this mode is utilized. Electronic publishing reduces the time to publication and increases accessibility of research findings. The mandate set by medical publishers (DeAngelis et al., 2004) to enroll in a registry of clinical trials if investigators desire to publish the results of their clinical trials in highly distinguished medical journals is also a step in the right direction.

Clinical research is costly. However, nurse-investigators' grant-writing skills and tireless efforts to pursue needed funds for investigative work pay off in the generation of advances in the field. Design skills that permit nurse investigators to effectively test interventions and advance clinical knowledge in the use of complementary therapies are critical. However, research conducted in non-clinical settings, including surveys of public use of complementary therapies, is also important. Nursing research is also needed to focus on the costs, relative cost benefits, and ethical issues surrounding access to and delivery of therapies.

Implications for Nursing Education

The implications of the increasing public use and the expanding knowledge base underlying complementary therapies has significance for nursing education. Nurses must become familiar with the wide range of practices in complementary therapies in order to safeguard the public and their patients. Nurses are often asked for advice regarding therapies. Curricula must therefore provide them with a general, working understanding of therapies and patient use, and knowledge about information resources for reference or for referral for patients' use (Chlan & Halcón, 2003). Further, the IOM report (IOM, 2004) recommends that all health professional schools incorporate information related to complementary therapies at all levels so that they may "competently advise their patients" about these therapies (p. 8). Nurses must prepare to access needed information electronically, to interpret information, and to apply that information to a range of patients and complex conditions. Well-honed critical thinking skills need to be informed by the best available knowledge base. Student nurses must explore the use of complementary therapies in patient histories and physicals so that the potential effects of the therapies on patients may be adequately determined. A case example of a CRNA who was prepared in a graduate curriculum that familiarized students with broad health care practices including complementary therapies illustrates the value of such a curriculum.

> In a county hospital where patients with a broad range of cultures and health practices are frequently encountered, a former graduate student reported that a patient presented for biopsy with her "healer." None of the anesthesia care providers were willing to incorporate the desire of the patient to have her healer in the operating room during the surgical procedure. The former student, familiar with a range of complementary therapies and having developed a level of comfort in the spectrum of health practices and choices from his curricular experience, accommodated the patient and agreed to provide anesthesia in the presence of the healer, who practiced a healing method with her hands throughout the surgery. The former student reported afterward that he had never experienced a case during which he had administered so little anesthesia and during which the patient's blood pressure remained so stable.

Exposure of health professional students to the public's interest in therapies and the broad range of therapies that are considered complementary will benefit them in their future practice. Such exposure can prepare nurses to expect, understand, and become more sensitive to cultural practices and preferences for and uses of culturally based complementary therapies. Knowledge of cultural practices helps to interpret findings in the physical assessment of patients. For example, moxibustion and coining, health-related practices used by some Southeast Asian cultures, leave marks on the body from rubbing or burning. Without health care professionals' appreciation of such cultural practices, these marks on patients' bodies are likely to be interpreted as some form of abuse.

Implications for Nursing Practice

Nursing is a practice discipline. The potential for nurses to encounter the use of complementary therapies by patients is significant and growing. Effective dialogue regarding the broad range of therapies available and used by patients requires clear and frank communication between providers and patients so that the integration of allopathic and complementary/alternative therapies can be safe and beneficial, leading to the achievement of mutually identified desired outcomes. With an exchange of information, patient education, and appropriate management of therapies, adverse or untoward effects of incompatible therapies and side effects of therapies may be prevented, detected early, or identified and effectively managed.

In practice, it is clear that the relationship between patient and provider must be a partnership. Patient disclosure of therapies used may help to elucidate any contributions of these therapies to the presenting condition; the potential of therapies to aid the patient can also be better evaluated. In the context of the patient–provider relationship, information can be exchanged to inform patients of potential risks and benefits of both allopathic and non-allopathic remedies. Patients' practices and preferences can be discussed and factored into the plan of care.

Health care providers have responsibilities to provide the public with guidance in use; to share information; to interpret scientific information; and to contribute to the knowledge base through investigation, research utilization, and patient counseling. Making optimal use of available knowledge and methods to disseminate research electronically and making information available at the point of care are important.

Nurses in practice settings are in key positions to assess patient needs and to administer complementary therapies judged, from the evidence base, to be beneficial. Nurses administer the therapies or refer patients to qualified providers to receive specific therapies. Boards of nursing across the United States have taken positions regarding nurses' use of complementary therapies in practice (Sparber, 2001). In Minnesota, the Board of Nursing recognizes that nurses are providers of complementary therapies and that they have been administering these therapies for hundreds of years. The State Practice Act is permissive of nurses' inclusion of complementary therapies. Recommendations of the Board for nurses' use of complementary therapies include, among other things: the willingness and consent of the patient and/or family, competence in administration of therapies, safe administration of therapies, and the sharing of the use of complementary therapies with other members of the health care team (Minnesota State Board of Nursing, 2003).

Teamwork, the exchange of information across providers, patient referral to specialized complementary care providers, and sharing experience of therapies between disciplines ensure that the care provided to the patient is coordinated across disciplinary lines. However, practice guidelines are clearly needed to set competency standards for appropriate use of complementary therapies (IOM, 2004).

Imagine the future with a new culture of care: one that is open and that offers patient-centered care, where care is viewed from the lens of the patient experience and couples the best of Western medicine with the best of available non-allopathic remedies. The exploration of therapeutic options includes the consideration of allopathic and non-allopathic remedies by patients and their providers, followed by the evaluation of the outcomes of the therapies selected. With the explosive increase in the use of complementary therapies, there will be new and interesting therapies explored and adopted based on evidence that supports their efficacy. Imagination aside, new information regarding the health practices of immigrant groups, increased global sharing of healing practices, and the public's appetite for new ways to achieve better health, to effect cures, or to forestall aging, all guarantee that the future of nursing practice will be interesting.

REFERENCES

Chlan, L., & Halcón, L. (2003). Developing an integrated baccalaureate nursing education program infusing complementary/alternative therapies into critical care curricula. *Critical Care Nursing Clinics of North America, 15*(3), 373–379.

DeAngelis, C. D., Drazen, J. M., Frizelle, F. A., Haug, C., Hoey, J., Horton, R., et al. (2004). Clinical trial registration: A statement from the International Committee of Medical Journal Editors. *Journal of the American Medical Association, 292*(11), 1363–1364.

Duley, L., & Farrell, B. (Eds.). (2002). *Clinical trials.* London: BMJ Books.

Fogg, L., & Gross, D. (2000). Threats to validity in randomized clinical trials. *Research in Nursing & Health, 23,* 79–87.

Gross, D. (2005). On the merits of attention-control groups. *Research in Nursing & Health, 28,* 93–94.

Gross, D., & Fogg, L. (2001). Clinical trials in the 21st century: The case for participant-centered research. *Research in Nursing & Health, 24,* 530–539.

Harrington, A. (1997). Introduction. In A. Harrington (Ed.), *The placebo effect: An interdisciplinary exploration* (pp. 1–11). Cambridge, MA: Harvard University Press.

Institute of Medicine. (2004). *Complementary and alternative medicine (CAM) in the United States* (Executive Summary, pp. 1–11). Washington, DC: The National Academies Press.

Institute of Medicine, Committee on the Use of Complementary and Alternative Medicine by the American Public. (2002). *Executive summary: Complementary and alternative medicine in the United States.* Washington, DC: National Academy Press. Retrieved from http://books.nap.edu/catalog/11182.html

Lindquist, R., Tracy, M. F., & Savik, K. (2003). Personal use of complementary and alternative therapies by critical care nurses. *Critical Care Nursing Clinics of North America, 15*(3), 393–399.

McKibbon, K. A. (1998). Evidence based practice. *Bulletin of the Medical Library Association, 86*(3), 396–401.

Minnesota State Board of Nursing. (2003). *Statement of accountability for utilization of integrative therapies in nursing practice.* Retrieved from www.state.mn.us/mn/externalDocs/Integrative_Therapies_Statement_050703032848_Accountabilies.pdf

National Center for Complementary and Alternative Medicine. (n.d.). *Executive summary: Our mission.* Retrieved May 29, 2005, from http://nccam.nih.gov/about/plans/2005/page2.htm

National Institutes of Health. (2004, February). NIH roadmap for medical research: A briefing by the NIH director and senior staff, February 27, 2004. Retrieved May 29, 2005, from http://nihroadmap.nih.gov/briefing/executive summary.asp

Pinn, G. (2001). Herbal medicine in oncology. *Australian Family Physician, 30*(6), 575–580.

Quinn, J. F., Smith, M., Ritenbaugh, C., Swanson, K., & Watson, M. J. (2003). Research guidelines for assessing the impact of the healing relationship in clinical nursing. *Alternative Therapies in Health and Medicine, 9*(3), SuppA65–79.

Sparber, A. (2001). State boards of nursing and scope of practice of registered nurses performing complementary therapies. *Online Journal of Issues in Nursing, 6*(3), manuscript 10. Retrieved from www.nursingworld.org/ojin/topics/tpc15_6.htm

Turner, J., Deyo, R., Loesser, J., Von Korff, J., & Fordyce, W. E. (1994). The importance of placebo effects in pain treatment and research. *Journal of the American Medical Association, 271*(10), 1609–1614.

World Health Organization. (2002). *WHO traditional medicine strategy: 2002–2005.* Geneva: World Health Organization. Retrieved May 29, 2005, from www.who.int/medicines/library/trm/trm_strat_eng.pdf

Index

Aboriginal peoples, native medicines, 15
Abstract, defined, 154
Accepting attitude, in therapeutic listening, 49
Acne, 345
Active imagery, 60
Active listening, 7–8, 35, 45–46
Active presence, 49
Activities of daily living (ADLs), 305–306
Acupressure
applications, 190, 264–266, 283, 285
client assessment, 261, 263
defined, 255–256
effects, evaluation of, 263
future research directions, 267
interventions, 261–263
point stimulation, 263–266
precautions, 266–267
scientific basis, 257–261
Traditional Chinese Medicine (TCM), 256–259, 261
Acupressure Potent Points, 266
Acupuncture
characterized, 8, 11, 16, 228, 259, 283
herbal medicines and, 352
insurance coverage, 6
points, 257
Acute care facilities, 177, 182, 291
Acute pain, 215, 343. *See also* Pain management; Pain reduction strategies

Adaptation, 85, 177
Adaptive coping, 122
Adaptive regression, 131
Addiction treatment, 82, 150, 249, 259
Adherence, 51
Adolescents
animal-assisted therapy, 178
aromatherapy, 343, 345–347
biofeedback techniques, 125–126
imagery sessions, 62–63
music interventions, 87
nutraceutical use, 375
overweight, 303–304
therapeutic listening, and, 50
utilization of complementary therapies, 5–6
Adoration prayers, 144
Adrenaline levels, 343
Adrenocorticothropin-releasing hormone (ACTH), 61
Adult-onset diabetes, 295
Advocacy, 11, 354
Aerobic exercise, 296, 300–302
Affective disorders, 304–305
African American population, storytelling, 153–154, 157
Age differences, music interventions, 83
Agency for Health Care Quality & Research, 386
Aggression, reduction of, 291
Agitation, 213, 216, 233, 343
Agoraphobia, 139
AIDS patients, 145, 243

Aikido, 130
Air, in traditional Chinese medicine, 16
Alcohol, terpenic, 336
Alcoholics Anonymous (AA), 161
Alcoholism, 145
Aldehydes, 336
Allergies, 339, 358
Allopathic therapies, 384–385, 392
Almond oil, 18
Alternate Nostril Breathing (ANB), 110
Altruism, 38
Alzheimer's patients, 178, 213, 232–233, 261–262, 345, 359
Ambulation, 177. *See also* Movement disorders
American Botanical Council, 356
American College of Sports Medicine, 299, 307
American Dietetic Association, 374
American Heart Association (AHA), 299, 307, 370
American Holistic Nurses Association (AHNA)
　Code of Ethics, 25
　functions of, 204, 219, 343
　Standards of Practice, 11
American Massage Therapy Association, 285
American Medical Association (AMA), 59
American Music Therapy Association, 82
American Nurses Association, Code of Ethics, 11
American Nutraceutical Association, 356
American Psychiatric Association, 59
Amyotrophic lateral sclerosis, 249
Anaerobic metabolism, 296
Anesthesia, 86
Angelica, herbal medicine, 345
Anger reduction, 209
Angina, 318
Animal-assisted therapy (AAT)
　animal qualification criteria, 182
　applications, 183–184

　benefits of, 175, 177
　defined, 176–177
　future research directions, 184
　guidelines for, 180–181
　historical perspectives, 175–176
　information resources, 184
　interventions, 179–182
　outcomes measurement, 180, 182
　patient qualification criteria, 181
　precautions, 182
　scientific basis, 177–179
Aniseed, 344
Ankh, 189, 206
Ankles, magnet therapy, 197
Antibiotics, 340, 351
Anticoagulants, 355, 359
Antidepressants, 344, 355, 361
Antiemesis, 259
Antihypertensives, 355
Anxiety reduction therapies
　benefits of, 16
　biofeedback benefits, 120
　exercise, 304–305
　Healing Touch (HT), 206, 208–209, 215–216
　imagery techniques, 60, 65
　journaling, 170–171
　meditation, 129, 137–139
　muscle relaxation, 328, 330
　music interventions, 83, 85–87
　prayer, 147, 150
　presence, 41
　reflexology, 277–279
　Reiki, 246, 249
　Saint John's wort, 360
　storytelling, 155, 160
　therapeutic listening, 51
　therapeutic humor, 99, 101–102
　Therapeutic Touch (TT), 229, 233–238
　yoga, 110
APIC-Infection Control and Applied Epidemiology, 182
Appetite, improvement of, 207, 279
Aquariums, benefits of, 179
Archetypal understanding, 30
Aromatherapy, *see* Essential oils
　applications, 343–347

benefits of, 9–10, 16, 333–334
clinical, 336
credentialing, 341
defined, 335–336
future research directions, 347
herbal medicines and, 352
historical perspectives, 335
information resources, 347
inhalation, 337–338
intervention, 337–343
massage therapy and, 285, 287, 292
outcomes measurement, 339–340
poisoning, accidental, 346
precautions, 340–341, 346
risks of, 341
topical applications, 338–339
Aromatherapy Registration Council, 341
"Around the platter," Tai Chi movement, 316–317
Arousal response, through massage, 287
Arrhythmia, 198, 300, 318
Arteriosclerosis, 276
Arthritis, 191, 196, 218, 235, 277, 319. See also Osteoarthritis; Rheumatoid arthritis
Arthrodesis patients, 197
Art therapy, 5
Asana, 108
Asian medical systems, traditional, 352. See also Traditional Chinese Medicine (TCM)
Aspirin, 351
Assessment skills, 8, 99–100, 146–147, 229–230, 236, 261, 263, 373
Association for Applied and Therapeutic Humor, 94
Asteraceae, 358
Asthma, 113, 120, 123, 137, 258–259, 265, 339, 345
Atherosclerosis, 370
Attention deficit disorder, 124
Attention deficit hyperactivity disorder (ADHD), 113, 347
Attention span, improvement techniques, 177

Attentiveness, in presence, 38–40
Auditory stimulation, 177
Auricular acupressure, 262
Auriculotherapy, 256, 259
Autism, 87, 183, 344
Autoimmune disease, 358
Autonomic nervous system (ANS), 85, 109, 118, 167
Autonomous nursing biofeedback, 119
Autonomy, 51
Availability-in-a-helping-way, 36
Awakening, in Tibetan medicine, 17
Awareness, with yoga, 108
Ayurvedic medicine, 5, 15, 17–18, 192

Baccalaureate nursing programs, 10
Back problems, relief from, 279. See also Low back pain
Back rub, see Massage
Bacterial infection, 344
Balance
   improvement therapies, 6, 113, 183, 196, 210, 214, 217, 279, 299, 315, 319
   in Native American traditions, 19
   in Tibetan medicine, 18
Balanced diet, significance of, 367–368. See also Functional foods; Nutraceuticals
Barbiturates, 340
Basic Healing Touch (HT) sequence, 209
Basil, in aromatherapy, 342, 345
Baystate Medical Center (Springfield, MA), 179
Beck's Depression Inventory, 214
Behavior patterns, 207
Behavioral problems, 344
Belladonna, 19
Belongingness, 160
Beneficence, 21
Bereavement, 233–234, 345
Bergamot, 340, 344
Beta-carotene, 359, 369
Bile, in traditional Tibetan medicine, 17

Biochemical changes, sources of, 61
Bioelectromagnetic therapies, 190
Biofeedback
    applications, 5, 124–126
    defined, 117–118
    efficacy research, 124–125
    future research directions, 126–127
    insurance coverage, 6
    intervention, 119–124
    outcome measurement, 122–123
    parameters used, 123
    protocol, 120–122
    scientific basis, 118
    technique, 119–120
Biofeedback Certification Institute of
        America (AAPB), 119, 123–124
Biofield therapies, see Energy/biofield
        therapies
Biologically-based therapies
    aromatherapy, 335–347
    functional foods, 367–376
    herbal medicines, 351–361
    nutraceuticals, 367–376
    overview of, 5, 333–334
Biomedical treatment settings, 249
Biomedicine, 15, 19
Biophysiological testing, 47
Black pepper, in aromatherapy, 344
Bleeding, internal, 211
Blood flow, 193
Blood glucose levels, 123, 213
Blood pressure, improvement
        therapies
    animal-assisted therapy (AAT),
        178, 180
    aromatherapy, 343
    biofeedback techniques, 122–123,
        126
    exercise program benefits, 298–299
    Healing Touch (HT) techniques,
        213
    meditation, 138
    massage, 286
    muscle relaxation, 324, 328–330
    presence, 37
    therapeutic humor, 97
    yoga, 113
    Tai Chi, 319
    yoga, 113

Body image, 184
Body postures, 18
Body scan meditation, 133
Body work, 5
Bone healing, 195–197
Bone marrow transplantation, 87,
        233
Botanicals, see Herbal medicines
Brain imaging, 131
Breast cancer, 277, 371
Breast-feeding, herbal medicines and,
        355, 361
Breathing
    breath control in yoga, 108–110
    deep, 315–316
    deep belly, 204
    disciplined, 17
    exercises, 62, 84
    Healing Touch (HT) techniques,
        209
    imagery technique, 66, 68
    muscle relaxation techniques,
        325–327
Breeding, 368
Bronchitis, 258, 265, 345
Buddhism/Buddhist meditation, 17,
        130
Burn care, 86–87, 233, 235, 266,
        345
Burnout prevention, 161, 250

Calcium, nutraceuticals, 368, 375
Cananga odorata, 347
Cancer patients
    acupressure, 267
    energy work with, 214
    functional foods/nutraceuticals,
        368, 374
    Healing Touch (HT) applications,
        206–208, 213, 215–216
    herbal medicines, 361
    imagery interventions, 69–71
    journaling, 171
    magnet therapy, 196
    massage therapy, 292
    meditation effects, 137
    muscle relaxation techniques,
        329–330

music interventions, 86–87
prayer effectiveness, 150
reflexology, 277–278
Reiki, 243, 248
storytelling techniques, 156–157
therapeutic humor, 98, 102
yoga, 113
Candida albicans, 346
Caraway, 344
Cardamom, 344
Cardiac output (CO), 297
Cardiac/cardiovascular patients
    animal-assisted therapy (AAT), 178
    aromatherapy, 344
    biofeedback, 123
    exercise programs, 304
    functional foods/nutraceuticals,
        368
    Healing Touch (HT) techniques,
        213
    herbal medicines, 353
    massage therapy, 286
    music interventions, 86–87
    prayer and, 145
    Tai Chi, 319
    therapeutic humor, 97–98
    Therapeutic Touch, 234
Cardiac rehabilitation (CR), 305,
    329–330
Care coordination, 161
Care planning, 37, 334
Caregiver(s)
    family as, 156
    prayer and, 150
    storytelling techniques, 156
    stress alleviation through yoga, 113
Caring, storytelling techniques,
    159–160
Caring-based approaches, 8
Carotid artery, 198
Carotid atherosclerosis, 137
Carpal tunnel syndrome, 113, 259
Cartesian philosophy, 6
Case-control studies, 387
Catecholamine levels, 97–98, 343
Cause-effect model, 217
Centering
    benefits of, 37, 39

Healing Touch (HT), 204
imagery techniques, 62
prayer, 132–134
Therapeutic Touch (TT), 228–229
Central nervous system, 315
Certification requirements, 9–10, 205
Ch'i, 244
Chakra, in Reiki, 247
Chakra Connection, 210
Chakra Spread, 210–211
Chamaemelum nobile, 347
Chamomile, aromatherapy, 342, 358
Change-oriented reflective listening,
    50
Chanting, 18
Chemical addictions, 82, 249
Chemotherapy, 86–87, 206, 259–
    260, 340, 361
Chen, Tai Chi style, 314
Cherokee Indians, 20
Chest pain/fullness/dyspnea, 125, 258
Chi, 206, 314
Children
    animal-assisted therapy, 178–179,
        182
    aromatherapy, 343–347
    biofeedback techniques, 124–126
    energy field of, 214
    exercise and, 296
    Healing Touch (HT) benefits, 207,
        216
    herbal medicine, 355
    hippotherapy, 183
    imagery applications, 60, 62–63,
        67
    juvenile diabetes, 372
    magnet therapy, 198
    music interventions, 85–87
    nutraceutical use, 375
    obesity in, 296
    overweight, 303–304
    storytelling techniques used with,
        156–157, 161
    therapeutic humor, 98
    therapeutic listening and, 50
    utilization of complementary thera-
        pies, 5–6
Chiropractic care, 5–6, 283

Cholesterol levels, 352, 368, 370
Chondroitin sulfate, 371
Christianity/Christian faith
  prayers for, 148
  spiritual direction, 28–29
Chronically ill patients, Healing
    Touch (HT), 214, 218
Chronic fatigue, 110. *See also* Fa-
    tigue; Sleep disorders
Chronic illness, 170–171, 214, 218,
    243, 319
Chronic obstructive pulmonary disor-
    der (COPD), 262, 319, 329
Chronic pain, *see* Pain management;
    Pain reduction therapies
  aromatherapy, 343
  biofeedback techniques, 122, 125
  Healing Touch (HT), 209, 215
  imagery effects, 60
  meditation effects on, 136–138
  muscle relaxation techniques, 330
  music interventions, 86
Chronic Pain Experience Instrument,
    214
Chronic pouchitis, 372
"Chuckle wagon," 100
Church attendance, 146
Circulatory system, 191, 336
Citrus bergamia, 340
Citrus peel oils, 336
Citrus reticulata, 347
Clary sage, aromatherapy benefits,
    342, 344–345
Classical music, 83–84
Classification for complementary ther-
    apies, 5
Classic of Internal Medicine, 191
Claudication, fitness walking pro-
    gram, 305–306
Clinical studies
  biofeedback, 124
  magnet therapy, 197
  meditation, 137
  music interventions, 88
  Therapeutic Touch (TT), 233
Clove, aromatherapy benefits, 344
Coca, 19
Cochrane Database of Systematic Re-
    views, 385

Coda, in storytelling, 154
Coenzyme Q10 (CoQ10), 371–372
Cohort studies, 386
Coining, 391
Colic, 344, 347
Collagen hydrolysate, 371
Colloquial prayer, 144
Colon cancer, 295
Colonoscopy, 87
Color therapy, 5
Colorado Center for Healing Touch,
    219
Coma, 346
Committee on the Use of Complemen-
    tary and Alternative Medicine,
    386
Common cold, 265
Communication Institute for Online
    Scholarship, 52
Communication skills
  storytelling, 157–159
  therapeutic humor and, 102
  therapeutic listening, 46–47
  verbalization, 177
Community, storytelling techniques,
    160
Community-dwelling adults/elderly,
    156, 178, 318–319
Community hospitals, 215
Comorbidity, 387
Companion animals, *see* Animal-
    assisted therapy (AAT)
Companion dogs, 183
Compassion, 28
Compassionate listening, 21
Complementary/alternative therapies,
    generally
  classification of, 4–5
  defined, 3–4
  efficacy of, 7
  goal of, 6
  implications for nursing, 8–12
  philosophical perspectives, 6
  utilization of, 4–8
*Complementary and Alternative Medi-
    cine in the United States,* 376
Complicating action, in storytelling,
    154

Compresses, hot/cold, 16
Concentration, in yoga, 109
Confidentiality, 51
Conflict, generally
  management, 171
  resolution, 161
Congestive heart failure (CHF), 371
Connective tissue, 192
Consciousness, 25, 226
Constipation, 125, 265, 344
Consumer information, resources for, 9
Continuing education programs, 10, 94
Conversational distance, 49
Cool down, exercise program, 301–302
Coping skills, development of, 95–96, 98, 122, 139, 183
Coronary artery disease, 137, 299
Coronary care units, 137
Coronary heart disease (CHD), 295, 305
"Corpse Pose," 110–111
Corticotropin-releasing hormone (CRH), 61
Cortisol levels, 238
Council for Responsible Nutrition (2004), 351–352
Counseling
  psychological, 176
  referrals to, 51
  stress-management, 119
Cramps, 344
Creative writing, 167, 170
Creativity, 159, 171
Cree Indians, 20, 157
Critical-care nursing, presence applications, 38, 41
Critical care patients, 179, 291
Critical thinking skills, 256, 391
Crohn's disease, 358, 372
Cultural differences
  acupressure, 259, 261
  biofeedback techniques, 126
  energy systems, 206
  music interventions, 81, 83–84
  in storytelling, 161–162

therapeutic humor, 101
therapeutic listening and, 51
Cun, in acupressure, 263
Curanderismo, 5
Curare, 19
Cycling, 300
Cyclosporine, 360
Cypress, 344–345
Cystitis, 344
Cytochrome P450, 360

Daisies, 358
Dalai Lama, 17, 28
Decision making, 6, 177
Deep breathing exercises, 84
Deep tissue massage, 286
Defense mechanisms, 102. See also
  Coping skills
Deficiency, in reflexology, 274
Degenerative diseases, 218
Delta Society, 182, 184
Dementia, 156, 213, 343, 358–359
Depression, symptom reduction
    therapies
  exercise, 304
  Healing Touch (HT), 213, 215, 217
  herbal medicines and, 357
  imagery techniques, 65, 70
  journaling, 171
  magnet therapy, 196
  meditation, 136–137, 139
  muscle relaxation, 329–330
  music intervention, 80
  prayer, 145–146, 150
  reflexology, 278
  Reiki, 248
  Saint John's wort and, 360
  therapeutic listening, 51
  yoga, 113
Dermatology problems, aromatherapy, 345
Desensitization, 131
Despair, 299
Detraining, in exercise program, 301
Dharana, 109
Dhyana, 109
Diabetes, generally

Diabetes, generally *(continued)*
  characterized, 113, 276, 295
  diabetic neuropathy, 243
  diabetic retinopathy, 359
  mellitus, 122–123
  mellitus, Type 2, 303
  Type II, 298
Diagnostic techniques
  in Ayuvedic medicine, 18
  meditation and, 137
  in Samoan medicine, 19
  in Tibetan medicine, 17
Dialogue, *see* Communication skills
  nurse-patient, 36–37
  writing, 169
Diaper rash, 344
Diaphragm
  movement, 315
  spasms, 258
Diaries, *see* Journaling
Diarrhea, 265
Diazepam, 336–337
Dietary foods/supplements, 367–368, 373
Dietary modification, 304
Dietary Supplement Health and Education Act of 1994 (DSHEA), 352
Dietary supplements, 5, 333, 354, 385
Diet therapy, 5, 16, 26, 334
Digestive system, 198
Digoxin, 351, 355, 360
Directed imagery, 64
Directed prayer, 144
Disease control, 51
Disease prevention strategies, 16, 284
Distance healing, 247, 250
Distraction strategies, 85–87, 102
Divine intervention, 20
Dizziness, 198, 359
Dog ownership, 178–179
Dopamine, 19, 61, 360
Doshas, in Ayuvedic medicine, 18
Double-blind clinical trials, 12
Dreams, 30–31
Drug(s)
  abuse/use, 137, 209

addiction, 125
  delivery, transdermal/patch, 198
Drumming circle, 16, 20, 82
Dualistic philosophy, 6
Duration, in music intervention, 80
Dying patients, 214, 345. *See also* Hospice; Palliative care
Dypsnea, 296
Dysmenorrhea, 261–262

Ear acupuncture, 256
Earth, perceptions of
  in Ayuvedic medicine, 18
  in Native American medicine, 19
  in Traditional Chinese medicine (TCM), 16
Eastern medicine, 217
Echinacea
  augustofolia, 353, 357–358
  characterized, 353, 357
  pallida, 353, 357–358
  purpurea, 353, 357–358
E. coli, 346
Ecosystem effects, 19
Ecstasy, with yoga, 109
EEG neurofeedback, 122
Effleurage, 288
Elderly patients
  acupressure, 261–262
  animal-assisted therapy, 178, 182
  aromatherapy, 345
  energy field of, 214
  exercise program benefits, 299, 304, 306–307
  Healing Touch (HT), 207, 216
  storytelling with, 156
  Tai Chi benefits, 317–318
  Therapeutic Touch (TT), 235–236
Electrocardiograms, 245
Electroencephalography (EEG), 47, 65
Electroencephalograms, 245
Electromagnetic fields, 192
Electromyogram (EMG), 119, 121
Electronic Communication Journal, 52
Elements of Tai Chi, The, 316
Elimination disorders, 124

Emotional, generally
  awareness, 61
  care, aromatherapy, 345
  distress, 248
  functioning, presence and, 40
  healing, 30
  intelligence, 50
  therapies, 19
Emotions, in Latino traditional medicine, 21
Empathy
  empathic listening, 45, 47
  empathic rapport, 47
  importance of, 45, 51
  storytelling techniques, 159
Empowerment, 6, 249
Endorphins, 258, 324
End-state imagery, 64
Energetic laser, 211
Energetic ultrasound, 211
Energy/biofield therapies
  acupressure, 190, 255–267
  benefits of, 5
  healing touch, 203–219
  magnet therapy, 191–198
  overview of, 189–190
  reflexology, 190, 271–280
  Reiki, 190, 243–251
  therapeutic touch, 189, 225–239
Energy blockages, Healing Touch
  (HT) techniques, 204, 210–211
Energy congestion, Healing Touch
  (HT) techniques, 204, 209–212
Energy exchange, 217, 226
Energy field(s)
  hand scan, 207, 210–213
  research studies, 217
  symmetrical, 230
  Therapeutic Touch (TT), 225–233
Energy flow
  Healing Touch (HT) techniques,
    210
  imbalance in, 227, 230–231
Energy healing therapies, 26. See also
  Energy/biofield therapies
"Energy medicines," 228
Energy patterns, 205, 211
Energy transfer, 226

Enlightenment, in Tibetan medicine,
  17
Entrainment, 80–81
Environmental sensitivities, 209
Environmental setting, significance of,
  8, 49, 84, 134, 147–148, 158–
  159, 249, 287
Ephedra, 357
Epilepsy, 125
Equilibrium
  as goal, 177
  in Tibetan medicine, 18
Esalen massage, 286
Essential oils
  antimicrobial action of, 346
  applications, 343–344
  carcinogenic, 340
  characterized, 18, 333–334,
    336–337
  commonly used, 342
  defined, 336
  generally regarded as safe (GRAS)
    status, 340
  guidelines for, 339–340
  herbal medicines and, 352
  names, common and botanical, 342
  plant taxonomy, 342
  safety considerations, 340–341,
    346
  teratogenic, 340
  topical applications, 337–340
Ether, in Ayurvedic medicine, 18
Ethics/ethical behavior, 28, 108, 204
Ethnic differences
  biofeedback techniques, 126
  humor, 96–97
  music inventions, 83
  in utilization of therapies, 6
Ethnic humor, 96–97
Eucalyptus, for aromatherapy
  characterized, 342, 344, 346
  globulus, 345
  smithii, 344–345, 347
Evaluation, in storytelling, 154
Evidence-based practice (EBP), 11,
  384–386
Excess, in reflexology, 274
Exercise

Exercise *(continued)*
  benefits, 26, 146, 283–284
  defined, 296
  fitness walking, 301–303
  future research directions, 308
  goals for, 301
  information resources, 308
  injury avoidance strategies, 307
  intervention, 298–308
  outcomes measurement, 306–307
  precautions, 307–308
  scientific basis, 297–298
  techniques, 299–303
  therapeutic benefits of, 295–296,
    298
  in Tibetan medicine, 17

Falls, impact on elderly, 304, 319
Family, generally
  as caregivers, 156
  relationships, 139
  therapy, 160–161
Fasting, 18
Fatigue, reduction therapies, 291,
  296, 343, 347
Fear reduction
  Healing Touch (HT) techniques,
    209
  imagery techniques, 60
  journaling, 171
  meditation, 139
  music interventions and, 83
  prayer, 147
  therapeutic humor, 101–102
Fecal elimination disorder, 125
Feet
  acupressure, 262
  magnet therapy, 196–197
  massage, 291–292
  reflexology, *see* Reflexology
  spasms in, 325
  Therapeutic Touch (TT), 231
  in Traditional Chinese Medicine
    (TCM), 273
Fennel, for aromatherapy, 342, 344
Fennel seed oil emulsion, 347
Fenugreek, 355
Fiber, dietary, 367–368

Fibromyalgia, 137–138, 197, 218,
  233, 238, 243, 259
Fight-or-flight response, 61, 324
Fire
  in Ayuvedic medicine, 18
  in traditional Chinese medicine
    (TCM), 16
First Nations of Canada, 20
Fitzgerald, William H., Dr., 274
Focused journaling, 167, 169–170
Focusing Institute, 52
Folk remedies, 19
Follow-up referrals, 160
Food, *see* Functional foods; Nu-
    traceuticals
  additives, 333–334
  as medicine, 18
  processing technologies, 368
  supplements, 5
Forbidden points, 257
Formal humor, 96, 99
Four Medical Tantras, 17
Fractures, 197, 211, 232, 295
Framing, through storytelling, 161
Frankincense, aromatherapy,
  344–345
Free-flow writing, 167–169
Friction strokes, in massage, 288
Fright-illness rituals, 20
Full body techniques, Healing Touch
  (HT), 209–211
Full presence, 37
Functional abilities, 183, 207, 216,
  237
Functional foods
  benefits of, 367
  defined, 368
  examples of, 369
Functional magnetic resonance im-
  aging (fMRI), 131
Fungal infection, 344

Gallows humor, 96–97
Gamma aminobutyric acid (GABA),
  337, 360
Gastrointestinal disorders, 264, 344
Gate control theory, 286
Gattefosse, Maurice, 335

Gender differences, 6, 157. *See also* Women's health
Generally Recognized as Safe (GRAS), essential oils and/or foods, 370
Genetic engineering, 368
Genuineness, importance of, 45
Geranium, for aromatherapy, 342, 344
Gerbera, 17
German chamomile, 345
Germs, Samoan treatment of, 19
Ginger, for aromatherapy, 17, 342, 344–345, 347
Gingko/*Gingko biloba,* 357–359
Glucosamine, 371
Glucose, anaerobic metabolism of, 296
Glycolysis, 296
God
  perception of, 143–144
  relationship with, 28–30
Government regulation, *see* Legislation
Great Spirit, Native American medicine, 20
Grieving, 102. *See also* Bereavement
Grounding process, 231
Group exercise, 304
Guided imagery, 11, 59, 63–64, 68, 71
Gynecological problems, aromatherapy, 344

Haemophilus influenza, 346
Haiku, 170
Hall effect, 193
Hallucination, 136
Hamilton Depression Scale, 360
Hand(s)
  acupressure, 264–265
  gestures, Healing Touch (HT) techniques, 207
  massage, 289–290
  reflexology, 272, 276
Happiness, 182
Harmony
  as goal, 6–7, 15–16, 18, 25, 182

meditation and, 139
in music intervention, 79–80, 84
through Tai Chi, 313, 316
through yoga, 107–108, 111
Hayashi, Chujiro, 244
Head, generally
  injury, 85–86
  lice, 347
Headache(s), 120, 122–125, 137, 233–234, 237, 259, 279, 329, 359
Healing ceremonies, Native American medicine, 20
Healing circle, 155
Healing meditation, 226, 229
Healing process, 7–8, 217
Healing rituals, 19
Healing touch, 5, 8–11, 189
Healing Touch (HT)
  applications, 215–217
  benefits of, 214–215
  client feedback, 219
  defined, 204
  goal of, 217
  historical perspectives, 203
  information resources, 217, 219
  instrumentation, 217
  intervention techniques, 207–213
  outcomes measurement, 208, 213–214
  patient response, 208
  practitioner role, 204–205, 207–208
  practitioner training, 218
  precautions, 214–215
  research studies, 215–219
  scientific basis, 205–207
  training for, 204–205
Healing Touch International, 217, 219
Health, generally
  history, 8
  insurance coverage, 126
  promotion, 7, 146, 161–162, 205, 284, 329
  Tai Chi benefits, 318–319
  with yoga, 108
Health care industry

Health care industry *(continued)*
  costs/cost containment, 6, 87–88
  medical pluralism, 15
Health care teams, 393
Health maintenance organizations
  (HMOs), 6
Healthy People 2010, 295, 298, 301
Heart disease, 267, 305, 307–308,
  374
Heart rate, influential factors
  exercise program, 296–297, 300,
    302
  massage therapy, 286–287
  muscle relaxation therapy, 328,
    330
  therapeutic humor, 97
Hematology, 249
Herbal extracts, 340
Herbalists, 19–20
Herbal medicines, *see* Aromatherapy;
    Essential oils
  applications, 357–361
  benefits of, 16–19
  defined, 352–353
  future research directions, 361
  information resources, 353, 356
  intervention, 354–357
  precautions, 354–357
  research studies, 12
  safety considerations, 385
  scientific basis, 353–354
  standardization of, 353
  technique, 354
  utilization survey, 351–352
Herbal pills, 17–18
Herbal preparations, 9, 333–334
Herb-drug interactions, 355
Herb-herb interactions, 355
Herb Research Foundation, 356
Herpes simplex viruses, 346
Hiccups, 258
High blood pressure, *see* Hy-
    pertension
Higher Being
  perception of, 143–144, 146–147
  relationship with, 28, 30
Hindu patients, prayers for, 148
Hip fractures, 295

Hippotherapy, 183
HIV/AIDS patients
  acupressure, 260
  aromatherapy, 346
  herbal medicines, 358
  journaling for, 167
  massage therapy, 292
  meditation, 137
  programs for, 248–249
  Reiki, 243
Holistic health care, 175
Holistic listening, 45
Holistic philosophy, 6, 10, 117–118,
  143, 149, 204, 214, 271
Holistic therapies, journaling, 166,
  287
Homeopathy, 5, 228
Hook and back up technique, re-
    flexology, 276–277
Hope, sources of, 161, 237
Horseback riding, therapeutic, 183
Hospice care
  animal-assisted therapy, 178
  Healing Touch (HT), 215
  reflexology, 278
  Reiki, 243, 248–249
  storytelling techniques, 156–157
Hospital setting, aromatherapy, 343
Hostility, 51
Hot/cold balance, 20
Hot flashes, 361
Humanistic nursing theory, 36
Humor
  applications, generally, 101–102
  assessment, 99–100
  benefits of, 5, 8, 26, 93–94
  effectiveness measurement, 101
  future research directions, 103
  incongruity theory, 95
  information resources, 100
  interview guide, 99
  laughter, benefits of, 93–96
  physiological effects, 94, 97, 101
  precautions, 101
  psychological perspectives, 98–99,
    102
  release theory, 95–96
  scientific basis, 97–99

spontaneous, 99–100
styles of, 96–97
surprise, 95
techniques, 100–101
therapeutic goals, 94
timing of, 101
Humor resource center, 100
Humors
  in Ayuvedic medicine, 18
  in traditional Tibetan medicine, 17
Huntington's disease, 371–372
Hydrolats, 345
Hydrotherapy, 5
Hypercholesterolemia, 352–353, 370
Hypericin, 360
Hypericum perforatum, see Saint
    John's wort
Hypertension
  acupressure, 267
  animal-assisted therapy, 178
  aromatherapy, 340, 344
  biofeedback techniques, 123, 125
  exercise program effects, 295,
    298–299
  functional foods, 340, 371
  herbal medicines, 353
  magnet therapy, 191
  meditation and, 137–138
  muscle relaxation, 329
  nutraceuticals, 368, 371
  yoga, 110, 113, 120
Hyperventilation, 125
Hypnosis/hypnotic abilities, 59, 64,
    71
Hypoglycemia, 123
Hypoglycemics, 355
Hypotension, aromatherapy, 344
Hypothalamic-pituitary-
    adrenocortical (HPA) axis, 131
Hyssop, 346

IARP International Association of Re-
    iki Practitioners, 251
Ice massage, 262
Idinavir, 360
IgA immune response, 372
Illness, *see* Chronic illness
  Mexican traditional medicine,
    20–21

in Native American medicine, 19
response to, 51
in Samoan medicine, 18–19
Therapeutic Touch (TT), 227
Imagery
  adverse events of, 66
  applications of, 59–60, 66–71
  biofeedback-assisted, 120
  characterized, 5, 8, 10, 59
  defined, 60
  future research directions, 71–72
  intervention techniques, 62–66
  scientific basis, 60–62
Immobile patients, 178, 304
Immune deficiency disorders, 218
Immune system, influential factors,
    61, 97–98, 111, 167, 213, 217,
    233–234, 249, 265, 324, 371
Immunizations, 87
Immunoglobulin levels, 235
Immunosufficiency syndrome, 150
Incantations, 18
Incontinence, 125, 277
Indigenous cultures, 153–155, 334
Indigestion, 344
Infants, *see* Neonatal Intensive Care
    Unit
  aromatherapy, 345–347
  colic, 344, 347
  diaper rash, 344
  energy work with, 214–215
  with G6PD deficiency, 346
  premature, 196
Infection
  acupressure and, 266
  aromatherapy and, 343–344
  control, 343
Infertility, 344
Inflammatory disorders, magnet ther-
    apy, 196–197
Information resources, *see specific
    types of therapies*
Ingham, Eunice, 274
Insomnia, 110, 125, 129, 329
Institute for Health and Healing, Ab-
    bott Northwestern Hospital
    (Minneapolis, MN), 11

Institute for the Advancement of the Studies of Complementary Studies, 248
Institute of Clinical Pharmacology, 360
Institute of Medicine (IOM), 386, 388
Institutionalized elderly, 235
Instrumentation, 217–218
Insulin, 136
Insurance coverage, 6
Integumentary system, 286
Intensive care patients, 171, 179–180
Intercessory prayer, 144–145, 148
Interdisciplinary teams, 12
Interleukin-1, 358
International Association of Yoga Therapists, 110
International Board Certified Lactation Consultants (IBCLC), 355
International Center for Reiki Training, 244, 251
International Communication Association, 52
International Institute of Reflexology, 272
International Journal of Listening, 52
International Listening Association, 52
Interval, in music intervention, 80
Intestinal cancer, 266
Iron supplements, 375
Irritable bowel syndrome, 120, 125, 137–138, 279, 344
Ischemic pain, 305

Jaw area pain, 125
Jewish faith, prayers for, 148
Jin si ju jitsyu, 255–256
Jogging, 300
Joint(s), generally
   injuries, Healing Touch (HT) techniques, 211
   mobility, 306
   pain, 277, 307
   swelling, 197
Jokes, 95, 101
Journaling

applications, 170–172
benefits of, 5, 8, 165–167
defined, 166
dreams, 31
future research directions, 172
guidelines for, 168
historical perspectives, 165
intervention techniques, 167–170
outcomes measurement, 170
precautions, 170
scientific basis, 166–167
types of, 168–170
Journal of Holistic Nursing and Complementary Therapies in Nursing & Midwifery, 8
Journal of the American Medical Association (JAMA), 227
Juniper, aromatherapy, 344–345
Juvenile diabetes, 372

Kapha, 18
Keating, Thomas, 133–134
Ketones, 336, 341
Ki, 189, 206
Ki energy, in Reiki, 247–248
Kirlian photography, 195
Kneading, massage strokes, 288
Knee pain, 125, 196–197, 236
Krieger, Dolores, Ph.D., R.N., 225–226
Kunz, Dora, 225–226
Kunz, Kevin and Barbara, 272, 280

Labor and delivery
   acupressure, 261–262
   aromatherapy, 343
   expedition of, 265
   induction of, 265
   Reiki, 249
Labov, William, 154
Lacerations, see Wound healing
Lactation, 355
Lactobacillus GG therapy, 372
Lactones, 336
Laetrile, 333
Lamentation, 144
Laughter
   benefits of, 93–95, 101

physiological effects, 97, 101
reasons/trigger for, 95–96
Lavandula angustifolia, 336–337, 340, 347
defined, 340
Lavender, aromatherapy, 336–337, 339–342, 344–347
LD$_{50}$, 358
Leadership roles, 12
Learning process, storytelling techniques, 160
Legal issues, 9
Legislation
Dietary Supplement Health and Education Act of 1994 (DSHEA), 352
Nutrition Labeling and Health Act of 1990, 353
State Practice Act, 392
Lemon, aromatherapy, 344, 346
Lemon eucalyptus, 344
Lemongrass, 342, 344–346
Length of stay, 51, 181, 184, 213, 218
Leukemia, 266
Level I/Level II/Level III Reiki, 245, 249
Licensure, 9
Lifestyle improvement, 18
Light/dark balance, 20
Lightheadedness, 198
Light therapy, 5
Limbic system, 336
Listening skills, storytelling techniques, 159
Living matrix, 192
Localized HT techniques, 211–213
Long-term care facilities, 161, 176, 215, 343
Longitudinal studies, yoga's long-term effects, 113
Lord's Prayer, 148
Low back pain, 113, 125, 197, 259, 262, 307, 319, 344
Low-energy emission therapy, 190
Lung(s)
cancer, 277
chronic conditions, 218

Lupus, 358
Lycopene, 369
Lymph system, 286

McGill Pain Questionnaire, 237–238
McGill-Mezack Pain Questionnaire, 214
Magnet therapy, *see* Therapeutic magnets
applications, 5, 195–197
commercial applications, types of, 195–196
defined, 192
effectiveness, measurement of, 195
historical perspectives, 191–192
information resources, 198
intervention, 193–195
precautions, 198
research questions, 198
scientific basis, 192–193
Magnetic beads, auricular, 262
Magnetic clearing, Healing Touch (HT), 209
Magnetic passes, 207
Magnetic resonance imaging (MRI), 131
Ma huang, 357
Maintenance, exercise program, 301
Mana, 206, 244
Mandarin, 344–345, 347
Manipulative and body-based therapies
exercise, 295–308
massage, 285–292
muscle relaxation techniques, 323–331
overview of, 5, 283–284
Tai Chi, 313–320
Manipulative medicine, 19
Mantra, 130, 133
MANTRA project, 145
Manuka, 344
Marjoram, aromatherapy, 341
Massage
applications, 290–292
benefits of, generally, 5, 8, 10–11, 16–18, 20, 238, 283
defined, 285–286

Massage *(continued)*
  essential oils application, 337
  future research directions, 292
  hand, 289–291
  historical perspectives, 285
  information resources, 292
  outcomes measurement, 290
  precautions, 290
  reflexology combined with, 276
  shoulder, 288–289
  strokes, 288
  types of, 286
Master's degree programs, 10
Mattress pads, 197
Maury, Marguerite, 335
Mayo Clinic, 374
Mayo Clinic Health Letter, 193
Meal rituals, 20
Medical clinics, 215
Medication(s)
  administration, 37
  impact on energy work, 214
  overdosage of, 136
  side effects of, 7, 279
Medicinal plants, 18–20
Medicine man, in Native American
    medicine, 19–20
Meditation
  in action, 132
  applications, 136–139
  benefits of, 5, 8, 16–18, 26, 129
  centering process, 204
  defined, 130–131
  efficacy of, 135
  future research directions, 139–140
  guidelines for, 134–135
  healing, 226, 229
  Healing Touch (HT) techniques,
    206
  historical perspectives, 126–130
  intervention, 132–134
  mindfulness, 27
  outcome measurement, 135
  prayer compared with, 144
  precautions, 136
  scientific basis, 131–132
  types of, 130, 133–134
  with yoga, 109, 111

Melaleuca alternifolia, 340, 343
Melissa, aromatherapy, 344, 346–347
Melissa officinalis, 347
Melody, in music intervention, 80, 84
Memory, *see* Alzheimer's patients;
    Dementia
  loss, 345
  recall, 177
Menopausal symptoms, 344, 353,
    361
Menstrual cramps, 259, 344, 353
Mental illness, 113
Mental repetition, in meditation, 130
Mentgen, Janet, 204
Menthol, 346
Mentoring, 204, 214
Meridians
  acupressure, 256–257, 259
  acupuncture, 352
  reflexology, 273, 275
  Tai Chi, 314
Mescaline, 19
Mesoamerican traditional medicine,
    19–20
Meta-analysis study
  imagery interventions, 70
  music intervention, 87
  Therapeutic Touch (TT), 232
Metabolic equivalents (METs), 296
Metabolic rate, 324
Metabolism, exercise program and,
    296
Metal, in traditional Chinese medi-
    cine, 16
Methicillin-resistant *Staphylococcus
    aureus* (MRSA), 343–344
Migraine headaches, 124–125, 233,
    237, 279, 344
Milieu treatment, 176
Mind-body intervention, 27, 71
Mind-body techniques, imagery,
    65–66
Mind Clearing, 211
Mind-body therapies
  humor, 93–103
  imagery, 59–72
  music intervention, 79–88
  overview of, 5, 57–58

Mind-body-spirit connection, 109, 244
Mindful hatha yoga, 133
Mindfulness meditation, 132–133, 138–139
Minerals, 352
Mobility improvement, 183, 213, 299. *See also* Movement disorders
Modified foods, 369
Mood, generally
    disturbance, 137, 237, 319
    state, improvement strategies, 343
Morale, 182
Morals, 161
Morbidity, 51
Motion gesture, Healing Touch (HT) techniques, 207
Motor skills, 177, 183
Movement disorders, 183, 276–277
Moxibustion, 17, 256, 391
Multi-infarct dementia, 359
Multiple sclerosis, 113, 218, 278–279, 358
Muscle(s), *see* Musculoskeletal system
    injury, 196
    pain, 307
    relaxation, *see* Muscle relaxation
    spasms, 232
    sprains, 191, 307
    strains, 307
    strengthening, 118–119
    tension/tension feedback, 124, 324
Muscle relaxation
    applications, 328–330
    benefits, 284
    defined, 323
    future research directions, 330–331
    historical perspectives, 323
    information resources, 325
    intervention, 325–328
    outcomes measurement, 328
    precautions, 328
    progressive (PMR), 323–324, 329–330
    relaxation response, 324
    scientific basis, 324–325
Musculoskeletal, generally

conditions, 232
disorders, 236
injury, 307
system, 286
Music intervention
    applications, 85–87
    benefits of, generally, 5, 8, 10, 81–83, 285
    defined, 79–80
    future research directions, 87–88
    group music making, 82
    guidelines for, 83–84
    individual music listening, 81–82
    with massage therapy, 292
    outcomes measurement, 84–85
    physical response to music, 81, 83
    precautions, 85
    scientific basis, 80–81
    techniques, 81–82
    timing of, 88
    types of music, 83
Music therapists, functions of, 80
Muslim patients, prayers for, 148
Mycotherapies, 352
Myocardial infarction, 299
Myocardial ischema, 318
Myofascial pain, 259
Myrrh, aromatherapy, 344–345

Naiouli, aromatherapy, 344–345
Narratives, humorous, 102
National Association of Holistic Aromatherapy (NAHA), 341, 347
National Center for Complementary/Alternative Medicine (NCCAM), 3–7, 9, 143, 189, 192, 243, 275, 283, 333, 356, 361, 385–386
National Center for Health Statistics, 5
National Communication Association, 52
National Institutes of Health (NIH)
    functions of, 3, 7, 69, 131, 243, 259, 298, 351, 374–375
    NCCAM, *see* National Center for Complementary and Alternative Medicine (NCCAM)
    Research Teams of the Future, 390

National Library of Medicine, 353
Native American medicine
    characterized, 5, 15, 17, 19–21
    spiritual direction, 28
Native American population
    prayers for, 148
    storytelling, 157
Nature, in self-healing process, 27
Naturopathy, 5
Nausea, 16, 259–260, 264, 329–330,
    343, 345, 347
Nei guan, 258
Neonatal intensive care unit (NICU),
    87, 213, 231–232
Neroli, for aromatherapy, 342
Nervous breakdown, 313
Nervous systems, 286, 336
Neural adaptation, 85
Neuralgia, intercostal, 258
Neuroendocrine stress hormones, 98
Neurological diseases/disorders, 196,
    276
Neuromuscular massage, 286
Neuroplasticity, 131–132
Neurotransmitters, 61
New Age music, 83
Newman, Margaret, 154
New York State Nurses Association,
    on use of complementary thera-
    pies, 11
Nightingale, Florence, 8, 79
Nightmares, 31
Nitric oxide, 359
Niyama, 108
Nondirected prayer, 144
Nonverbal communication, 48–49
Nonverbal response, 37
Noradrenaline, 360
North American native healing, 19
Notes on Nursing (Nightingale), 8
Nurse Healers, The, 239
Nurse midwives, 343
Nurse-patient relationship
    presence, 35–41
    therapeutic listening, 45–53
Nursing care satisfaction, 51
Nursing education
    autonomous nursing biofeedback,
    119

communication skills, therapeutic,
    46–47
curriculum, 8–10, 144
experiential learning, 10
future directions for, 390–392
Healing Touch (HT) techniques,
    204
nurse as healer, see Self as healer
prayer, 144
therapeutic communication skills,
    46–47
Nursing practice, future directions
    for, 392–393
Nursing research, 7–8, 11–12, 88,
    389–390
Nursing shortage, 28
Nutmeg, aromatherapy, 17
Nutraceuticals
    applications, 374–376
    assessment guide, 373
    benefits, 333, 352, 368
    defined, 368–369
    future research directions, 376
    information resources, 374
    intervention, 372–374
    outcomes measurement, 372–373
    precautions, 373–374, 385
    safety considerations, 385
    scientific basis, 369–372
Nutritional therapies, see Nu-
    traceuticals
Nutrition consultation, 11
Nutrition Labeling and Health Act of
    1990, 353

Obesity, 295
Observation research, 386
Observation skills, 40
Obsessive-compulsive disorder
    (OCD), 113
Occupational therapists, 183
Ojibwa Indians, 20, 157
Oncology, aromatherapy, 345. See
    also Cancer patients
Opioid systems, 258
Oral contraceptives, 360
Oregano, 44, 346
Organic chemicals, 336

Organ transplantation, 137
Orientation, in storytelling, 154
Origanum marjoranum, 341
Ornish diet, 5
Orthomolecular medicine, 5
Osteoarthritis, 113, 197, 236, 259, 344, 371
Osteopathy, 283
Osteoporosis, 306, 368
Outcome imagery, 64
Oxides, 336
Oxygen consumption, 297–298, 324

Pain Drain, 211
Pain management therapies
    acupressure, 258, 265
    aromatherapy, 343–344
    biofeedback, 120, 125
    characterized, 16, 190
    Healing Touch (HT), 206–207, 209–210, 212–213, 215, 217
    imagery, 60, 65–71
    magnet therapy, 190–191, 193, 195–197
    massage, 285–286, 291–292
    meditation, 136–138
    muscle relaxation, 328–330
    music interventions, 86
    reflexology, 277–279
    Reiki, 243, 248–249
    therapeutic humor, 102
    Therapeutic Touch (TT), 233, 236–238
Pain reduction therapies, *see* Pain management therapies
Pain Visual Analog Scale, 214
Palliative care, 233, 243, 248–249, 345
Palma rosa, for aromatherapy, 342, 344
Panic attacks, 139
Panic disorder, 139
Paresthesia, 279
Parkinson's disease, 359, 372
Partial presence, 37
Passive imagery, 60
Patchouli, aromatherapy, 345
Patella, subluxication of, 125

Pathogens, 343
Patient(s), *see specific types of patients*
    bill of rights, 9
    education, 392
    relationship with doctor, 6, 46, 392
    satisfaction, 46–47, 208
Patient-doctor communication, 46
Patient-provider relationship, 392
Pawnee Indians, 20
Pediatrics, *see* Adolescents; Children; Infants
Peer review, 386
Pelvic pain, 196
Peppermint/peppermint oil, for aromatherapy, 342, 344, 346
Perceived exertion, in fitness walking program, 303
Percussion strokes, in massage, 288–289
Peripheral artery disease (PAD), 305–306, 358
Peripheral vascular disease, 359
Personal growth, sources of, 171
Pertussis, 258
Petition prayer, 144
Pet ownership, 178–179
Pet visitation, 176. *See also* Animal-assisted therapy (AAT)
Petrissage, 288
Phantom limb pain, 125
Pharmacotherapy, 305
Phenols, 336, 340
Philosophical perspectives, 6, 10–11
Phlegm, in traditional Tibetan medicine, 17
Physical Activity Readiness Questionnaire (PAR-Q), 307
Physical presence, 36–38, 41
Physical repetition, in meditation, 130
Physical therapists, 183
Physician-patient relationship, 6
Physician utilization, 178
Phytochemicals, 367, 369
Phytomedicines, 353
Phytotherapies, *see* Herbal medicines

Pilgrimages, 18, 20
Pine, in aromatherapy, 345
Pitch, in music intervention, 79, 83
Pitta, 18
Placebo effect, 190, 387
Plant-based therapies, see Herbal
  medicine
Pluralism, 15
Poetry, journaling guidelines, 170
Polysomnography, 195
Positron emission tomography (PET),
  131
Post-anesthesia patients, 209
Posture
  implications of, 183
  -related pain, 125
  relaxation technique, 327
  in yoga, 108
Powerlessness, 102
Practice settings, 10–11. See also Environmental settings
Prana, 189, 192, 244
Pranayama, 108–109
Pratyahara, 109
Prayer, see Spirituality
  applications, 149–150
  centering, 132–134
  ceremony, Mesoamerican tradi-
    tional medicine, 20
  circles/chains, 148
  defined, 144
  effectiveness of, 5, 10, 16–18, 26,
    29, 145, 150, 204
  examples of, 148
  future research directions, 150
  information resources, 147–148
  intervention techniques, 146–149
  meditation and, 144
  outcome measurement, 149
  perceptions of, 143
  popularity of, 149
  precautions, 149
  spiritual assessment, 146–147
  types of, 144–145, 148
Pregnancy
  acupressure, 257, 259–260, 266
  aromatherapy and, 340
  Healing Touch (HT) and, 214

herbal medicines, 355
  magnet therapy and, 198
  nutritional needs, 375–376
  Therapeutic Touch (TT), 232
Premenstrual symptoms/syndrome,
  279, 344
Prescription medications, 9, 351,
  357, 360
Presence
  applications, 41
  attributes of, 38
  benefits of, 37
  centering, 39
  defined, 35–36
  effectiveness measurement, 40
  future research directions, 41
  Healing Touch (HT), 218
  importance of, 2, 7–8, 38
  intervention, 38–41
  precautions, 40–41
  scientific basis, 36–38
  storytelling techniques, 159
  technique, 39–40
Pressure points, stimulation of, 190
Pressure ulcers, 345
Prison population, 178, 183–184
Pritkin diet, 5
Probiotics, 372
Problem concentration, in meditation,
  130
Procedural pain, 60
Process imagery, 64
Professional associations, functions
  of, 9. See also specific profes-
  sional associations
Profile of Mood States, 213
Progressive muscle relaxation (PMR)
  defined, 323–324
  effects of, 324, 329–330
  technique, 325–327
Prostate cancer, 243
Pseudohypericin, 360
Psoriasis, 137, 345
Psudomonas auruginosa, 346
Psychiatric crises, 51
Psychological counseling, 176
Psychological presence, 37
Psychoneuroimmune response, 70–71

Psychosis, 112
Psychosocial functioning, presence and, 40–41
Psychotherapy, 137, 183
Public health nursing, 343
Public Radio Music Source, 82
PubMed web site, 353
Pulsating electromagnetic field therapy (PEFT), 197
Puns, 96
Purification ceremonies, 18–19

Questionnaires
  McGill-Melzack Pain Questionnaire, 214, 237–238
  Physical Activity Readiness (PAR-Q), 307
  Situational Humor Response (SHRQ), 101
  Stanford Health Assessment, 236
  State-Trait Anxiety Inventory (STAI), 328
Qi, 16, 189, 192, 206, 256–258, 265, 273, 275, 352
Qi Gong, 5, 11, 16–17, 206
Qi Qong, 228
Quality of care, 161
Quality of life (QoL), 7, 71, 156, 213, 216, 233, 237, 260, 278, 305
Quinine, 19
Qur'an, 148

Racial differences
  biofeedback techniques and, 126
  meditation effects, 138
  in storytelling, 153–154
  in utilization of therapies, 6
Radiation therapy, 345, 361
Ragweed, 358
Rand, William, 244
Randomized clinical trials, 386
Ravansara, 344–345
Raynaud's Syndrome, 125
Reach for Recovery, 161
Recognition, 160
Reconnective healing, 11

Reductionistic biomedical health care system, 26
Referrals, 8–9, 51, 160, 248, 392
Reflective holistic nursing, 25
Reflexology
  applications, 11, 190, 277–279
  classification of, 283
  defined, 271–273
  future research directions, 279–280
  information resources, 280
  intervention, 275–277
  as massage, 286
  outcomes measurement, 276
  popularity of, 271
  precautions, 276–277
  scientific basis, 273–275
  techniques, 276–277
  Traditional Chinese Medicine (TCM), 273–274
  Zone Therapy, 273
Rehabilitation facilities, 183
Reiki
  applications, 248–249
  attunements, 245, 247
  characteristics of, 5, 11, 190, 243
  defined, 244–245
  full hands-on sessions, guidelines for, 247, 250
  future research directions, 250–251
  goals of, 250
  historical perspectives, 243–244
  information resources, 251
  interventions, 246–248
  outcomes measurement, 247–248
  practitioners of, 246, 249–250
  precautions, 248
  scientific basis, 245–246
  self-treatment, 249–250
  technique, 246–247
Reiki Page, 251
Relaxation strategies, see Muscle relaxation techniques
  animal-assisted therapy, 179
  aromatherapy, 343, 345
  biofeedback response, 118–119, 120, 123–124
  through Healing Touch (HT), 207, 209, 212, 216

Relaxation strategies *(continued)*
massage, 285–287, 291
meditation, 132, 134, 138
music intervention, 79, 81–84
reflexology, 278–279
Reiki, 248
response to, generally, 132, 134,
286–287, 324
techniques, generally, 11, 62
Therapeutic Touch (TT), 231, 233,
237
yoga, 107, 109–111
Reliefband®, 259
Relief Brief®, 262
Religion/religious influences, *see*
Prayer; Spirituality
Reminiscence, 8
Renal transplantation, 150
Research, generally
current state of, 388–389
designs, 386–388
future directions, 383–384
implications of, 389–393
Resolution, in storytelling, 154
Respiratory illness, aromatherapy,
345
Respiratory problems, 191
Respiratory rate, 324, 328
Respiratory system, 97, 177–178,
337
Rest, 26
Restrained patients, 86
Reversibility, exercise program, 301
Rheumatoid arthritis, 344, 358
Rhythm, in music intervention, 80,
83–84
RICE (rest, ice, compression, eleva-
tion) therapy, 307
Ringworm, 346
Rites of passage, aromatherapy, 345
Rituals
in Native American medicine,
19–20
prayer(s), 18, 144
Rolfing, 5, 283
Roman chamomile, 344–345, 347
Rosa damascena, 347
Rose, aromatherapy, 341–342,
344–346

Rosemary, 340, 344–345
Rose otto, 347
Rosewood, for aromatherapy, 342

Sacrificial offerings, 20
Sage, for aromatherapy, 342, 344
Saint John's wort, 8, 357, 359–361
Salivary immunoglobulin A (S-IgA),
97–98, 213
Samadhi, 109
Samoan medicine, 15–16, 18–19
Sandalwood, in aromatherapy, 18,
342, 345–346
Sarcastic humor, 96
Savory, for aromatherapy, 344
Scars, 266
Scented oils, 18
Schizophrenia, 136, 178
SeaBands®, 259
Sedative-hypnotics, 355
Sedatives, 136
Sedentary lifestyle, 296, 300,
306–307
Seizure disorders, 125, 329–330, 340
Self as healer
dreams, 30–31
future research directions, 31
self-care, 26–27
spiritual direction, 28–30
transformational journey, 27–28
Self-awareness, 25
Self-care, 17, 26–37, 94
Self deprecating humor, 96
Self-disclosure, 159
Self-discovery, 47
Self-esteem, influential factors, 170,
279, 287
Self-expression, 47
Self-healing journey
barriers, 27–28
becoming a healer, 27
needs, 27–28
nurse's role in, 25, 204
stressors, 27–28
Self-help groups, 161
Self-help treatments, 195
Self-hypnosis, 59
Self-knowledge, 25, 160

Self-reliance, 166
Self-study modules, 10
Self-understanding, 49
Sensory imagery, 60
Sensory inhibition, in yoga, 109
Serotonin levels, 61, 131, 360
Sesame oil, 18
Severe depression, 136. *See also*
    Depression
Sexually transmitted diseases, 266
Shaman(s), 19–20, 59, 352
Shamanism, 27
Sharing, storytelling techniques, 160
Sharing circle, 155
Shark cartilage, 333
Shiatsu, 255–256, 286
Shock humor, 95
Silence, therapeutic listening tech-
    niques, 49
Simple touch, 285
Singing, 16, 19–20
Sinusitis, 345
Sitting meditation, 133
Situational humor, 86
Situational Humor Response Ques-
    tionnaire (SHRQ), 101
Skiing, cross-country, 300
Skin, *see* Dermatology
    disease, 266
    injury, 359
Slapstick humor, 95
Sleep, generally
    behavior, 26, 207, 261–262
    disorders, 195, 360
    disturbance, improvement thera-
        pies, 86, 291, 344
    improvement therapies, 278–279,
        284–285, 291, 328, 339, 343
    quality of, 319
Smoking cessation, 139, 171, 343
Smudging, 20
Social isolation, 102, 160
Social support
    systems, 26
    theory, 177
Soft tissue
    massage techniques, 286
    sprains, 191

Solar plexus, in reflexology, 275
South American healing, 19
Soy protein, 368
Spasms, improvement with reflexol-
    ogy, 279
Spasticity, 279
Spearmint, 347
Special foods, 19
Spielberger's State-Trait Anxiety In-
    ventory, 213
Spike lavender, 341, 344–345
Spiritual advice, 16, 18
Spiritual care, aromatherapy, 345
Spiritual development, 28
Spiritual directors, role of, 29–30
Spiritual Directors International, 29
Spiritual functioning, presence and,
    40
Spirituality
    assessment of, 146–147
    church attendance, 146
    implications of, 28–30, 143
    spiritual growth, 171–172
    storytelling and, 160
    yoga and, 108
Spontaneous humor, 99–100
Spontaneous storytelling, 159
Sports massage, 286
Sprains, 191, 232, 307
Stanford Health Assessment Question-
    naire, 236
Stanols, dietary plant, 368, 370
Staphylococcus aureus, 343–344, 346
Statement clarification, 49
State Practice Act, 392
State-Trait Anxiety Inventory (STAI),
    328
Steady state exercise phase, 298
Sterols, dietary plant, 370
Stimulation, through music interven-
    tion, 86
Storytellers, training for, 160
Storytelling
    applications, 160–161
    benefits of, 16, 19, 153–154, 157
    components of, 154
    defined, 154–155
    future research directions, 161–162

Storytelling *(continued)*
  intervention techniques, 158–160
  outcomes measurement, 160
  precautions, 160
  scientific basis, 155–157
Strains, 232
Stress management, 26, 93–94, 119.
    See also Stress reduction
    therapies
Stress Reduction Clinic, University of
    Massachusetts Medical Center,
    133
Stress reduction therapies
  acupressure, 261–262
  animal-assisted therapy, 183
  benefits of, 60, 284
  Healing Touch (HT), 208–210,
    215–216
  magnet therapy, 191, 195
  massage, 291
  meditation, 129, 131, 138–139
  mindfulness-based (MBSR), 133
  muscle relaxation, 329–330
  music interventions, 85–86
  Reiki, 246, 248–249
  yoga, 107, 109
Stress response, 60–62, 324
Stretching exercises, 300
Stroke patients, 113, 150, 218, 249,
    259, 374
Stump pain, 125
Subconscious mind, 59
Substance abuse, 113, 125
Suicide, 136
Sulforaphane, 369
Sun, Tai Chi style, 314
Superconducting quantum interfer-
    ence device (SQUID), 195, 206,
    245
Superiority laughter, 95
Supernatural, 19
Support groups, 8
Support system, significance of, 145
Surgery
  Native American medicine, 19
  patients, *see* Surgical patients
  simple, 18
  stress reduction techniques, 85–87

Surgical intensive care units (SICU),
    179–180
Surgical patients
  acupressure, 260
  Healing Touch (HT) techniques,
    210, 215–216, 218
  massage therapy, 292
  muscle relaxation, 329
  Reiki, 243, 248–249
  stress reduction techniques, 86–87
  Therapeutic Touch (TT), 233–235
Survival rates, influential factors, 160
Sweat baths, 20
Sweat lodge
  ceremony, 20
  purification, 16
Swedish massage, 286, 291
Sweet marjoram, in aromatherapy,
    344–345
Swimming, 300
Sympathetic nervous system, 97, 287
Symptom management, music inter-
    vention, 85–87
Systemic disease, 209

Tactile stimulation, 177
Tai Chi
  applications, 16, 130, 318–319
  "Around the platter" movement,
    316–317
  benefits of, 5, 16, 283–284, 313
  class selection factors, 318
  defined, 313–314
  future research directions, 319–320
  guidelines for, 316–317
  information resources, 316
  interventions, 315–318
  outcomes measurement, 317
  precautions, 317–318
  scientific basis, 314–315
  styles of, 314
  techniques, 315–316
Tai Chi Chih, 314
*Tai Chi Chuan for Health and Self-
    Defense,* 316
Tai Chi Transcendent Art, 316
Takata, Mrs. Hawayo, 244
Talking circles, 16, 20, 155, 157–159

Talk test, 302
Tamanu carrier oil, 345
Tanka, 170
Taoism, 256
Target heart rate, 302
Tarragon, 344
Teas, benefits of, 19
Tea tree, in aromatherapy, 340,
    344–347
Tea tree oil, 343
Temperature feedback, 119, 122
Temporomandibular disorders, 125
Tendonitis, 307
Tennis elbow, 259
Tension headaches, 124–125,
    233–234
Tension reduction therapies
    Healing Touch (HT), 209
    muscle relaxation, 330
    music interventions, 83, 85–86
    reflexology, 279
    storytelling, 161
Terminally ill patients, 210
Terpenes, 336
Tertiary care, 215
Thanksgiving prayer, 144, 147
Theophylline, 355, 360
Therapet, 182, 184
Therapeutic listening
    applications, 2, 51–52
    defined, 45–46
    future research directions, 53
    guidelines for, 48–50
    information resources, 52
    interventions, 48–51
    outcome measurement, 50–51
    precautions, 51
    scientific basis, 46–48
    technique, 49
Therapeutic magnets
    application of, methods and dura-
        tion, 194–195
    permanent, 196
    strength of, 194
    types of, 193–194
Therapeutic presence, 36–37
Therapeutic Touch (TT)
    applications, 232–233

assessment goal, 229–230
balancing, 231
characterized, generally, 5, 11, 189
defined, 225–226
energy direction for healing,
    230–231
energy field clearing and mobiliza-
    tion, 230
future research directions, 233–239
historical perspectives, 225–226
information resources, 239
interventions, 228–232
outcomes measurement, 231–232
practitioner's role, 226–227,
    229–231
precautions, 232
scientific basis, 226–228
Therapeutic Touch Network Ontario,
    239
Therapist, see specific types of
    therapies
    credentials of, 9
    roles, 6, 120, 124
Thistles, 358, 361
Thumb walking technique, 276–277
Thyme, 344, 346
Thymus mastichina, 341
Tibetan medicine, 15–17
Tinnitus, 329, 359
T-lymphocytes, 98
Toenail fungus, 344
Tone of voice, therapeutic listening,
    49
Topical journaling, 167, 169–170
Touch, see Healing Touch (HT); Ther-
    apeutic Touch (TT)
    benefits of, 8
    therapeutic listening guidelines, 49
Traditional Chinese medicine (TCM),
    5, 15–17, 189–190, 192, 256–
    259, 261, 273–274, 334
Traditional healing systems, 15
Trager body work, 283
Transcendent presence, 36–37
Transcendental meditation (TM),
    132–133, 138, 178
Transcutaneous electrical nerve stimu-
    lation (TENS), 190

Transdermal drug delivery, 198
Trauma, treatment of, 19, 209
Traumatic brain injury, 125
Tricyclic antidepressants, 360
Trinity Mother Frances Health System (Tyler, TX), 179
Trust development, 94
Tsubo, 255
Tuberculosis, 113, 266
Tui na, 255
Tumor-necrosis factor-alpha (TNF-α), 358
Tumors, 340
Type 2 diabetes mellitus, 298, 303

Ulcers, 266, 345
Ultrasound, energetic, 211
Ultraviolet light, 340
Uncertainty, 28
U.S. Food and Drug Administration (FDA), 197, 352–354, 356, 367–368, 374
Universal energy, 26
Universal order, 217
"Universal source" of energy, 208
University of Minnesota Center for Spirituality and Healing, 10
Unlicensed therapies, 9
Unruffling, 230
Upper respiratory illness, 358
Urinary system
  elimination disorders, 125
  incontinence, 119, 123, 125
  problems, aromatherapy for, 344
  symptoms, 279
Usui, Mikao, 244, 247
Usui Reiki, 245, 251
Utilization of therapies
  age differences, 5–6
  educational attainment and, 6
  ethnic differences, 6
  gender differences, 6
  growth of, 4–5
  patient demand and, 11
  racial differences, 6

Validation, 160
Valnet, Jean, 335

Vata, 18
Ventilator-dependent patients, 86–87
Ventricular contractions, 324
Verbal aggression, 101
Verbalization skills, 177
Verbal stimulation, 177
Vertigo, 359
Vibration strokes, in massage, 288
Violence prevention education programs, 156
Vipassana meditation, 132
Viral infection, 344
Virtue, 17, 28
Visual concentration, in meditation, 130
Visualization, 16, 60
Vital energy, defined, 192
Vital signs, 37
Vitamins
  A, 376
  benefits of, 334, 352
  E, 359
Vomiting, 258–259, 329–330
Vulvar vestibulitis, 125

WakeMed Hospital (Raleigh, NC), 179
Walking exercise program, 300–303
Warfarin, 360
Warmth, importance of, 45
Warm-up phase, in exercise program, 299–300, 302
Water
  in Ayuvedic medicine, 18
  retention, 344
Web sites, as information resource
  aromatherapy, 347
  generally, 9
  Healing Touch (HT), 217, 219
  herbal medicines, 353, 356
  magnet therapy, 198
  massage, 292
  muscle relaxation, 325
  music interventions, 82
  nutrachemicals, 374
  prayer, 184
  reflexology, 280
  Reiki, 251

Tai Chi, 316–317
therapeutic listening, 52
Therapeutic Touch (TT), 239
Weight control, 139, 299
Weight gain, prevention of, 300
Well-being
    enhancement of, 317
    as goal, 20
    influential factors, 61, 85, 94, 129, 139, 149, 157, 160, 171, 177, 183, 205, 207, 209, 213, 216–217, 287, 304, 324, 351
Wellness, in Tibetan medicine, 18
Western biomedical model, 1
Western biomedicine, 4
Western Medicine, 6–7, 12, 217, 257–259, 265, 357, 361, 393
Western science, 217
West Haven-Yale Multidimensional Pain Inventory, 236
Wholeness, 25
Widows/widowhood, 157
Wind, in traditional Tibetan medicine, 17
Wisdom
    attainment with yoga, 107, 111–112
    spiritual, 244
    storytelling techniques, 160
Women's health
    breast cancer, 277, 371
    breastfeeding, 355, 361
    gynecological problems, 344
    labor and delivery, 249, 261–262, 265, 343
    menopausal symptoms, 344, 353, 361
    menstrual cramps, 259, 344, 353
    nutritional needs, 375–376
    pregnancy, 214, 232, 257, 259–260, 266, 340, 355
    premenstrual symptoms, 279
    premenstrual syndrome, 344
Wood, in traditional Chinese medicine, 16
Woodwinds Health Campus (Woodbury, MN), 11

Work environment, 28. See also Environmental settings; Practice settings
Workshops
    Healing Touch (HT), 205
    humor, 94
    indigenous healing, 155
World Religions, 147
Worry reduction, Healing Touch (HT) techniques, 209
Wound healing
    aromatherapy, 343
    acupressure and, 266
    energy and biofield therapies, 190
    Healing Touch (HT) techniques, 209, 211, 213, 218
    magnet therapy, 196–197
Wound Sealing, 213
Wu, Tai Chi style, 314

Yakima Indians, 157
Yama, 108
Yang, Tai Chi style, 314
Yin/yang, 16, 256, 258
Ylang-ylang, aromatherapy, 342, 344–345, 347
Yoga
    applications, 112
    benefits of, 5, 16–18, 107–109, 112–113
    defined, 108–109
    future research directions, 112–113
    Healing Touch (HT) techniques, 206
    intervention, 110–112
    mindful hatha yoga, 133
    overview of, 107–108
    polarity of, 107
    precautions, 112
    scientific basis, 109–110
Yoga Alliance, 110
Yoga Sutra, 108
Yogi, Maharishi Mahesh, 133
Yogurt, 372
Young adults
    animal-assisted therapy, 178
    Therapeutic Touch (TT), 234–235

Zen Buddhism, 28, 130
Zinziber officinali, 347
Zone Therapy, 273

SPRINGER PUBLISHING COMPANY

Teaching Evidence-Based Practice in Nursing

Rona F. Levin, PhD, RN
Harriet R. Feldman, PhD, RN, FAAN, Editors

"In their outstanding book, Rona Levin and Harriet Feldman...capture creative approaches to teaching evidence-based practice. This book includes comprehensive and unique strategies for teaching evidence-based practice for all types of learners across a variety of educational and clinical practice settings. The concrete examples of teaching assignments provided in the book bring the content alive and serve as a useful, detailed guide for how to incorporate this material into meaningful exercises for learners. Levin and Feldman's book is a truly wonderful, necessary resource for educators working in all healthcare professional programs as well as clinical settings." —From the Foreword by
Bernadette Mazurek Melnyk, PhD, RN, CPNP/NPP, FAAN, FNAP

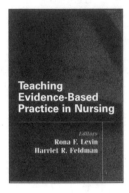

Based on the idea that nursing students and nurses at all levels can contribute to the development of a scientific base for nursing practice by critiquing and questioning guidelines, treatments, and outcomes of their own practice, this book examines the ways in which the teaching and learning of evidence-based practice (EBP) occurs. The book provides useful strategies for educators and facilitates the work of faculty to develop curricula that incorporate EBP and the work of nurses in the clinical setting to implement it.

Partial Contents

Part I: Setting the Stage

Part II: The Basics of Teaching/Learning Evidence-Based Practice

Part III: Teaching/Learning Evidence-Based Practice in the Academic Setting

Part IV: Teaching/Learning Evidence-Based Practice in the Clinical Setting

2006   400 pps   0-8261-3155-7   softcover

11 West 42nd Street, New York, NY 10036-8002 • Fax: 212-941-7842
Order Toll-Free: 877-687-7476 • Order On-line: www.springerpub.com